W9-DEC-287

Shoulder Arthroscopy

Shoulder
Arthroscopy

Gary M. Gartsman, MD

Clinical Professor
Department of Orthopaedic Surgery
University of Texas Health Science Center
at Houston Medical School
Fondren Orthopedic Group
Houston, Texas

SAUNDERS
An Imprint of Elsevier

SAUNDERS
An Imprint of Elsevier

The Curtis Center
Independence Square West
Philadelphia, Pennsylvania 19106

SHOULDER ARTHROSCOPY   ISBN 0–7216–9488–8

Notice

Arthroscopy is an ever-changing field. Standard safety precautions must be followed but as new research and clinical
experience broaden our knowledge, changes in treatment and drug therapy may become necessary or appropriate.
Readers are advised to check the most current product information provided by the manufacturer of each drug to be
administered to verify the recommended dose, the method and duration of administration, and contraindications. It is
the responsibility of the treating physician, relying on experience and knowledge of the patient, to determine dosages
and the best treatment for each individual patient. Neither the Publisher nor the editors assumes any liability for any
injury and/or damage to persons or property arising from this publication.

The Publisher

Library of Congress Cataloging-in-Publication Data

Gartsman, Gary M.
    Shoulder arthroscopy/Gary M. Gartsman.—1st ed.
      p. ; cm.
    ISBN 0–7216–9488–8
      1. Shoulder joint—Endoscopic surgery. I. Title.
      [DNLM: 1. Shoulder joint—surgery. 2. Arthroscopy—methods.
    WE 810 G244s 2003]
    RD557.5.G376 2003
    617.5'72059—dc21   2002191102

Publishing Director, Surgery: Richard Lampert
Acquisitions Editor: Hilarie Surrena
Project Manager: Tina Rebane
Book Designer: Gene Harris

RDC/DNP

Printed in China

Last digit is the print number: 9   8   7   6   5   4   3

Preface

Ten years have passed since the publication of *Arthroscopic Shoulder Surgery and Related Procedures.* Harvard Ellman and I coauthored that text in an attempt to bridge the gap between traditional open operations and newer arthroscopic approaches. Much has happened in the past decade that has created the need for a new and different textbook. Knowledge in shoulder anatomy, pathogenesis, diagnosis, and treatment has expanded greatly. Paralleling this increase in information has been an explosion of arthroscopic techniques, procedures, instruments, implants, and devices.

Arthroscopic shoulder operations are no longer limited to procedures of bone and soft tissue removal. In the 1980s the vast majority of arthroscopic shoulder operations were diagnostic glenohumeral examination, removal of loose bodies, subacromial decompression, and distal clavicle resection. The 1990s witnessed the transition of arthroscopic shoulder surgery to repair and reconstruction. Arthroscopic techniques are now used to repair full-thickness rotator cuff tendon tears, to correct glenohumeral instability, to reattach labrum lesions, and to manage refractory shoulder stiffness.

The purpose of this textbook is to present the current state of arthroscopic shoulder surgery as seen by one author. There are, of course, many different methods to treat shoulder lesions with arthroscopy but I have chosen to present my own views and trust that the reader will also seek out the opinions of others. My focus in this book is primarily on operative technique and my goal is to present an approach to arthroscopic shoulder operations in enough detail so that the reader can manage both the routine and complex problems he or she encounters. This required that I exclude some important nonsurgical material.

There are a number of texts currently available that devote hundreds of pages to patient history, diagnosis, pathogenesis, physical examination, rehabilitation, and imaging studies. Their bibliographies are complete and extensive. One such text is *The Shoulder* by Rockwood and Matsen. I see no need to duplicate their efforts, and I recommend that all who are seriously interested in shoulder problems study their text thoroughly.

So what kind of textbook is this? This is a book for orthopedic surgeons who want to perform reconstructive arthroscopic shoulder surgery. In order to do this the surgeon needs to understand why certain procedures are performed and to have them described in adequate detail. I have tried to take the reader through the operations in stepwise fashion; however, for complex procedures text is not sufficient. State-of-the-art communication in arthroscopy involves more than thoughts and words on a printed page. The accompanying CD-ROM contains videos that illustrate the concepts and techniques that I describe in the text.

Since 1982 I have been privileged to instruct hundreds of residents, fellows, and visiting orthopedic surgeons in shoulder arthroscopy. I have tried to adopt a tone that captures the many conversations we have had. Imagine that you and I are in the operating room performing shoulder arthroscopy. You can ask any questions you wish and I have all the time in the world to answer. Let's begin!

Gary M. Gartsman, MD

To my wife Carol,
Who helped make this book come to life.
Who makes it all worthwhile.

Contents

THE BASICS

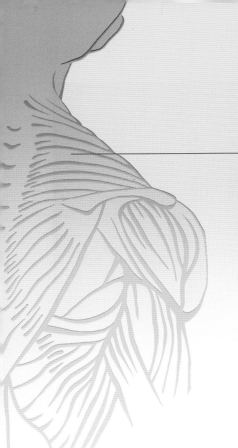

Making the Transition

1

I believe it is helpful for surgeons considering making the transition from open shoulder surgery to arthroscopic shoulder surgery to develop a plan or framework. There are two basic areas of knowledge: intellectual skills and technical skills. Currently, orthopedic surgeons learn the basic skills of shoulder arthroscopy during their residency or fellowship, but more advanced reconstructive surgical techniques require sufficient time with an experienced mentor. This experience varies widely among training programs. How does the orthopedic surgeon acquire the necessary intellectual and technical skills?

Intellectual Skills

The fundamental decision is whether or not to perform shoulder arthroscopy or continue with open repair techniques. Most surgeons are comfortable with open procedures. If they are satisfied with their patient outcomes, they do not find any reason to change. Surgeons have various reasons for deciding to learn or advance their arthroscopic skills, however. These reasons include the belief that arthroscopic techniques result in improved results, peer pressure, their desire to learn new concepts and techniques, and patient demand.

Various publications and presentations have documented equal or superior results with arthroscopic technique for the treatment of arthroscopic subacromial decompression for stage 2 impingement, arthroscopic acromioclavicular joint resection for acromioclavicular joint arthritis, and arthroscopic rotator cuff repair. The results of arthroscopic treatment for glenohumeral instability are approaching or even surpassing those of open technique.

Orthopedic surgeons are also subject to peer pressure. When they talk among themselves about various shoulder conditions and their treatment, surgeons who perform open operations exclusively can feel they are "behind the times." Orthopedic surgeons are in general conditioned to learn new approaches to patient care, and many surgeons with whom I have spoken about this particular issue believe that although their results from open repair are good, they want to "try something new."

Because of the dramatic increase in knowledge available, many patients are now aware of newer arthroscopic techniques and will ask their surgeons whether they perform the procedure arthroscopically or with open technique. Patients have the perception that arthroscopic procedures produce less pain, smaller scars, and more rapid rehabilitation, and they are increasingly insistent on finding surgeons who can meet their needs. Strong arguments can be made to refute all three of the foregoing assertions, and it is not my position that any or all of them are valid. Nonetheless, the foregoing remarks reflect the opinions of orthopedic surgeons I have questioned about this issue.

Before embarking on acquiring shoulder arthroscopy skills, I believe the orthopedic surgeon must evaluate his or her practice pattern. Do you perform a sufficient number of shoulder operations to justify learning a new skill? I believe all orthopedic surgeons should be comfortable with diagnostic glenohumeral joint arthroscopy, but not everyone needs to learn more advanced techniques. If you perform fewer than 20 to 30 shoulder procedures per year and are comfortable with open technique, I would not advise investing the time and effort required to do these few procedures arthroscopically. Do you have the emotional stability to handle periods of frustration when you attempt to perform procedures arthroscopically? Remember, you are attempting to move from the familiar and comfortable to something that is new and awkward. If you cannot perform routine arthroscopic subacromial decompression in 30 minutes or less, you do not have the arthroscopic skills required to perform more complicated reconstructive arthroscopic procedures. Improve your skills until your speed increases before taking on a bigger challenge. How do you acquire the necessary skills? Each surgeon should develop a plan for learning that is focused on two central issues. You must develop a plan that allows you to master both the intellectual and technical skills required. In reality, it is hard to separate intellectual and technical skills. Learning how to pass a suture through the anterior inferior glenohumeral ligament won't be very helpful if you don't learn when this step is necessary.

Technical Skills

Improve your arthroscopic skills. Most orthopedic surgeons learn the basics of shoulder arthroscopy during residency or fellowship, but those who do not have other resources available to them. The Orthopedic Learning Center is one such resource. Developed and administered by the American Academy of Orthopedic Surgeons and the Arthroscopy Association of North America, the Orthopedic Learning Center in Rosemont, Illinois, hosts numerous courses each year that cover both basic and advanced shoulder arthroscopy. Didactic lectures, panel discussions, and video demonstrations are presented in state-of-the-art lecture halls. The center also houses a wet cadaveric laboratory with 48 workstations so that participants can learn and practice with cadaver specimens and arthroscopic instruments. Although this is a successful technique for learning basic shoulder arthroscopy, many surgeons are not satisfied with this approach to learn more complex procedures such as arthroscopic rotator cuff repair or glenohumeral reconstruction.

There are several reasons for this. Generally, the courses are 2 to 3 days long and cover a broad range of topics. A typical Orthopedic Learning Center course may include lectures and cadaver instruction on arthroscopic subacromial decompression, distal clavicle excision, open and arthroscopic rotator cuff repair, and open and arthroscopic glenohumeral reconstruction. Not enough time is allowed for participants to become comfortable with all procedures. Because of the breadth of subjects covered, it is unusual for each instructor to be an expert on all the topics. Participants also demonstrate a great disparity in arthroscopic skill. One surgeon interested in learning arthroscopic rotator cuff repair may be paired with a beginner who wants to focus on glenohumeral joint inspection.

The Arthroscopy Association of North America also offers more individualized instruction through their Masters Series, and those with whom I have spoken about their experience with this series found it extremely worthwhile. James Esch has been active in shoulder arthroscopy education for years and annually organizes a superior course that combines lectures and cadaver work. Stephen Snyder has a wonderful facility in California that combines state-of-the-art video learning with an opportunity to watch a superb surgeon at work. My approach to the issue of surgeon education has been to offer a small course limited to 12 registrants that focuses solely on one topic, arthroscopic rotator cuff repair. I restrict the enrollment to surgeons with

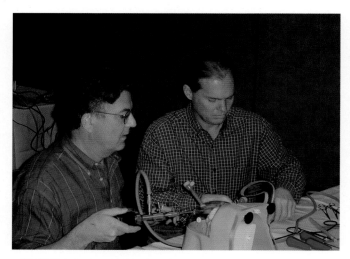

FIGURE 1–1. Joe W. King Invitational Rotator Cuff Repair Course.

advanced arthroscopic skills. Over a 2-day period, techniques using arthroscopic instruments and video arthroscopy are gradually introduced to repairs on anatomically detailed plastic shoulder models, to give everyone ample opportunity to master the required intellectual and technical skills (Fig. 1–1).

You can also advance your arthroscopic skills by focusing on the details of open repairs. First, take the opportunity to perform arthroscopy during all your open rotator cuff repairs and glenohumeral reconstructions before you perform the open repair. Learn what the typical glenohumeral joint looks like in a 63-year-old patient with a full-thickness rotator cuff repair. From the glenohumeral joint, try to identify the tear. Move the arthroscope into the subacromial space. Identify the rotator cuff tear, and estimate its size and shape. Ask the circulating nurse to write down these measurements. Now open the shoulder and record the size and shape of the tear. With practice, you will find that you can accurately assess rotator cuff tear size and shape. Before performing an open Bankart repair, use the arthroscope to identify the Bankart lesion and to estimate its size, and compare these findings with your impression during the open repair.

As your experience increases, become more precise with your observations. When you are viewing the rotator cuff tear from the subacromial space, insert a probe and use it to measure the length and width of the rotator cuff tear. Insert a grasper and determine the tear's reparability. Grasp different portions of the tear edge and advance them to different locations near the greater tuberosity. This will help you learn to appreciate tear geometry and repair geometry as viewed through the arthroscope. Make note of the tendon quality. After you perform the open repair and close the skin, reinsert the arthroscope into the subacromial space and observe how a completed repair appears.

As you can appreciate from the foregoing description, I believe that the transition from open to arthroscopic repair proceeds slowly as the surgeon makes incremental improvements in technical skill and adds to his or her knowledge base. I consider it extremely difficult for any surgeon to learn about an arthroscopic rotator cuff repair and then try to perform one from beginning to end the next day. I spent 1 year making the transition using the approach I just described.

At the same time your arthroscopic skills are improving and your knowledge is increasing, learn the principles and technical steps needed for an arthroscopic repair. An arthroscopic rotator cuff repair consists of the following elements: glenohumeral joint arthroscopy, subacromial bursectomy, coracoacromial ligament release, and acromioplasty. You should be expert in this portion of the procedure. You must be able to identify the tear size, geometry, and reparability. Next, an arthroscopic rotator cuff repair requires that you insert suture anchors, pass sutures through the tendon, manage sutures, and tie secure knots. Fortunately, you can master these techniques before you enter the operating room.

Suture Anchors

Ask your local representative of the instrument manufacturer for a spare suture anchor, and familiarize yourself with its characteristics. Are the sutures preloaded, or must they be loaded in the operating room? Are the sutures desirable for your rotator cuff repair? If not, can they be switched? Will the suture anchor accept multiple sutures or just one? If the anchor has two sutures, how are they arranged? Which suture do you have to tie first? Practice inserting the anchor into a board or sawbones, and learn how much force is required. Learn how to orient the eyelet so that the sutures will slide easily. You should practice reloading the anchor in case you pull out the sutures (Figs. 1–2 to 1–4).

Sutures Through Tendon

There are two basic methods of passing a braided suture through a tendon or ligament, and you should familiarize yourself with both. The direct method involves using an instrument to pierce the ligament or tendon and pulling or pushing the suture through it.

The indirect method requires that you use some sort of monofilament suture passed through the tendon. This monofilament suture is then used to pull the braided suture through the soft tissue. The surgeon can attach a piece of felt or foam rubber to a wooden board and can practice using instruments to pass sutures (Figs. 1–5 to 1–10).

Suture Management

Suture management is critical to reconstructive arthroscopic shoulder operations. Whether the surgeon is operating in the subacromial space for a rotator cuff repair or in the glenohumeral joint for a glenohumeral reconstruction, the fundamental problem is too many sutures in too little space. There are two basic approaches to this issue: tie the sutures as you insert them, or move the sutures out of the way through cannulas. Every surgeon will have to experiment with both techniques and determine which one is most satisfactory. Even if you tie the sutures after you insert each one, suture management is important. To insert sharp instruments through cannulas without nicking the suture (and risking suture breakage), a basic principle is to keep the working cannula free of sutures. Percutaneous anchor

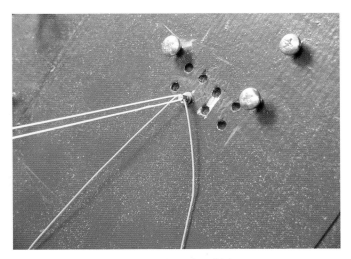

FIGURE 1–2. Suture orientation in anchor. White sutures on top, green sutures below.

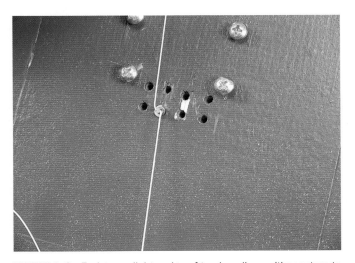

FIGURE 1–3. Eyelet parallel to edge of tendon allows either suture to slide freely.

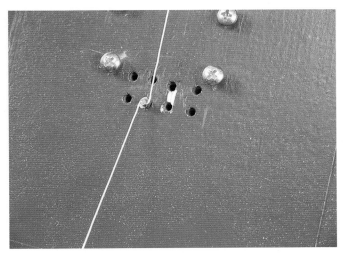

FIGURE 1–4. Eyelet parallel to edge of tendon allows either suture to slide freely.

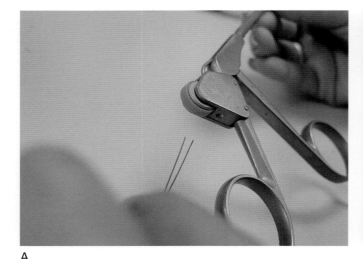

A

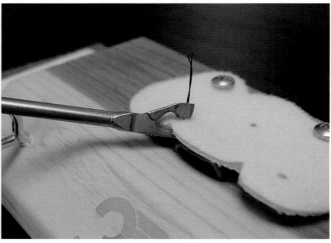

FIGURE 1–6. Two free ends of nylon suture placed through felt.

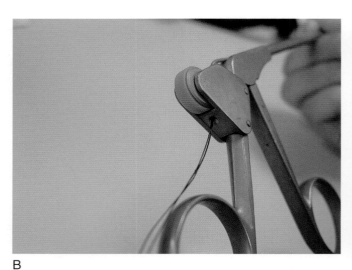

B

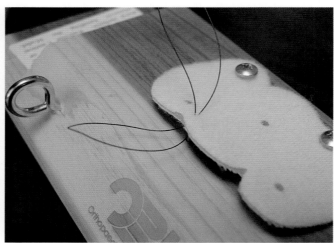

FIGURE 1–7. Remove Caspari suture passer. Nylon suture remains in felt.

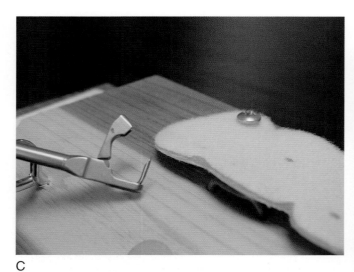

C

FIGURE 1–5. A, Two free ends of 2-0 nylon suture folded in half. B, Two free ends are inserted into back hole of Caspari suture passer. C, Loaded Caspari suture passer and tying board.

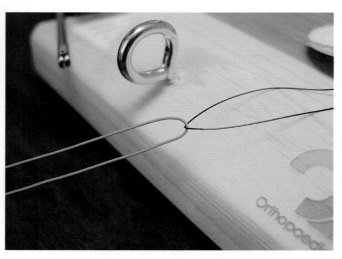

FIGURE 1–8. Loop braided through looped end of nylon suture.

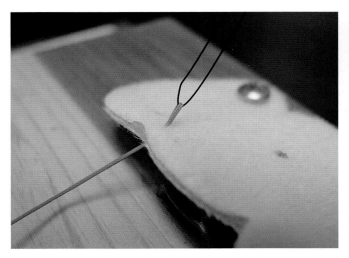

FIGURE 1–9. Pull on free ends of nylon suture and pull braided suture through felt.

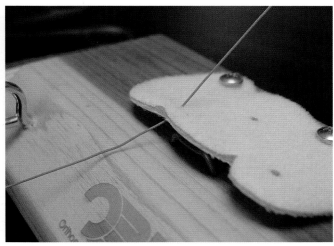

FIGURE 1–10. Braided suture passed through felt.

insertion is an option in the subacromial space but not in the glenohumeral joint because of the mass of soft tissue the anchor must penetrate.

You can practice suture management in two ways. Write out in detail each step of the operation and decide when you must move sutures. For example, the steps for a rotator cuff repair are as follows:

Arthroscopic Rotator Cuff Repair

Insert anchor No. 1, anterior position, through the lateral cannula.
Use a crochet hook to pull green and white sutures out through the anterior cannula.
Use a Caspari **suture passer** with 2-0 looped nylon inserted through the lateral cannula.
Grasp the tendon.
Check to see that the needle hole is clear
Advance the nylon suture.
Use a crochet hook to pull the two strands of nylon out through the anterior cannula and apply a hemostat.
Release the Caspari from the tendon and withdraw it out through the lateral cannula while advancing the hemostat.
Remove the Caspari from the nylon suture.
Use the crochet hook from the lateral cannula to retrieve one limb of the green suture.
Loop the grasper from the lateral cannula to untangle sutures.
Pass 6 cm of suture through the nylon loop.
Pull on the hemostat and nylon suture to bring the green suture through the tendon.
Apply the hemostat to the two green sutures.
Caspari with 2-0 looped nylon inserted through lateral cannula.
Grasp the tendon.
Check to ensure that the needle hole is clear.
Advance the nylon suture.
Use the crochet hook to pull the two strands of nylon out through the anterior cannula and apply a hemostat.

Release the Caspari from the tendon and withdraw it out through the lateral cannula while advancing the hemostat.
Remove the Caspari from the nylon suture.
Use the crochet hook from the lateral cannula to retrieve one limb of the white suture.
Loop the grasper from the lateral cannula to untangle the sutures.
Pass 6 cm of suture through the nylon loop.
Pull on the hemostat and nylon suture to bring the white suture through the tendon.
Apply the hemostat to the two white sutures.
Remove the hemostat from the white sutures.
Crochet hook from the lateral cannula retrieves both white sutures from the anterior cannula.
Loop the grasper to untangle.
Tie the white sutures.
Remove the hemostat from the green sutures.
Loop grasper to untangle.
Tie the green sutures.

For a glenohumeral reconstruction, some of the steps are as follows:

Arthroscopic Bankart Repair

Insert the arthroscope posteriorly.
Use a spinal needle to identify the anterior-superior portal immediately superior to the subscapularis tendon.
Insert an 8-mm cannula.
Use a spinal needle to identify the anterior-inferior portal near the biceps exit from the rotator interval.
Insert a 5.5-mm cannula.
Insert a probe through the anterior-superior cannula to determine the extent of the Bankart lesion.
Insert a shaver through the anterior-superior cannula to debride soft tissue from the anterior scapular neck.
Insert a bur to decorticate the anterior scapular neck.
Remove the anterior superior cannula.

Insert a metal cannula and trocar into the anterior-superior portal.

Observe the anterior scapular neck decortication.

Determine how many anchors are required to repair the Bankart lesion.

Move the arthroscope to the posterior portal.

Reinsert the 5.5-mm cannula anterior-superiorly.

Insert a drill through the anterior-superior cannula to drill anchor holes.

Insert an anchor through the anterior-superior cannula and place it in the most inferior drill hole.

Remove the inserter.

Two suture strands from the inferior anchor are exiting the anterior-superior cannula.

Insert a **spectrum** suture passer through the anterior-inferior cannula and pierce the capsule and labrum.

Advance the free ends of the nylon suture into the joint.

Retrieve the free ends of the nylon suture with a crochet hook placed in the anterior superior cannula.

Apply a hemostat to the tips of the nylon suture.

Place the tip of the hemostat at the entrance of the anterior-superior cannula to decrease the tendon on the nylon suture.

Remove the Spectrum suture passer from the anterior-inferior cannula.

Nylon loop is outside of the anterior-inferior cannula.

Use Prolene suture to reverse the direction of the loop.

Loop of Prolene is outside of the anterior-superior cannula.

Assistant holds one limb of each anchor suture in each hand.

Insert a crochet hook through the anterior-inferior cannula and retrieve one limb of the anchor suture from the anterior superior cannula to the anterior inferior cannula.

Place 6 cm of anchor suture through Prolene loop (anterior superior cannula).

Apply traction to the hemostat and pull the anchor suture from the anterior superior cannula into the joint, through the labrum and out through the anterior-inferior cannula.

Two anchor sutures are now through the anterior-inferior cannula.

Tie the sutures.

Repeat steps from additional anchors as needed.

If you write out the operative steps in detail, you will have an accurate impression of how many manipulations of sutures are needed.

You can then practice these steps before you get to the operating room. Get a 12- by 12-inch board, and insert picture eyelets to simulate portal location. Place cannulas through the eyelets, and insert and anchor them in the center. Practice moving the sutures from cannula to cannula until the motions are automatic.

I drew out the essential steps of the operation on a piece of paper and practiced the required maneuvers until I felt comfortable. Borrow a suture passer, knot pusher, crochet hook, loop grasper, sutures, and hemostats from the operating room. This should not prove difficult. In my hospital I merely gave the operating room head nurse my photo identification, a major credit card, the deed to my home, and my automobile.

I have included the drills I used and encourage you to rehearse the procedure with your assistant until both of you are familiar with your roles and the necessary steps. Although this may seem time-consuming, this level of preparation yields great dividends during the actual operation. Drill 1 simulates a one-anchor, two-suture rotator cuff repair. Drill 2 simulates a two-anchor, four-suture rotator cuff repair. Drill 3 simulates a three-anchor, six-suture complex rotator cuff repair. Drill 4 simulates a Bankart repair.

Drill 1

This is shown in Figures 1–11 to 1–21.

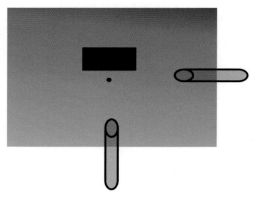

FIGURE 1–11. Drill 1 simulating a right shoulder. Anterior cannula on the right, lateral cannula in the center. Black felt represents rotator cuff tendon.

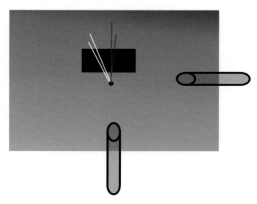

FIGURE 1–12. Insert anchor with two sutures. Four suture strands.

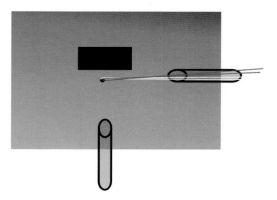

FIGURE 1–13. Pull four suture strands out the anterior cannula.

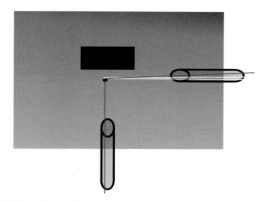

FIGURE 1–14. Pull one green strand through lateral cannula.

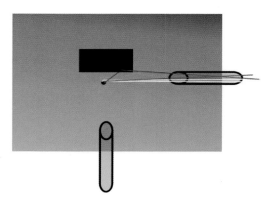

FIGURE 1–15. Place it through felt with a suture passer.

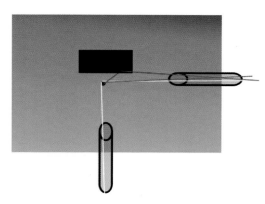

FIGURE 1–16. Pull one white suture strand through lateral cannula.

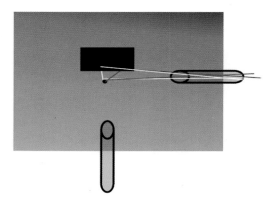

FIGURE 1–17. Place it through felt with a suture passer.

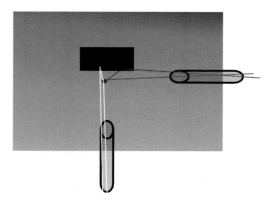

FIGURE 1–18. Retrieve both white suture strands from anterior cannula to lateral cannula.

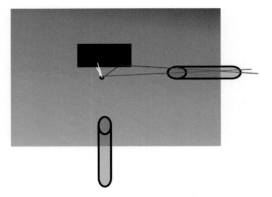

FIGURE 1–19. Tie white sutures.

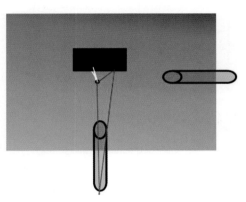

FIGURE 1–20. Retrieve green suture strands from anterior cannula to lateral cannula.

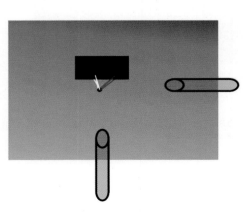

FIGURE 1–21. Tie green sutures.

Drill 2

This is shown in Figures 1–22 to 1–40.

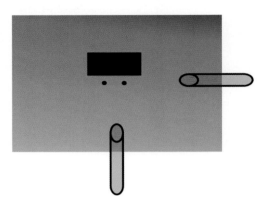

FIGURE 1–22. Drill 2 simulating a right shoulder. Anterior cannula on the right, lateral cannula in the center. Black felt represents rotator cuff tendon. Two drill holes for anchors.

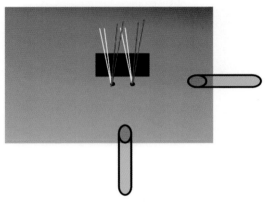

FIGURE 1–23. Insert two anchors. Four sutures, eight suture strands.

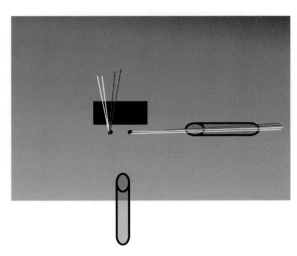

FIGURE 1–24. Pull sutures from anterior anchor out anterior cannula. Apply hemostat.

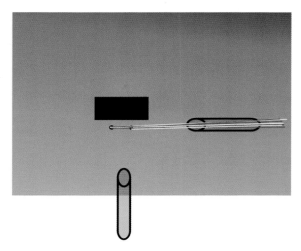

FIGURE 1–25. Pull sutures from posterior anchor out anterior cannula. Apply hemostat.

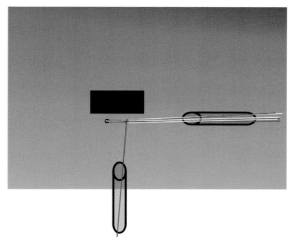

FIGURE 1–26. Retrieve one green suture strand from anterior anchor and bring it out lateral cannula.

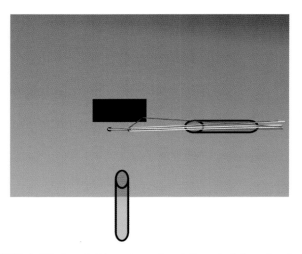

FIGURE 1–27. Insert this suture strand through felt and pull out anterior cannula.

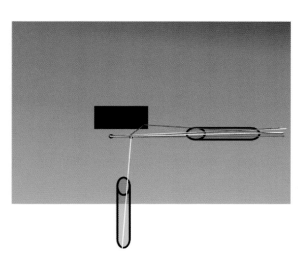

FIGURE 1–28. Retrieve one white suture strand from anterior anchor and bring it out lateral cannula.

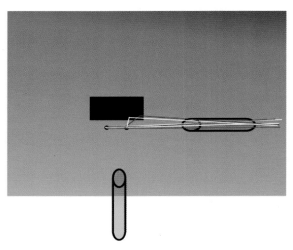

FIGURE 1–29. Insert this suture strand through felt and pull out anterior cannula.

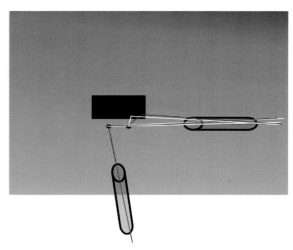

FIGURE 1–30. Retrieve one green suture strand from posterior anchor and bring it out lateral cannula.

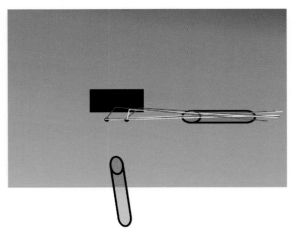

FIGURE 1–31. Insert this suture strand through felt and pull out anterior cannula.

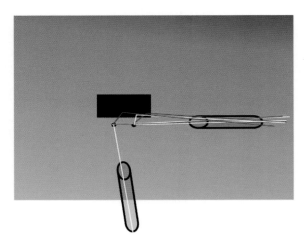

FIGURE 1–32. Retrieve one white suture strand from posterior anchor and bring it out lateral cannula.

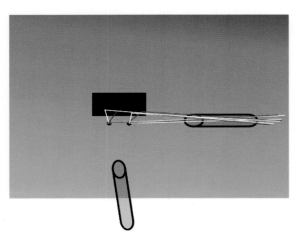

FIGURE 1–33. Insert this suture strand through felt and pull out anterior cannula.

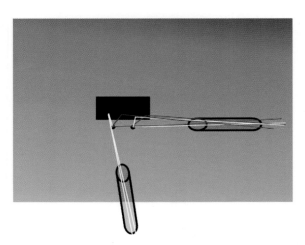

FIGURE 1–34. Retrieve both posterior anchor white strands from anterior cannula and pull out lateral cannula.

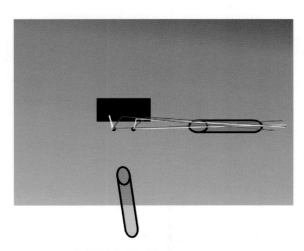

FIGURE 1–35. Tie these sutures.

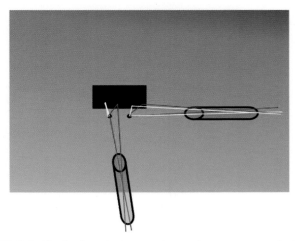

FIGURE 1–36. Retrieve both posterior anchor green strands from anterior cannula and pull out lateral cannula.

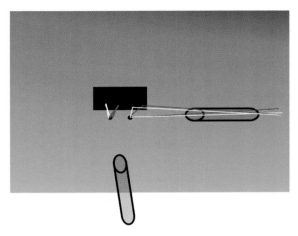

FIGURE 1–37. Tie these sutures.

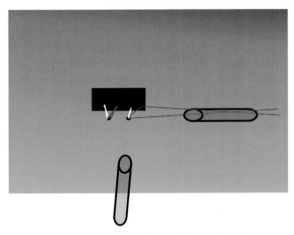

FIGURE 1–38. Repeat steps for anterior anchor white suture.

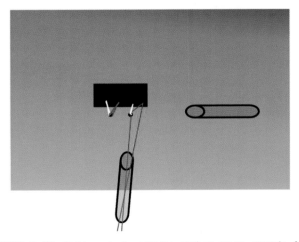

FIGURE 1–39. Retrieve both anterior anchor green strands from anterior cannula and pull out lateral cannula.

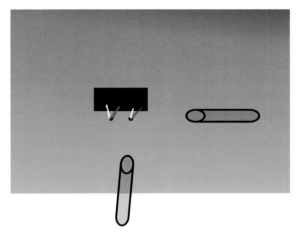

FIGURE 1–40. Tie sutures. Repair complete.

Drill 3

This is shown in Figures 1–41 to 1–73.

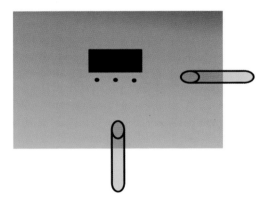

FIGURE 1–41. Drill 3 simulating large or massive rotator cuff repair. Three anchor holes.

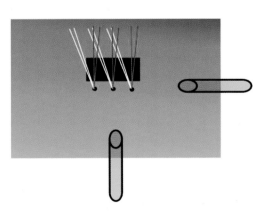

FIGURE 1–42. Three anchors. Six sutures and 12 suture strands.

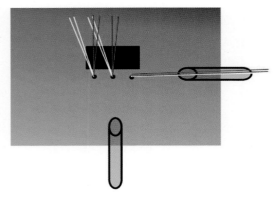

FIGURE 1–43. Pull anterior anchor sutures out anterior cannula.

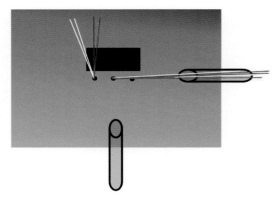

FIGURE 1–44. Pull middle anchor suture strands out anterior cannula.

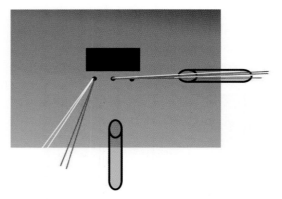

FIGURE 1–45. Move posterior anchor strands to left or lateral cannula simulating removing these through a posterolateral percutaneous stab wound.

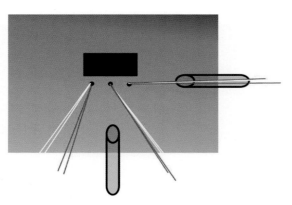

FIGURE 1–46. Move middle anchor sutures from anterior cannula simulating an anterolateral percutaneous stab wound.

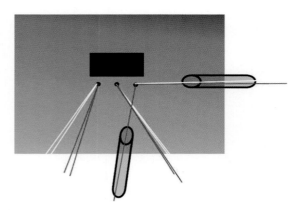

FIGURE 1–47. Retrieve one green suture from anterior anchor from anterior cannula and out lateral cannula.

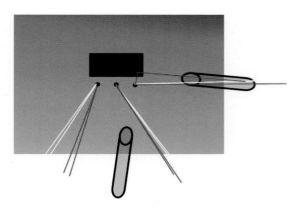

FIGURE 1–48. Place this suture through felt and withdraw it out anterior cannula.

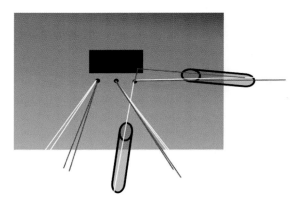

FIGURE 1–49. Retrieve one white suture from anterior anchor from anterior cannula and out lateral cannula.

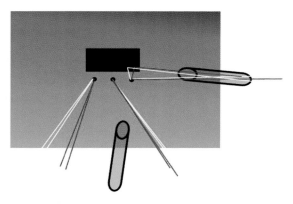

FIGURE 1–50. Place this suture through felt and withdraw it out anterior cannula.

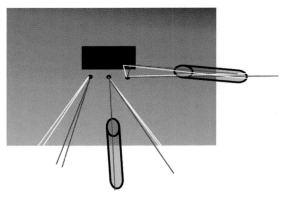

FIGURE 1–51. Retrieve one green suture from middle anchor from anterolateral stab wound and withdraw it out lateral cannula.

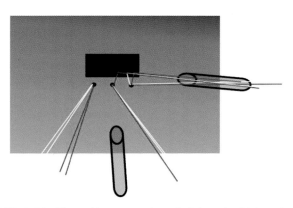

FIGURE 1–52. Place this suture through felt and withdraw it out anterior cannula.

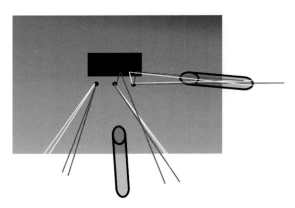

FIGURE 1–53. Withdraw suture strand that is through felt and pull it out anterolateral stab wound.

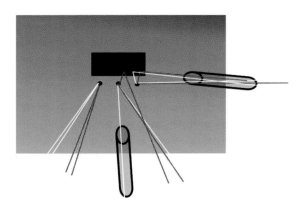

FIGURE 1–54. Retrieve one white suture from middle anchor from anterolateral stab wound and withdraw it out lateral cannula.

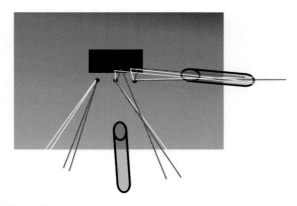

FIGURE 1–55. Place this suture through felt and withdraw it out anterior cannula.

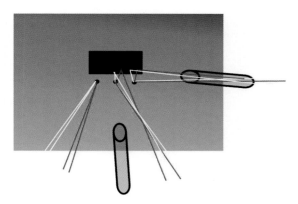

FIGURE 1–56. Withdraw suture strand that is through felt and pull it out anterolateral stab wound.

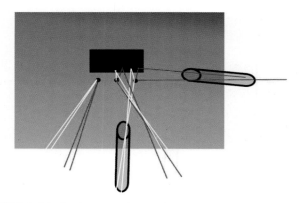

FIGURE 1–57. Retrieve anterior anchor white suture strands from anterior cannula out lateral cannula.

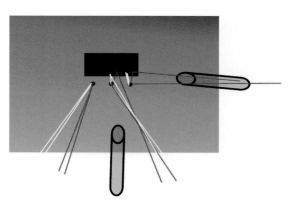

FIGURE 1–58. Tie sutures.

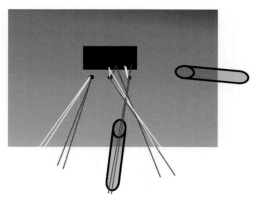

FIGURE 1–59. Retrieve anterior anchor green suture strands from anterior cannula out lateral cannula.

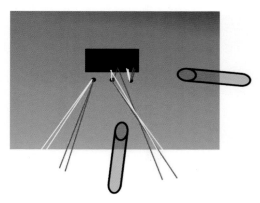

FIGURE 1–60. Tie sutures.

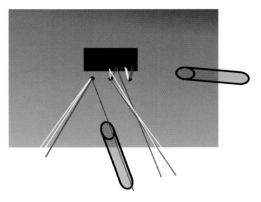

FIGURE 1–61. Withdraw posterior anchor green suture strand from posterolateral stab wound and withdraw it out lateral cannula.

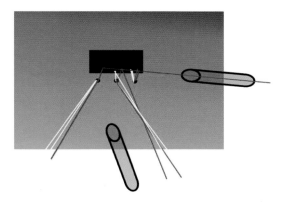

FIGURE 1–62. Place this suture through felt and withdraw it out anterior cannula.

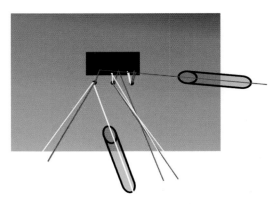

FIGURE 1–63. Withdraw posterior anchor white suture strand from posterolateral stab wound and withdraw it out lateral cannula.

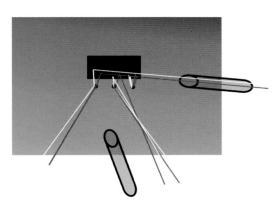

FIGURE 1–64. Place this suture through felt and withdraw it out anterior cannula.

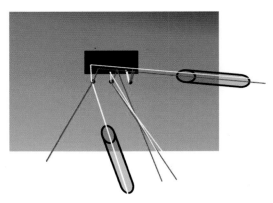

FIGURE 1–65. Retrieve posterior anchor strand from posterolateral stab wound and withdraw it out lateral cannula.

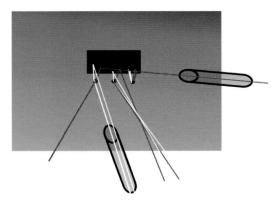

FIGURE 1–66. Retrieve posterior anchor strand from anterior cannula and withdraw it out lateral cannula.

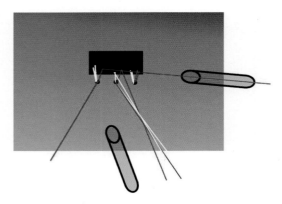

FIGURE 1–67. Tie white sutures from posterior anchor.

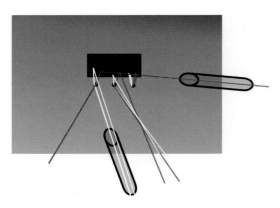

FIGURE 1–68. Retrieve both posterior anchor green sutures and withdraw them out lateral cannula.

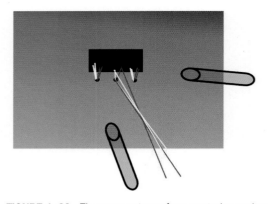

FIGURE 1–69. Tie green sutures from posterior anchor.

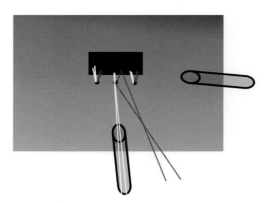

FIGURE 1–70. Retrieve both middle anchor white sutures and withdraw them out lateral cannula.

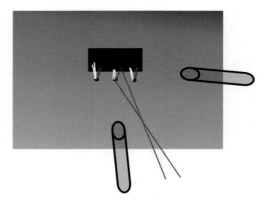

FIGURE 1–71. Tie middle anchor white sutures.

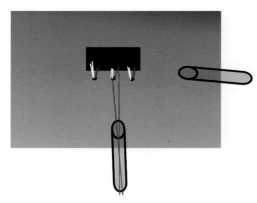

FIGURE 1–72. Retrieve both middle anchor green sutures and withdraw them out lateral cannula.

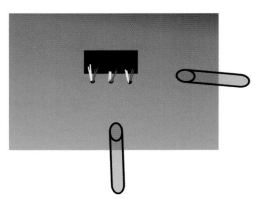

FIGURE 1–73. Tie middle anchor green sutures.

Drill 4

This is shown in Figures 1–74 to 1–83.

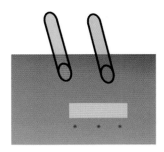

FIGURE 1–74. Drill 4. Right shoulder Bankart repair with three suture anchors. Green cannula is anterior inferior. Orange cannula is anterior superior.

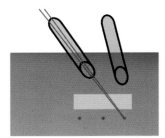

FIGURE 1–75. Insert inferior anchor and withdraw sutures out orange cannula.

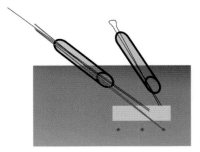

FIGURE 1–76. Place nylon passing suture through green cannula. Two free ends are exiting orange cannula and looped end is exiting green cannula.

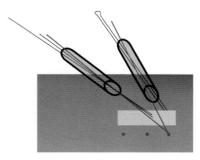

FIGURE 1–77. Pull one suture strand from orange cannula out green cannula.

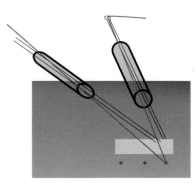

FIGURE 1–78. Place end of green suture through looped end of nylon suture.

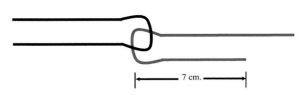

FIGURE 1–79. Close-up view.

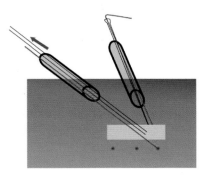

FIGURE 1–80. Pull on two free ends of nylon suture.

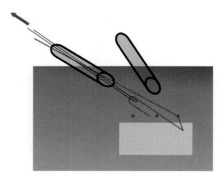

FIGURE 1–81. Pull green suture from green cannula through felt.

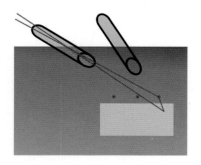

FIGURE 1–82. Continue to pull on nylon suture and bring green suture out orange cannula.

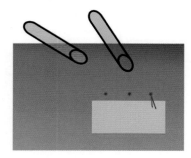

FIGURE 1–83. Tie suture. Repeat for two additional anchors.

KNOT TYING. Because reconstructive arthroscopic shoulder surgery involves soft tissue repair, knot tying is a critical skill. Failure to master this skill leads many surgeons to alter fundamental principles of an operation. An example of this is thermal capsulorrhaphy for gleno-

humeral instability. A surgeon who cannot tie secure knots will rely too heavily on thermal techniques. Failure will inevitably occur because capsular tightening is usually only one part of the repair. Thermal capsulorrhaphy cannot repair Bankart or SLAP (superior labral anterior and posterior) lesions and, perhaps most important, cannot shift the capsular tissue in different directions. These deficiencies are not a failure of the device or thermal technique but represent a failure of the surgeon to appreciate what steps are necessary to balance the lax soft tissue system.

The difficulties surgeons have with arthroscopic knot tying are real, but these difficulties can be overcome with instruction and practice. Surgeons tie knots in open surgery on a daily basis. The arthroscopic knots are identical, except the knot pusher replaces the surgeon's index finger.

The surgeon should learn two basic knots: an overhand knot and a sliding knot. Although there are many knot variations, only these two basic knots are necessary. When one is learning to tie knots, it is easier to see the required steps with clothesline, rather than with surgical suture. All the knots described here are shown on video.

Knot Tying

OVERHAND KNOT. After the suture has been inserted through the soft tissue, the surgeon should verify that no tangles exist. Use the loop grasper and encircle one suture limb and withdraw the instrument. Perform this step before tying every knot. Tie a half hitch with either two-handed or one-handed technique. Place one limb of the suture through the knot-tying instrument. Apply a hemostat to the suture strand that is through the knot pusher so that you have something to pull against as you push the knot down the cannula. Gently push the half hitch down the cannula. Slowly place tension on the two strands and observe which strand must be pushed away for the knot to lie flat. If you push the other strand away, the knot will not lie flat. It is not important whether the first throw is overhand or underhand, but it is important for the surgeon always to tie the knots with the same technique. Use the knot pusher to past point. This allows you to pull the suture strands tight with a 180-degree angle. Place another throw in the same direction as the first, past point, and tighten the knot. Now reverse the direction of the throw and place a third hitch. Reverse the post of the knot for greater knot security, and place a fourth throw. Reverse the post and the direction of the throw for the fifth half hitch.

It is critical that the surgeon become skilled in tying a knot with one-handed technique. Gradually incorporate arthroscopic knot tying into surgery by first tying knots with the knot pusher during an open repair and moving to arthroscopic knot tying as your skills increase. The steps are shown in Figures 1–84 to 1–96.

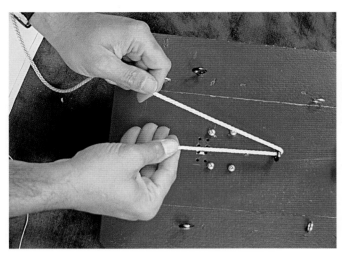

FIGURE 1–84. One-handed knot.

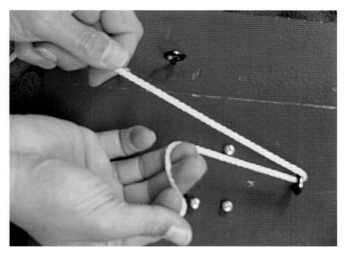

FIGURE 1–85. One-handed knot.

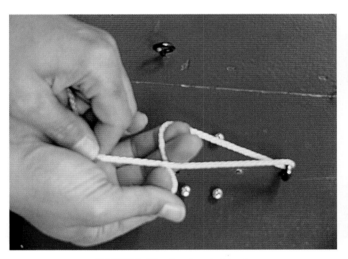

FIGURE 1–86. One-handed knot.

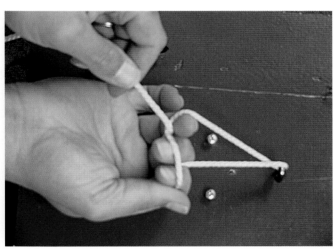

FIGURE 1–87. One-handed knot.

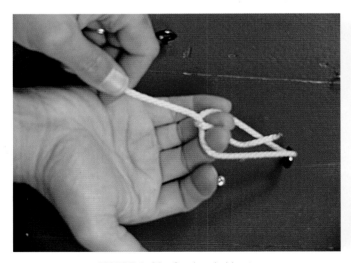

FIGURE 1–88. One-handed knot.

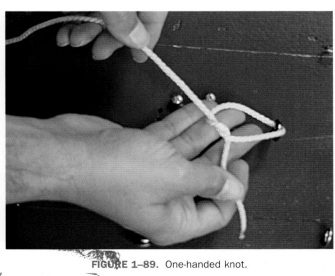

FIGURE 1–89. One-handed knot.

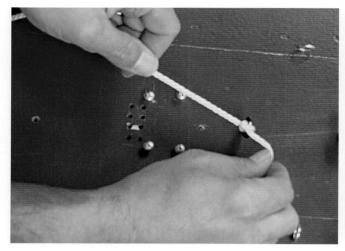

FIGURE 1–90. One-handed knot.

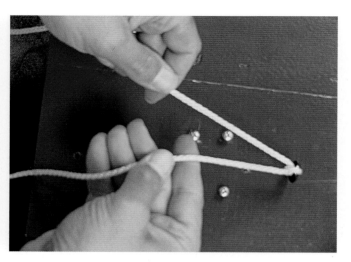

FIGURE 1–91. One-handed knot.

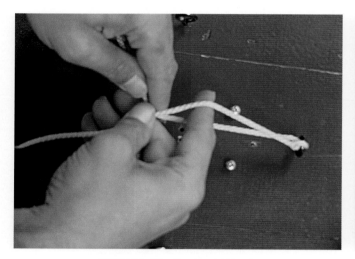

FIGURE 1–92. One-handed knot.

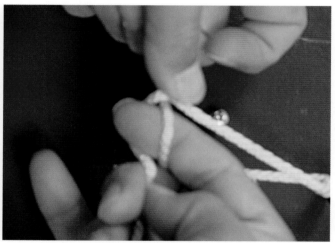

FIGURE 1–93. One-handed knot.

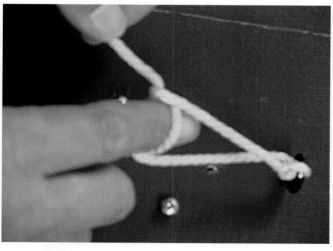

FIGURE 1–94. One-handed knot.

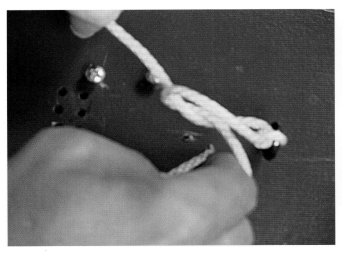

FIGURE 1–95. One-handed knot.

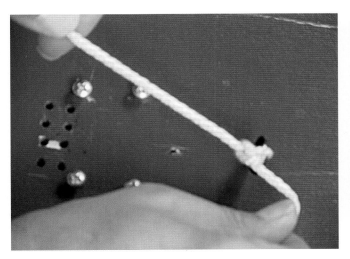

FIGURE 1–96. One-handed knot.

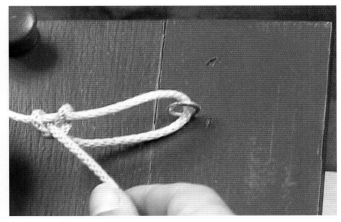

FIGURE 1–97. Slipping second throw. Two half-hitches in same direction.

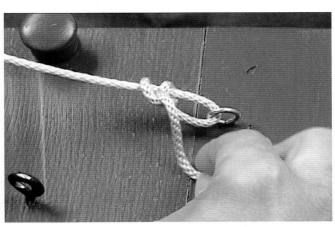

FIGURE 1–98. Pull on post limb. No tension on other suture limb.

An additional skill that I believe is critical is learning to slip the second throw. Most of the time, the tendon or ligament that is to be tied is under tension and will retract slightly after the first knot throw. One method to deal with this problem is to eliminate the tension on the soft tissue by having an assistant hold the soft tissue with a tissue grasper. Another method is to place a traction suture through the soft tissue. A third method (and the one I prefer) involves slipping the second throw. Tie the first throw routinely. Make a second half hitch in the same direction and slowly advance it down the cannula. Check to see that the suture is not tangled. Pull on the post limb, and release all tension on the other limb. The knot will slide down to the soft tissue without locking and will enable you to approximate the soft tissue. Past point and lock the second throw. Finish the remaining throws, and complete the knot (Figs. 1–97 to 1–99).

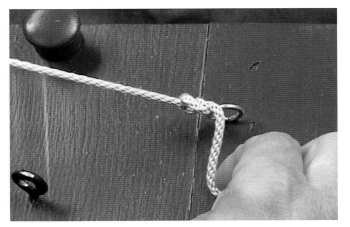

FIGURE 1–99. Knot slides down. Place remaining throws.

Sliding Knot

There are literally dozens of sliding knots, but I believe it is necessary to learn only one at first. After you have placed the suture through the soft tissue, grasp both ends and confirm that the suture slides freely. Pull on one end so that it becomes the shorter one. Make a loop with the longer strand, and pinch it between your thumb and index finger. Pass the longer suture over the shorter one four times. Bring the end of the longer suture strand up through the loop to complete the Duncan loop. Freshen the knot by applying tension to each strand. Pull on the shorter strand to advance the knot. Place three alternating half hitches to secure the knot (Fig. 1–100).

Intellectual Skills

Intellectual skills can be honed by attending instructional courses that are presented by the American Academy of Orthopedic Surgeons, the American Shoulder and Elbow Surgeons, and the Arthroscopy Association of North America. These courses are held throughout the United States. A full day of current shoulder information is given at the open meeting of the American Shoulder and Elbow Surgeons that is held at the annual American Academy of Orthopedic Surgeons meeting.

Excellent textbooks are available, such as *The Shoulder*, by Rockwood and Matsen. Subscribe to the *Journal of Shoulder and Elbow Surgery and Arthroscopy*. Both are sources of current thought on shoulder problems.

Perhaps the most important intellectual tool that the surgeon can possess is a plan to master reconstructive arthroscopic operations. As a general approach, I recommend the following: learn the individual steps of the arthroscopic repair, practice these techniques outside the operating room, gradually incorporate these techniques into the open repair, perform the arthroscopic repair and open the shoulder, and finally perform the operation exclusively with arthroscopic technique. I have spoken with physicians who decided to make the transition to arthroscopic repair in one step. Although theoretically this seems reasonable, in practice it can result in a 6-hour rotator cuff repair that benefits neither patient nor surgeon. I followed (and advise) a more gradual transition.

Establish time limits for your arthroscopic procedures. Give the circulating nurse authority to inform you that 1 hour has passed and it is time to open the shoulder. Listen to that person! Consider a plan similar to the one I followed and describe here.

Arthroscope all rotator cuff tears before performing an open repair.

STAGE 1

1. Arthroscope glenohumeral joint.
2. Enter subacromial space and expose tear with bursectomy.
3. Measure length and width (retraction).
4. Use grasper and estimate reparability and what goes where.

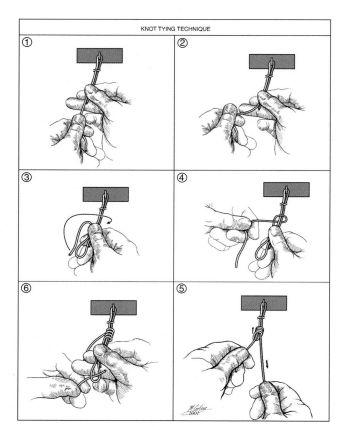

KNOT TYING TECHNIQUE

FIGURE 1–100. Technique for sliding knot.

5. Perform arthroscopic decompression.
6. Open and repair rotator cuff tear.

Repeat this sequence with each rotator cuff repair. When you can perform steps 1 to 5 in 30 minutes, advance to next stage.

STAGE 2

1. Arthroscope glenohumeral joint.
2. Enter subacromial space and expose tear with bursectomy.
3. Measure length and width (retraction).
4. Use grasper and estimate reparability and what goes where.
5. Perform arthroscopic decompression.
6. Measure length and width.
7. Use round bur to abrade rotator cuff tear repair site.
8. Open and repair rotator cuff tear.

Repeat this sequence with each rotator cuff repair. When you can perform steps 1 to 7 in 30 minutes, advance to the next stage.

STAGE 3

1. Arthroscope glenohumeral joint.
2. Enter subacromial space and expose tear with bursectomy.

3. Measure length and width (retraction).
4. Use grasper and estimate reparability and what goes where.
5. Perform arthroscopic decompression.
6. Use round bur to abrade rotator cuff tear repair site.
7. Insert anterior anchor and pull sutures out anterior cannula. Apply hemostat.
8. Insert posterior anchor and pull sutures out anterior cannula. Apply hemostat.
9. Open and repair.

Repeat this sequence with each rotator cuff repair. When you can perform steps 1 to 8 in 35 minutes, advance to the next stage.

STAGE 4

1. Arthroscope glenohumeral joint.
2. Enter subacromial space and expose tear with bursectomy.
3. Measure length and width (retraction).
4. Use grasper and estimate reparability and what goes where.
5. Perform arthroscopic decompression.
6. Use round bur to abrade rotator cuff tear repair site.
7. Insert anterior anchor and pull sutures out anterior cannula. Apply hemostat.
8.. Insert posterior anchor and pull sutures out anterior cannula. Apply hemostat.
9. Pass anterior anchor sutures through tendon.
10. Pass posterior anchor sutures through tendon.
11. Open and complete rotator cuff repair.

Repeat this sequence with each rotator cuff repair. When you can perform steps 1 to 10 in 45 minutes, advance to the next stage.

STAGE 5

1. Arthroscope glenohumeral joint.
2. Enter subacromial space and expose tear with bursectomy.
3. Measure length and width (retraction).
4. Use grasper and estimate reparability and what goes where.
5. Perform arthroscopic decompression.
6. Use round bur to abrade rotator cuff tear repair site
7. Insert anterior anchor and pull sutures out anterior cannula. Apply hemostat.
8. Insert posterior anchor and pull sutures out anterior cannula. Apply hemostat.
9. Pass anterior anchor sutures through tendon.
10. Pass posterior anchor sutures through tendon.
11. Tie knots.

Instrument Handling

Reconstructive shoulder arthroscopic operations are complex, and success is built on certain small details. One area that surgeons often overlook is the appropriate handling of arthroscopic instruments. Correct hand positions and movements are elements that all surgeons can master with very little effort.

Arthroscope

The surgeon should practice holding and manipulating the arthroscope with both the right and the left hands. If you can hold the arthroscope with only one hand, operating on the opposite shoulder will force you into awkward positions. Practice with both hands during a diagnostic glenohumeral arthroscopy until you can smoothly and rapidly maneuver the arthroscope and view all critical areas of the joint.

A second skill is arthroscope rotation. Many surgeons rotate the arthroscope with the opposite hand. This may be satisfactory during the diagnostic phase, but when the surgeon has an instrument in the opposite hand, this becomes difficult. Learn to rotate the arthroscope by using the index finger of the hand holding the arthroscope.

Caspari Suture Punch

You should learn to use the Caspari suture punch with either hand, and you can master this skill on a practice station. It is also necessary to advance the suture with the thumb of the hand holding the instrument so you are not forced to use your opposite hand.

The scrub nurse will hand you the Caspari numerous times during an arthroscopic repair, and this phase of instrument transfer can be awkward or smooth. Rehearse the instrument transfer with your scrub nurse so that both of you are familiar with the correct technique (Figs. 1–101 to 1–103).

Spectrum Suture Passer

Familiarize yourself with the proper handling and transfer of this instrument. Have the scrub nurse load the looped

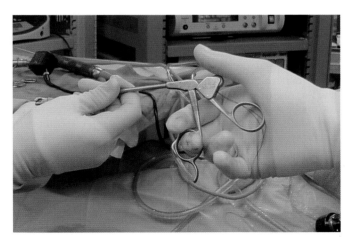

FIGURE 1–101. Incorrect handling of Caspari suture passer. Nylon suture will get caught in your palm.

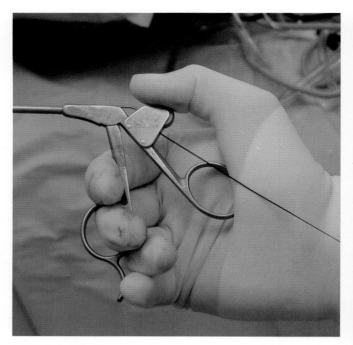

FIGURE 1–102. Correct position of nylon loop. Hold the Caspari suture passer against your thenar eminence and control the orange wheel with your thumb.

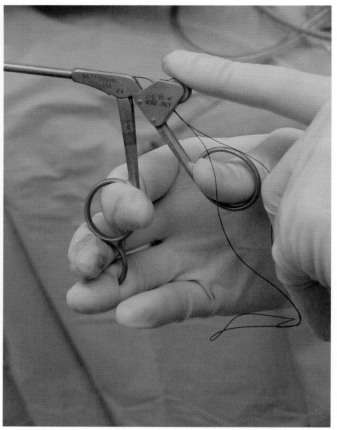

FIGURE 1–103. Incorrect use of Caspari suture passer. Two hands are required.

nylon suture from the opposite side of the thumb so that the suture will not become tangled as you advance it.

Knot Pusher

Various knot-tying instruments are available, and surgeons should examine them and determine which one feels most comfortable. I prefer a simple instrument and view the tip of the instrument as an arthroscopic projection of my index finger (Fig. 1–104).

The surgeon should determine what shaft length is most comfortable. This is done by trial and error. I have shortened the standard shaft length to fit my thumb motion during the tying maneuver.

My experience is that many surgeons underestimate the level of skill required to perform complicated arthroscopic reconstructive operations. Many, but not all, of the necessary skills can be mastered before the surgeon enters the operating room.

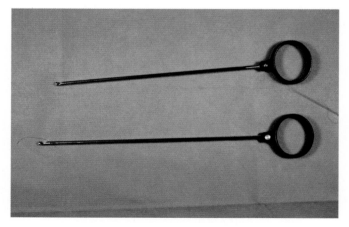

FIGURE 1–104. Knot pushers.

2

Operating Room Setup

The essential elements of this chapter are general operating room organization, anesthesia, patient positioning, hand instruments, power instruments, fluid management, and image capture.

I find it helpful to bring a copy of my patient record to the operating room. This allows me to compare the examination performed while the patient was under anesthesia with the examination I documented in the office. For patients with glenohumeral instability, I can compare the patient's history of which activities or motions produce pain with the amount of translation observed during examination performed with the patient under anesthesia. The patient record also includes my summary of the pertinent findings of the magnetic resonance imaging or computed tomography scans so that I can compare these with the findings at arthroscopy. I also display the relevant radiographic study so that I can review it if necessary (Figs. 2–1 and 2–2).

Operating Room Setup

The room organization is shown in Figure 2–3. There must be adequate space between the head of the table and the anesthetist to allow me sufficient space to maneuver (Fig. 2–4). I have the cart with the arthroscopy equipment angled toward me so I can see all gauges (Fig. 2–5). Similarly, the arthroscopic pump and fluid bags should be visible so that I can see the pressure and flow at any time (Figs. 2–6 and 2–7). I also request theanesthetist to rotate the blood pressure monitor to enable me to check it during the procedure without disturbing his or her concentration. An absorbent mat to collect fluid is placed on the floor under my feet (Fig. 2–8). I arrange the foot pedals that con-

trol the power instruments and the cautery to permit easy access (Fig. 2–9).

Operating Room Tables

The shoulder preparation table contains the skin razor and adhesive tape for removing hair. We use an iodine-based product (Duraprep). For patients with iodine allergy, we use a Hibiclens (chlorhexidine gluconate) scrub followed by an isopropyl alcohol solution. I prefer to have the patient's hair shaved from the area that will be covered by the bandage. I have not found it necessary to shave the axilla.

Only those instruments required for the operation are placed on the Mayo stand (Figs. 2–10 and 2–11). The back table contains rarely used instruments and the postoperative dressing (Fig. 2–12).

Anesthesia

Our routine is to perform an interscalene block in the preoperative holding area. The patient is then moved to the operating room, where general anesthesia is started. The interscalene block has no direct effect on blood pressure. With sensory input blocked, there is no sympathetic response to the otherwise painful stimuli, and catecholamine release is avoided. The beta-antagonistic effects (vasodilatation and bradycardia) of the general anesthetic agents are then more pronounced without the pain response to offset them. These effects cause relative bradycardia and hypotension. The result is improved visualization. Because the operated area is anesthetized, only light general anesthesia is necessary, thus minimizing postopera-

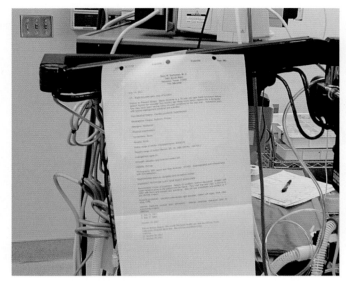

FIGURE 2–1. Patient record.

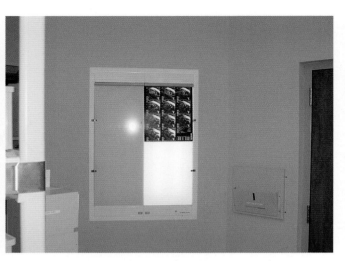

FIGURE 2–2. Radiographic display.

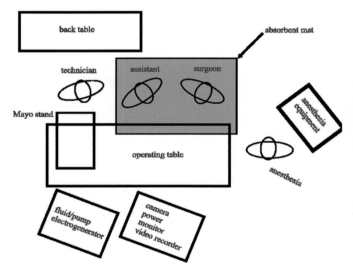

FIGURE 2–3. Operating room setup.

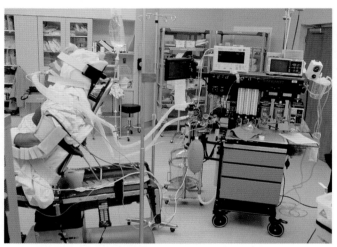

FIGURE 2–4. Equipment position.

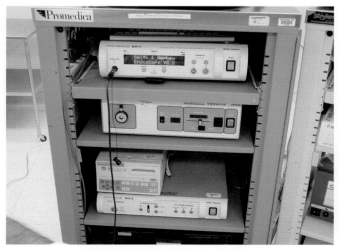

FIGURE 2–5. Equipment cart.

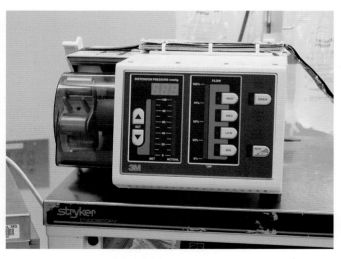

FIGURE 2–6. Arthroscopic pump.

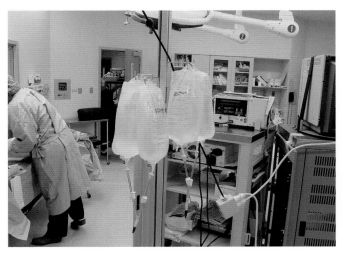

FIGURE 2–7. Fluid bags.

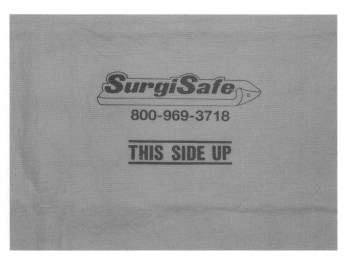

FIGURE 2–8. Absorbent mat.

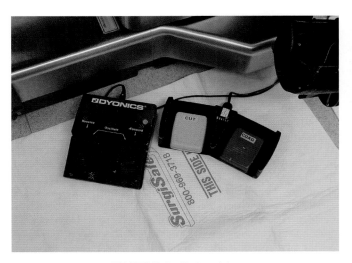

FIGURE 2–9. Foot pedals.

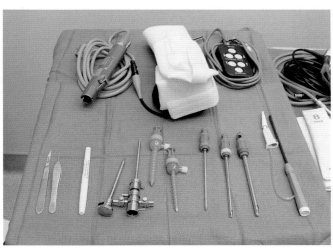

FIGURE 2–10. Mayo stand.

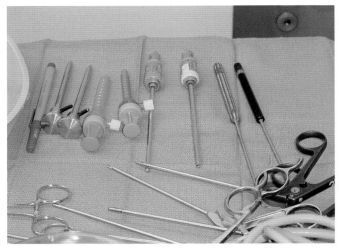

FIGURE 2–11. Mayo stand.

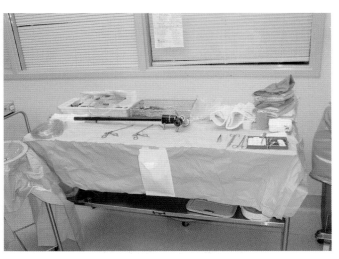

FIGURE 2–12. Back table.

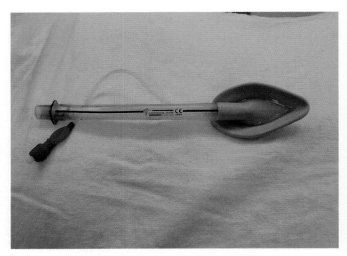

FIGURE 2–13. Laryngeal mask airway tube.

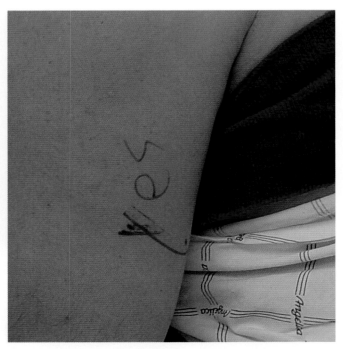

FIGURE 2–15. Skin marking.

tive nausea. Our anesthesiologists prefer a laryngeal mask airway, which eliminates the need for endotracheal intubations. Immediate postoperative pain is well controlled. Because many patients find remaining motionless in the seated position uncomfortable and I find patient movement distracting, I prefer to use general anesthesia in these patients, rather than operating using regional block alone (Figs. 2–13 and 2–14).

To minimize "wrong-site" surgery, we confirm with the patient which shoulder is to undergo the surgical procedure. We use a surgical marking pen to write "yes" on that shoulder and "no" on the contralateral shoulder (Fig. 2–15).

Patient Positioning

A successful shoulder arthroscopy is the result of advanced planning and organization. Many seemingly minor details

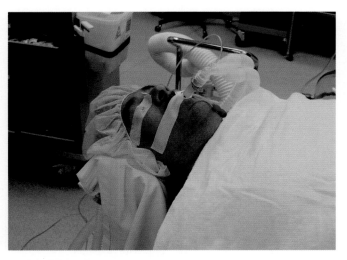

FIGURE 2–14. Laryngeal mask airway tube secured with tape.

have a profound effect on the procedure, and I encourage all surgeons to invest the necessary time to prepare the operating room and surgical staff adequately.

Surgeons position patients in either the lateral decubitus or the sitting (beach-chair) orientation. Each position has its advantages and disadvantages, and surgeon preference should dictate the choice. I believe that both diagnostic and reconstructive shoulder arthroscopy can be successfully performed with the patient in either position. I pay considerable attention to patient positioning because this aids in portal placement and facilitates the procedure. Incorrect positioning adds complexity to an already difficult procedure.

Lateral Decubitus Position

The lateral decubitus position offers excellent access to the posterior shoulder and allows arm suspension (and distraction as necessary) without the need for an assistant. The surgeon can choose to terminate the arthroscopic procedure and perform open operations in the subacromial space easily. Disadvantages include the need to lift and turn the patient into the lateral decubitus position, the possibility of excessive distraction across the glenohumeral joint and possible nerve injury, limited access to the anterior shoulder, and the need to reposition the patient if an open anterior glenohumeral reconstruction is required. Another potential disadvantage is the tendency for the suspension apparatus to place the arm in internal rotation. This is important in glenohumeral reconstruction when shoulder repair of the glenohumeral ligaments or rotator interval in internal rotation may result in permanent loss of external rotation. The surgeon can overcome all these difficulties with appropriate care.

TABLE 2–1. TABLE POSITIONING AIDS: DECUBITUS
1. U-shaped Vacupak beanbag, 3 feet long
2. Axillary roll
3. Kidney rest supports for operating room table (2)
4. Contoured foam head-and-neck support
5. Arm board
6. Pillows (2)
7. Foam pads for ankles, knees, and arms
8. 3-inch-wide cloth adhesive tape

Before the patient is brought to the operating room, a vacuum beanbag is placed on the operating table and is smoothed (Table 2–1). The patient is assisted onto the table and is centered on the beanbag. The cephalad edge of the beanbag should be level with the patient's upper thorax, not high enough to protrude into the axilla. After general endotracheal anesthesia has been established, the tube is secured on the side of the patient's mouth away from the surgical side. Both shoulders are examined for range of motion and translation. The patient is then turned over on the unaffected side, and the pelvis and shoulders are placed perpendicular to the table. The beanbag is gathered up around the patient and is deflated until it is firm. The operating table is tilted 20 to 30 degrees posteriorly so that the glenoid is parallel to the floor. Considerable attention is given to protecting the neurovascular structures, soft tissues, and bony prominences. A soft sheet is rolled into a cylinder approximately 6 inches in diameter and is placed under the upper thorax to raise the patient's chest off the table, thereby minimizing pressure on the neurovascular structures within the axilla. The roll should not be placed in the axilla. A 1-L intravenous bag wrapped in a towel also works nicely. The downside hip and knee are slightly flexed to stabilize the patient. Place pillows between the legs to protect the ankles, knees, and peroneal nerves. Breasts are also carefully padded. Kidney rests are useful to support the beanbag, and broad adhesive tape may be used to stabilize the patient further. The cervical spine must be supported to prevent any hyperextension or lateral angulation during the procedure. An electrosurgical grounding pad is placed over the muscular area of the lateral thigh. The surgeon should inspect the position of the patient carefully and should check each pressure area to make sure it is adequately padded.

The circulating nurse prepares the patient's entire shoulder, arm, and hand. An assistant then grasps the patient's wrist with a sterile towel, and the surgeon and scrub nurse place the lower U-drape over the patient. The patient's forearm and hand are then placed in the traction device. Carefully pad the wrist to avoid pressure to the sensory branch of the radial nerve. The arm is then placed on the lower drape, the upper drape is put into position, and the fluid collection pouch is applied. The arm is then attached to the suspension device. Usually, 10 pounds of weight is all that is necessary, but the weight may be increased slightly for larger patients. The surgeon should think of the suspension device as a stabilizing mechanism, rather than a

method to produce traction. The patient's shoulder is positioned in 60 degrees of abduction and 10 degrees of flexion.

Sitting Position

I prefer the term *sitting position* over the historical term *beach-chair* position because the patient's thorax must be placed 70 to 80 degrees perpendicular to the floor. This upright position is needed to place the acromion parallel to the floor and to allow access to the posterior shoulder. A more recumbent position forces the surgeon to "work uphill" and makes entry into the inferior posterior shoulder difficult if such a portal is required for glenohumeral reconstruction. The advantages of the sitting position are that it is similar to that used during traditional open operations and conversion from an arthroscopic to an open rotator cuff repair or glenohumeral reconstruction does not require a change in patient position. The anterior shoulder is more approachable than in the lateral decubitus position because the surgeon need not lean over the patient to gain anterior access. The arthroscopic orientation seems more familiar to most surgeons, with the vertical orientation of the glenoid similar to that seen during physical examination or radiographic review. Shoulder distraction is not continuous, a feature that minimizes the chance of neurologic injury, and the assistant can provide distraction force during the brief periods when this is needed. A mechanical arm holder can maintain the patient's shoulder in external rotation during glenohumeral reconstruction and in elevation during rotator cuff repair. I use the McConnell arm holder (Table 2–2) (McConnell Orthopedics, Greenville, TX). A disadvantage of the sitting position is that although devices that position and hold the patient are useful, such devices are expensive. I currently use the Schloein patient positioner (Orthopedic Systems, Inc., Union City, CA).

Before the patient is brought to the operating room, the mechanical support is positioned and is secured to the operating table. The patient is assisted onto the operating table, and general anesthesia is induced. The back of the mechanical support is then raised, a small amount of Trendelenburg positioning is applied, and the legs are lowered. The position is adjusted until the patient's acromion is nearly parallel to the floor. This places the patient in a vertical sitting, rather than a semirecumbent beach-chair, position. I believe it is important to select a mechanical patient positioner that allows the 70 to 80 degrees of sitting necessary. The head and neck are positioned for patient comfort and are secured. Pillows are placed under the patient's knees, and a foam pad protects the contralateral elbow. I check to make sure no pads or drapes interfere with access to the anterior or posterior shoulder.

The shoulder, arm, and hand are prepared, and an assistant grasps the patient's wrist while the scrub nurse positions the bottom drape. The hand-wrist support is attached, and the forearm is placed on the patient's lap. The upper drape is applied, and the suction drainage bag is affixed around the shoulder. The applicable surface anatomy is drawn, and the surgical procedure may begin (Figs. 2–16 to 2–28).

I used the lateral decubitus position for 10 years and found it very satisfactory for diagnostic arthroscopy, arthro-

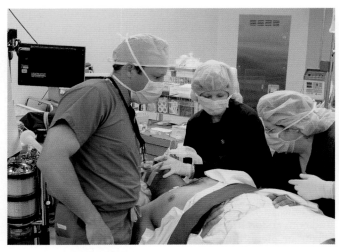

FIGURE 2–16. Positioning the patient.

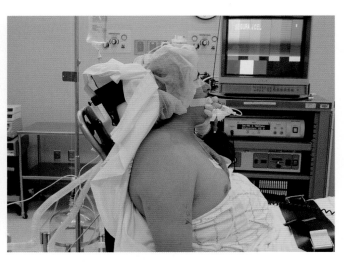

FIGURE 2–17. Patient in sitting position.

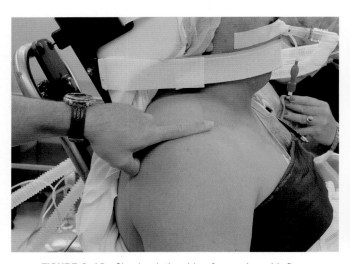

FIGURE 2–18. Check relationship of acromion with floor.

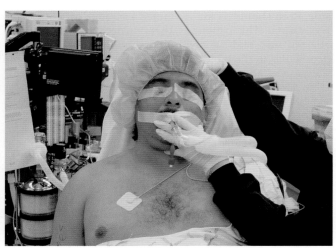

FIGURE 2–19. Secure breathing tube.

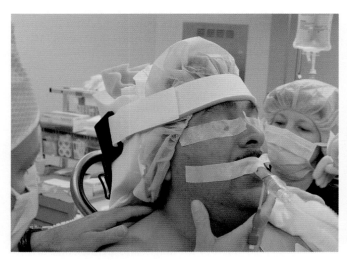

FIGURE 2–20. Position cervical spine.

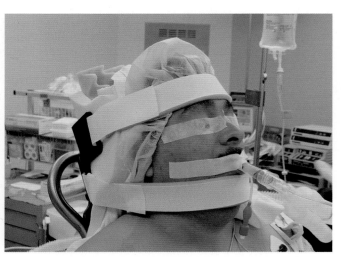

FIGURE 2–21. Secure cervical spine with chin strap.

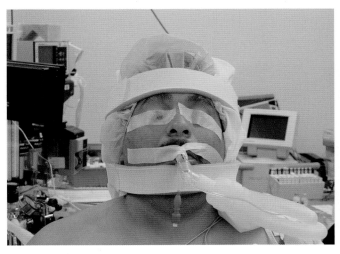

FIGURE 2–22. Check cervical spine alignment.

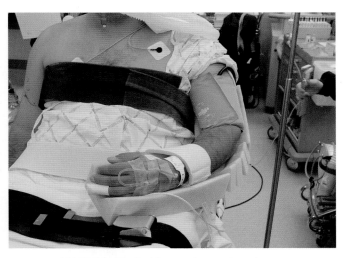

FIGURE 2–23. Pad legs and contralateral arm.

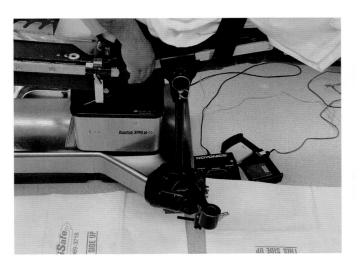

FIGURE 2–24. Base of McConnell arm holder.

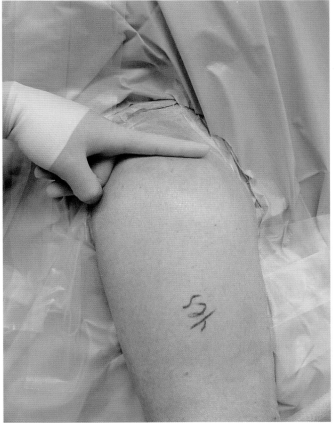

FIGURE 2–25. Recheck position of acromion.

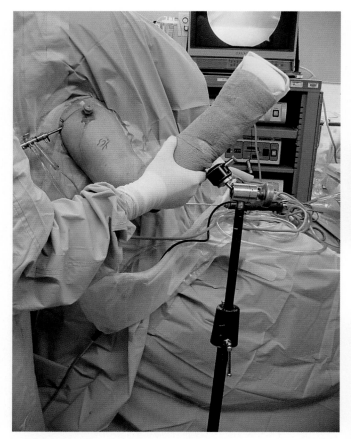

FIGURE 2–26. Positioning the shoulder with the McConnell arm holder.

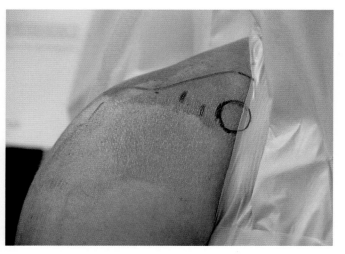

FIGURE 2–27. Access to anterior shoulder.

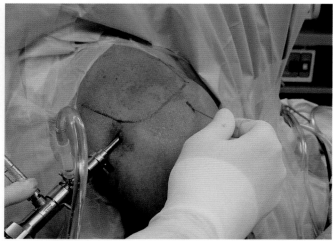

FIGURE 2–28. Access to posterior shoulder.

scopic subacromial decompression, and acromioclavicular joint resection. As I began to perform rotator cuff repair and glenohumeral reconstruction, however, I found that the disadvantages of the lateral position became more noticeable, and I made the transition to the sitting position, which I have used exclusively for the past 10 years.

Equipment

Arthroscope

I use a standard 4.0-mm arthroscope with a 30-degree angled lens for all shoulder arthroscopy. I have not found it necessary to use a 70-degree arthroscope. The increased lens angle may be useful when, while viewing from the posterior portal, you wish to see more of the anterior glenoid during a Bankart repair. I prefer to move the arthroscope to

an anterior superior portal during this portion of the procedure. The minor increase in time to move the arthroscope is more than offset by the superior view with the 30-degree arthroscope as compared with the distorted view of the 70-degree arthroscope.

Suture through Soft Tissue

Sutures are passed through soft tissue either directly or indirectly. Direct methods involve two mechanisms. One instrument passes the suture through the tendon or ligament in a manner similar to that of a standard needle such as the Cuff-Sew (Smith & Nephew Endoscopy, Andover, MA) (Figs. 2–29 to 2–34). Another method involves piercing the soft tissue with an instrument and then grabbing the suture and pulling it back through the soft tissue (Figs. 2–35 and 2–36). The indirect method involves placing a passing suture through the soft tissue and using this transport suture to pull the repair suture through the

TABLE 2–2. **TABLE POSITIONING AIDS: SITTING**
1. Mechanical patient positioner (Schloein, Steris)
2. McConnell foam wrist support and pole
3. Foam pads for ankles, knees, and arms

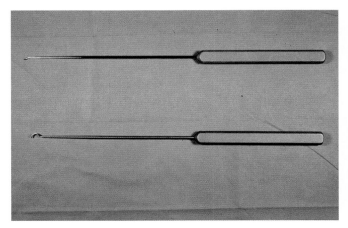

FIGURE 2–29. Straight Cuff-Stitch.

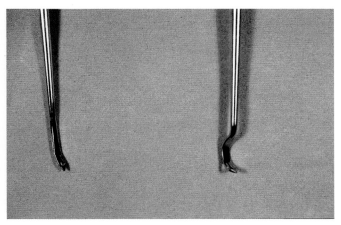

FIGURE 2–30. Instrument tips.

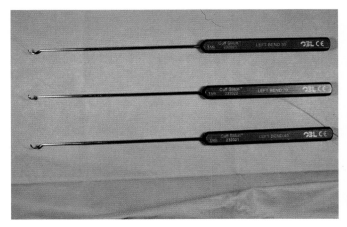

FIGURE 2–31. Left-angled Cuff-Stitch.

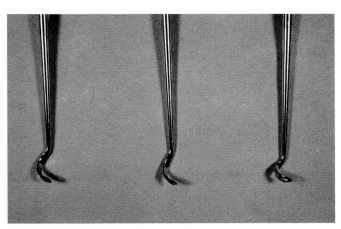

FIGURE 2–32. Instrument tips.

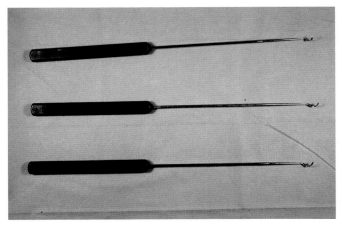

FIGURE 2–33. Right-angled Cuff-Stitch.

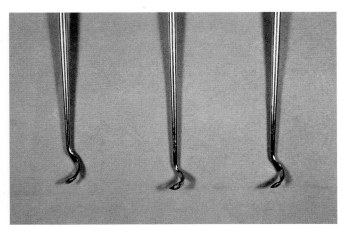

FIGURE 2–34. Instrument tips.

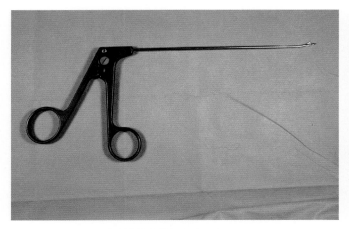

FIGURE 2–35. Arthropierce.

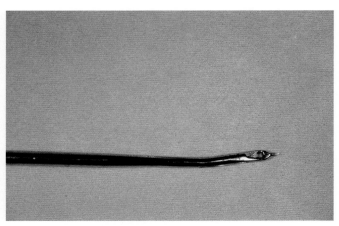

FIGURE 2–36. Instrument tip.

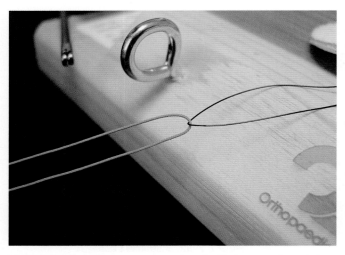

FIGURE 2–37. Indirect suture passing. Braided suture through loop end of 2-0 nylon.

soft tissue. The Linvatec shuttle relay (Linvatec, Largo, FL) is one transfer suture, but I prefer a standard 2-0 nylon suture. I cut the needle off and place the two ends together. This forms a loop on the other end that will transfer the repair suture. The cost saving is significant. My preference is for the indirect method because I believe it offers me more flexibility. The problem with the direct suture instruments is that once the instrument is through the soft tissue, the instrument's maneuverability is extremely limited. Unless the desired repair suture is directly in line with the instrument, I cannot retrieve it. With the indirect method, I can place the transfer suture at the exact point required. I then retrieve the repair suture with a crochet hook and use the transfer suture to place the repair suture through the soft tissue. This is a personal preference, and other surgeons may find another method superior (Figs. 2–37 to 2–39).

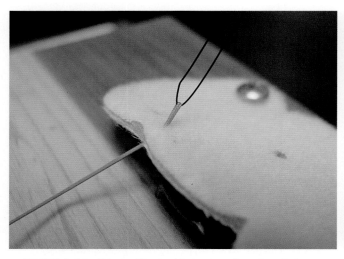

FIGURE 2–38. Nylon pulling braided suture through soft tissue.

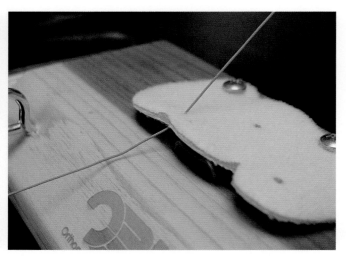

FIGURE 2–39. Braided suture passed through soft tissue.

Hand Instruments

I use several hand instruments during reconstructive shoulder surgery. I use the Caspari suture punch (Linvatec) to pass sutures through the rotator cuff during repair. Snyder modified this suture punch so that the upper front jaw is open to allow intra-articular removal of the shuttle suture from the instrument. I further modified this suture punch by increasing the length of the needle tip from 4 to 5 mm. I found that the 4-mm tip is often too short to pass through a rotator cuff tendon, and the small increase in length solved this problem. The Cuff-Stitch (Smith & Nephew Endoscopy) is a device that allows the surgeon to pass a suture directly through the tendon, ligament, or labrum and is preferred by some surgeons. The Arthropierce (Smith & Nephew Endoscopy) can either pass or retrieve sutures during margin convergence in rotator cuff repair or in rotator interval repair. I find the Spectrum instruments (Linvatec) especially useful during glenohumeral reconstruction for instability. These instruments function like the original Caspari suture punch but are angled so that the surgeon can reach inferiorly to grasp the capsule or labrum (Figs. 2–40 to 2–53).

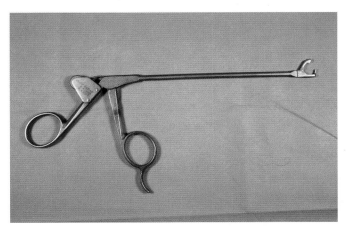

FIGURE 2–40. Caspari suture passer.

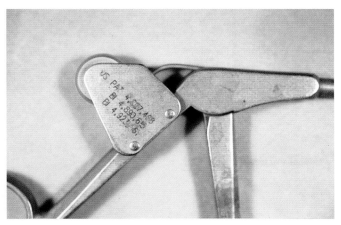

FIGURE 2–41. Close-up view.

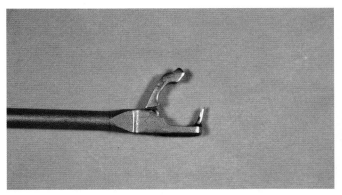

FIGURE 2–42. Caspari suture passer jaws open.

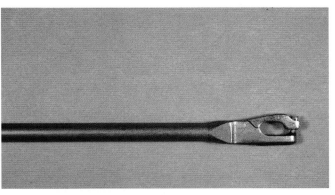

FIGURE 2–43. Jaws closed.

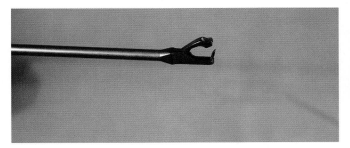

FIGURE 2–44. Open-ended jaws.

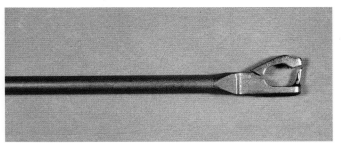

FIGURE 2–45. Jaw angle.

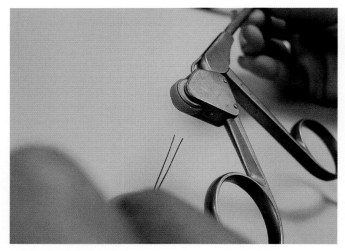

FIGURE 2–46. Place two free ends of folded 2-0 nylon in starter hole.

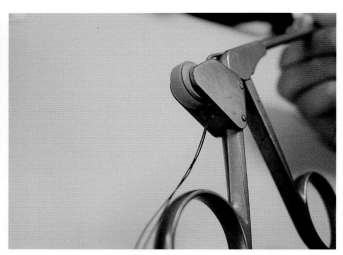

FIGURE 2–47. Advance nylon by turning orange wheel.

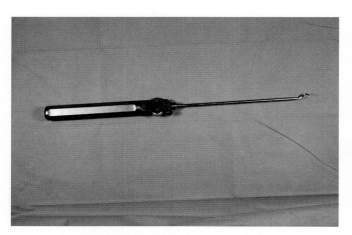

FIGURE 2–48. Spectrum suture passer.

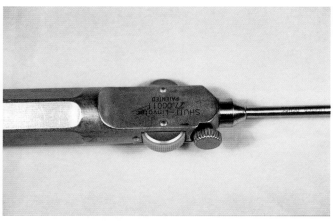

FIGURE 2–49. Close-up view.

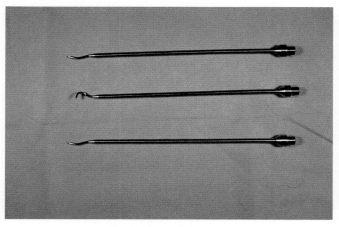

FIGURE 2–50. Straight tips.

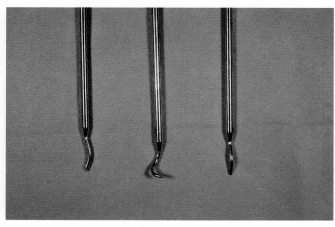

FIGURE 2–51. Close-up view.

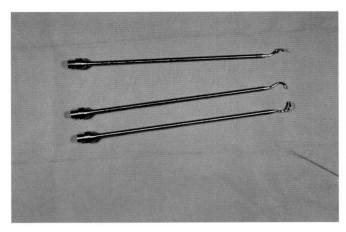

FIGURE 2–52. Curved tips.

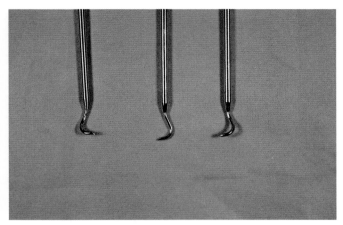

FIGURE 2–53. Close-up view.

Soft Tissue Management

I use a soft tissue grasper to test the tension of the gleno-humeral ligaments before instability repair and also to evaluate the excursion and reparability of a torn rotator cuff. Regular and locking graspers are helpful. One of the graspers has less aggressive teeth so that I can pull on sutures without shredding them. A blunt probe is useful to evaluate for the presence of a subtle Bankart or SLAP (superior labrum from anterior to posterior) lesion. When a Bankart lesion has healed with a fibrous union, the lesion may not be apparent, and a sharp chisel dissector can peel the labrum off the anterior glenoid. To ensure that the capsule does not remain adherent to the subscapularis, I use a blunt soft tissue instrument to dissect between the two structures. A large soft tissue punch is useful to excise portions of contracted capsule during contracture release. I have found the capsular punches designed by Harryman to be the most effective instruments for capsular release in patients with shoulder stiffness. I have modified two of the instruments so that they bend downward rather than upward because I am more comfortable with this angle of approach to the capsular tissue (Figs. 2–54 to 2–70).

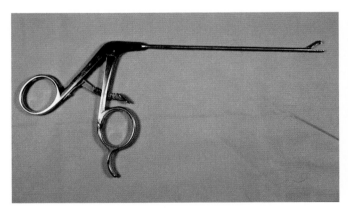

FIGURE 2–54. Soft tissue grasper, locking.

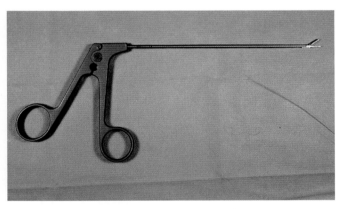

FIGURE 2–55. Soft tissue grasper.

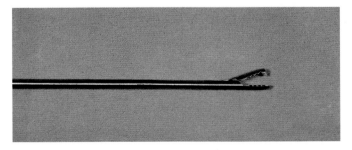

FIGURE 2–56. Close-up view.

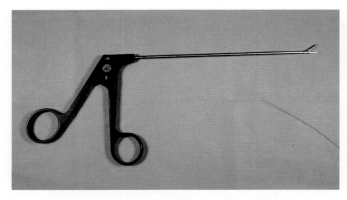

FIGURE 2–57. Soft tissue grasper, less aggressive.

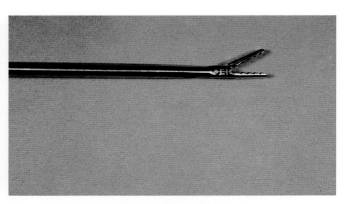

FIGURE 2–58. Close-up view.

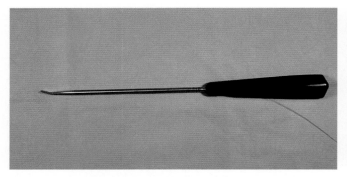

FIGURE 2–59. Chisel dissector.

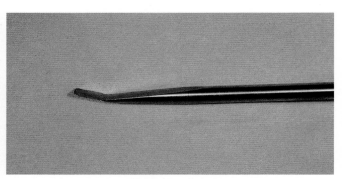

FIGURE 2–60. Close-up view.

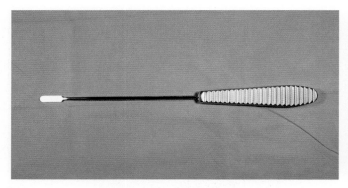

FIGURE 2–61. Blunt dissector.

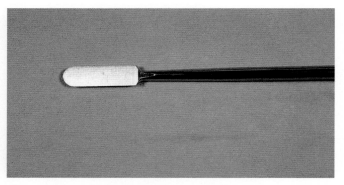

FIGURE 2–62. Close-up view.

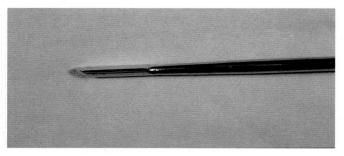

FIGURE 2–63. Close-up view.

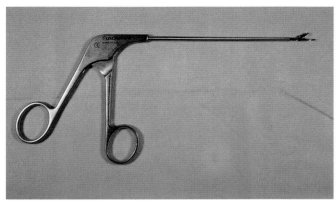

FIGURE 2–64. Capsular resection punch, straight.

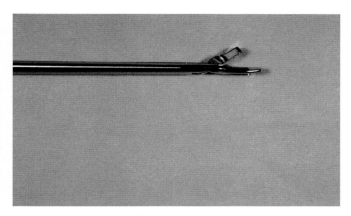

FIGURE 2–65. Close-up view.

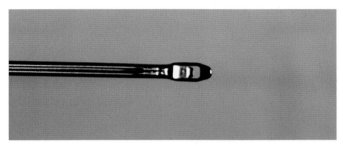

FIGURE 2–66. Jaw width.

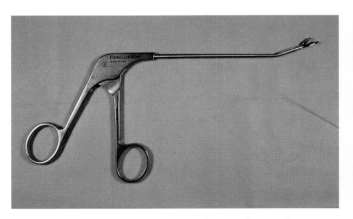

FIGURE 2–67. Capsular resection punch, curved.

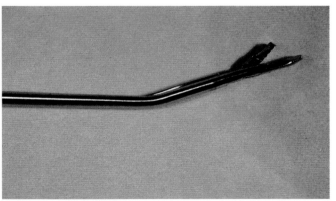

FIGURE 2–68. Close-up view.

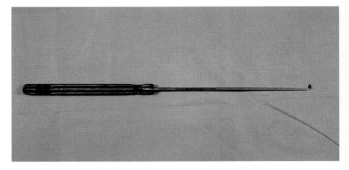

FIGURE 2–69. Blunt probe.

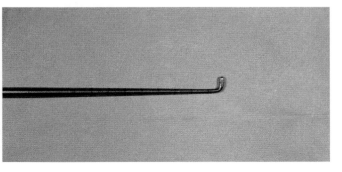

FIGURE 2–70. Blunt probe measuring guide markings.

Suture Management

A crochet hook is used to retrieve sutures from within the subacromial space or glenohumeral joint. If a suture remains caught in the tendon or labrum, I prefer to use a finer-toothed crochet hook that does not damage the suture. I use a looped suture grasper to ensure that no suture tangles exist within the working cannula before I tie each suture. The larger instrument is used during rotator cuff repairs, whereas the smaller size is easier to maneuver within the glenohumeral joint. Numerous knot-tying instruments are available, but I prefer a single-lumen knot pusher, which can double both as a knot pusher and as a knot puller. I have modified the length of the instrument to fit my hand comfortably. Arthroscopic scissors are needed to cut suture and soft tissue. I have an additional type of end-cutting scissors that I use when I cannot see the knot during a rotator interval repair (Figs. 2–71 to 2–84).

Suture

I use several different sutures during shoulder arthroscopy. The 5-mm rotator cuff anchor is preloaded with No. 2 Ethibond (No. 2 nonabsorbable braided suture), and the 2.8-mm anchor is preloaded with No. 1 Ethibond (No. 1 nonabsorbable braided suture). I use 2-0 nylon as a transfer suture to bring the braided sutures through the rotator cuff or glenoid labrum. If I am repairing from tendon to tendon, I may use, instead of the No. 2 Ethibond, No. 1 PDS (No. 1 absorbable monofilament suture) or No. 1 Prolene (No. 1 nonabsorbable monofilament suture). I use 3-0 Monocryl (3-0 absorbable monofilament suture) for the subcutaneous skin closure for the portal incisions.

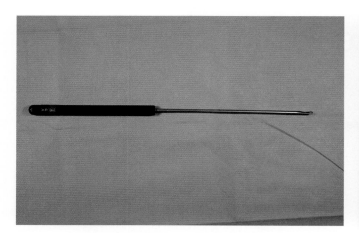

FIGURE 2–71. Crochet hook.

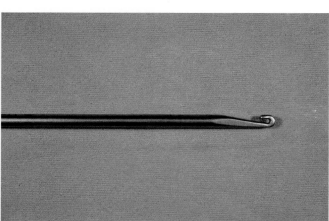

FIGURE 2–72. Close-up view.

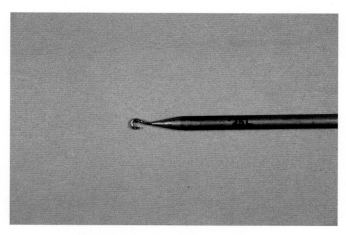

FIGURE 2–73. Crochet hook, fine tooth.

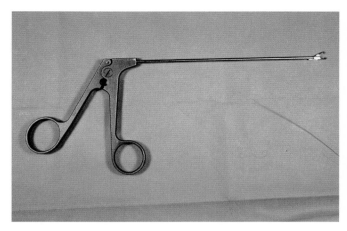

FIGURE 2–74. Loop grasper, large.

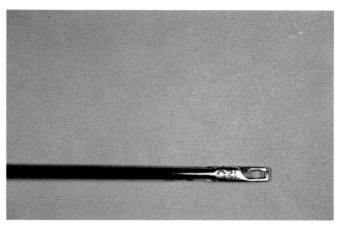

FIGURE 2–75. Close-up view.

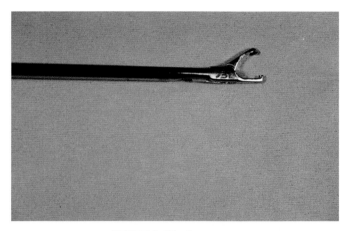

FIGURE 2–76. Jaws open.

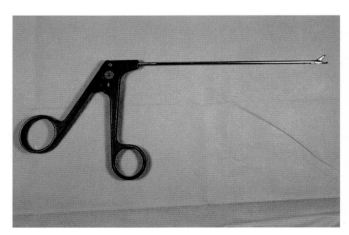

FIGURE 2–77. Loop grasper, small.

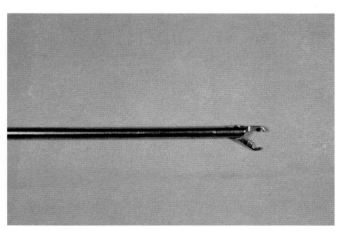

FIGURE 2–78. Close-up view.

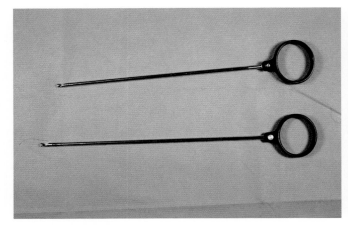

FIGURE 2–79. Knot pusher.

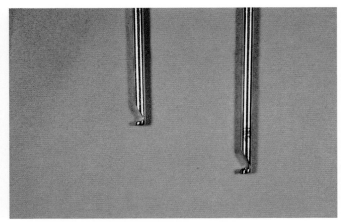

FIGURE 2–80. Close-up view.

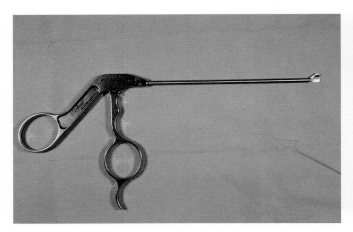

FIGURE 2–81. Scissors.

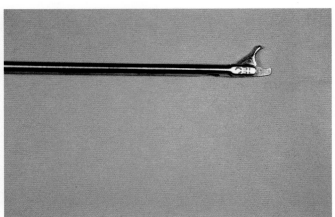

FIGURE 2–82. Close-up view.

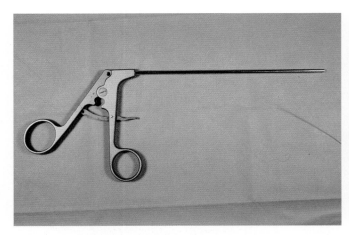

FIGURE 2–83. Scissors, end-cutting.

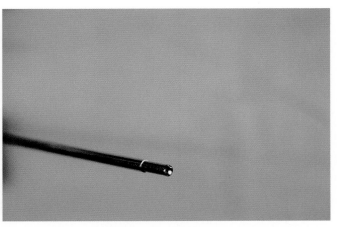

FIGURE 2–84. Close-up view.

Power Instruments

Relatively few power instruments are needed. I use a 4.0-mm shaver, a 5.0-mm shaver, a 4.0-mm round bur, and a 5.5-mm acromionizer bur. The 4.0-mm shaver and round bur are used within the glenohumeral joint for glenohumeral instability and SLAP repair. I use a power drill to predrill holes for the bone anchors for glenohumeral instability and SLAP repair. The larger shaver is used for removing bursal tissue during arthroscopic subacromial decompression, and I use the acromionizer for acromioplasty. I use the round bur within the subacromial space to prepare the repair site during rotator cuff repair (Figs. 2–85 to 2–90).

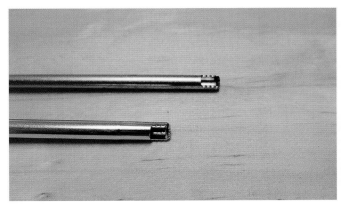

FIGURE 2–85. Shaver.

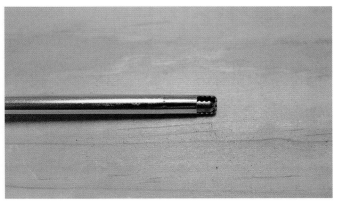

FIGURE 2–86. Close-up view.

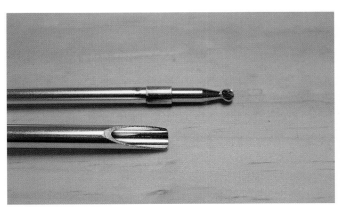

FIGURE 2–87. Round bur.

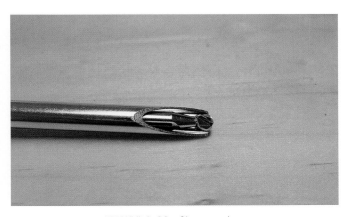

FIGURE 2–88. Close-up view.

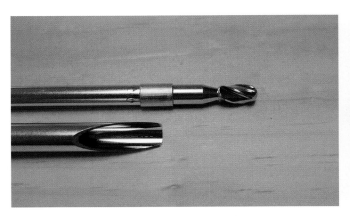

FIGURE 2–89. Acromionizer bur.

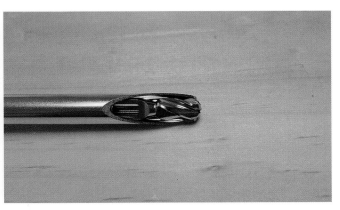

FIGURE 2–90. Close-up view.

Thermal Instruments

I use two types of thermal instruments during shoulder arthroscopy. The first instrument can cauterize or ablate tissue. I use the ablation setting during arthroscopic subacromial decompression to remove soft tissue from the undersurface of the acromion. I use the coagulation setting to control bleeding from branches of the coracoacromial artery or from vascularized bursal tissue. I prefer a probe with an attached suction device so that the bubbles produced during ablation or coagulation are removed from the operative field. The second instrument is a capsulorrhaphy probe that I use during glenohumeral reconstruction. I prefer a monopolar probe, but other surgeons obtain excellent results with a bipolar instrument. I do not consider this factor critical because I believe that several considerations are more important, as discussed in Chapter 4 (Glenohumeral Instability).

Fluid Management

I believe that an arthroscopic pump system for delivering fluid to the shoulder is a valuable asset. A pump system eliminates the need to hang bags of irrigating fluid high above the floor and allows the surgeon to increase pump pressure and flow rate when bleeding is encountered. I use lactated Ringer's solution. I do not use epinephrine because I have not noticed any major improvement in visualization. If the surgeon finds epinephrine helpful, I would advise adding it to every other bag of Ringer's solution to minimize any potential cardiotoxic effects.

Cannulas

The metal cannula that I use for the arthroscope has ports for inflow, outflow, and pressure. In addition to the metal cannula and blunt trocar for the arthroscope, I have found three additional plastic, translucent cannulas vital when I perform reconstructive arthroscopic shoulder surgery. During anchor insertion or knot tying, I often use the cannula to prevent adjacent soft tissue from interfering with the procedure. Because the cannula is translucent, I can insert an anchor or tie a knot with the cannula covering the involved area. The 8-mm cannula is large enough to accommodate the power tools and large suturing instruments. The 6-mm cannula is used for the anterior superior portal during glenohumeral reconstruction or SLAP repair because it is large enough to accept the 4-mm round bur. The 5-mm cannula is placed anteriorly during rotator cuff repair as both an outflow cannula and a retrieval cannula for the bone anchor sutures (Figs. 2–91 to 2–93).

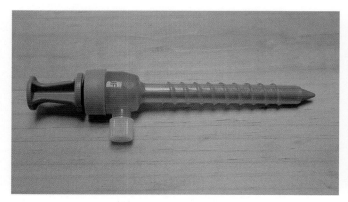

FIGURE 2–91. 8-mm cannula.

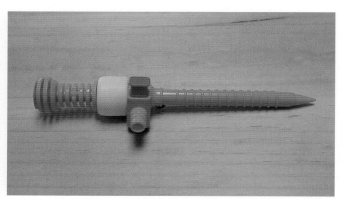

FIGURE 2–92. 5.5-mm cannula.

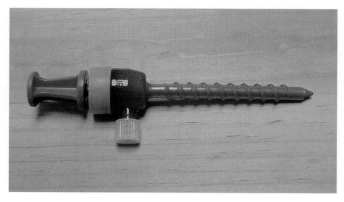

FIGURE 2–93. 5-mm cannula.

Transfer Rods

Surgeons who prefer to create portals with the inside-out technique find the Wissinger rod useful, and I describe its use in Chapter 3. Switching rods are blunt on both ends and are used to maintain the cannula position when the arthroscope is moved from one position to another (Figs. 2–94 to 2–96).

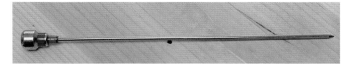

FIGURE 2–94. Wissinger rod.

Image Capture

I find it extremely helpful to record intraoperative photographs. Pictures record the lesions found during operation more precisely than the operative notes. They have the added advantage of documenting normal findings that we commonly omit from our operative record. Most arthroscopy systems have the capability to record photos during surgery with the use of a foot switch or a control button on the camera. The photos can be printed directly, or they can be stored on recordable media or on a computer hard drive.

Since I began performing shoulder arthroscopy, I have taken still photos, but I recently added video recording. I bring my digital video camera to the operating room and connect it to the S-video output of the arthroscopic camera box. I record the entire operation and then bring the camera back and disk (for still photos) to my office and select which portions of the operation I wish to keep. Typically, I save approximately 30 to 45 seconds of video imaging; this includes the lesions found at operation and their appearance after correction. The video is captured in AVI format, and I use another software program to compress it to MPEG1 or MPEG2. This step converts the data so that the computer hard drive can hold 10 times as much video. I create an electronic folder with the patient's name, and place the desired still photos and completed video in it. I have found it helpful to review the video and photos of patients who are doing either extremely well or poorly because it allows me to recollect the details of the operation. I do not routinely provide patients with still pictures or videos, but I will do so if they request it.

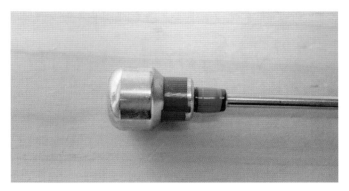

FIGURE 2–95. Handle.

Dedicated Team

I cannot emphasize enough the advantages of having a trained, dedicated operating room team. Reconstructive shoulder arthroscopy is complicated, and it is helpful when the scrub nurse, assistant, and circulating nurse can perform their jobs without instruction from the surgeon. The surgical nurse can load the Caspari or Spectrum suture instruments so they are ready for the next step, clean shavers and burs so they function appropriately, and have the next instrument ready so the operation runs smoothly.

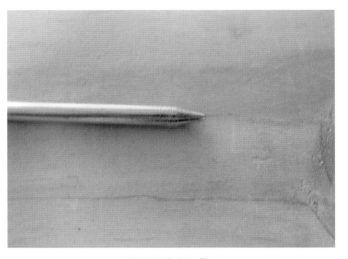

FIGURE 2–96. Tip.

3

Diagnostic Arthroscopy and Normal Anatomy

Only through an understanding of normal glenohumeral joint and subacromial space anatomy can the surgeon appreciate which structures are damaged.

Diagnostic Glenohumeral Arthroscopy

I believe that portal placement is critical and spend sufficient time to make the portal sites precisely. Draw the bone outlines of the acromion, distal clavicle, and coracoid with a surgical skin marker. Be careful not to draw the most superficial bone landmarks, but rather their inferior surfaces (to take into account the bone thickness), because portal entry points are referenced from these surfaces (Figs. 3–1 and 3–2).

Although trocar entry into the glenohumeral joint is simple and almost intuitive for the expert, surgeons beginning their arthroscopic experience may find joint entrance difficult. The standard advice of "start in the soft spot and aim for the coracoid" is only slightly helpful. The actual joint entry requires that the surgeon be very precise. Small deviations of 3 to 5 mm from the desired portal location make the operation more difficult. Complicating this process must be the realization that the portals vary from patient to patient because they are related to the patient's position on the operating table as well as patient size, rotundity, and kyphosis. The ideal portal location changes throughout the operation as soft tissue swelling increases and thus alters the local anatomy. Portal placement is also affected by the underlying diagnosis. My posterior portal for an acromioclavicular joint resection is different from my posterior portal placement for a SLAP (superior labrum from anterior to

posterior) lesion repair. There are no absolute rules, but there are certain guidelines that I find helpful.

I have found that the most reliable landmarks are bone. Anteriorly, I outline the coracoid process, the acromioclavicular joint, and the anterior acromion. Laterally, I identify the lateral acromial border, and, posteriorly, I outline the posterior acromion. My most important landmark is the posterolateral corner of the acromion because I can palpate it even in larger patients. I base my measurements from this point (Fig. 3–3).

Posterior Portals

Traditionally, surgeons describe the location of the posterior portal in the "soft spot" located approximately 2 cm inferior and 2 cm medial to the posterolateral acromial edge. Although I believe this location is adequate for glenohumeral joint arthroscopy, it is not optimally located for more complex reconstructive operations. If you make the incision in the traditional soft spot, you will enter the joint parallel to the glenohumeral joint line and slightly superior to the glenoid equator. This location allows you to enter the glenohumeral joint adequately, but the soft-spot entry site places the surgeon at a disadvantage if the same incision is now used to enter the subacromial space. Once the surgeon inserts the cannula into the subacromial space, the soft-spot portal directs the cannula superiorly and medially and causes two problems. Because the arthroscopic view is now directed medially, the lateral insertion of the rotator cuff is more difficult to visualize. The superior angle of the arthroscope also makes it difficult to look down on the rotator cuff tendon and to appreciate the geometry of rotator cuff

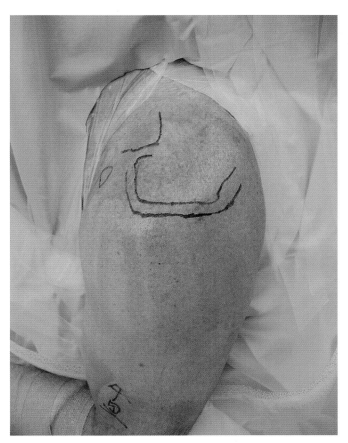

FIGURE 3–1. Bone landmarks.

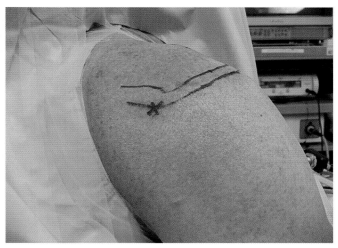

FIGURE 3–3. Posterolateral acromial corner.

terolateral acromion. The more superior and lateral location minimizes these difficulties. The superior entry allows the cannula to enter the subacromial space immediately beneath the acromion, parallel to its undersurface. This approach maximizes the distance between the arthroscope an the rotator cuff. The greater separation between the arthroscope and the rotator cuff gives the surgeon a better appreciation of rotator cuff lesions. The superior position (parallel and immediately inferior to the acromion) also facilitates acromioplasty because the surgeon is afforded a better view of the acromial shape. The more lateral position (immediately medial to the lateral acromion) places the arthroscope in line with the rotator cuff tendon insertion.

For operations restricted to the glenohumeral joint, such as Bankart or SLAP lesion repair, I enter the joint more medially than I do for those operations primarily involving the subacromial space, such as rotator cuff repair, that

lesions (Figs. 3–4 and 3–5). One solution to this problem is a second posterior portal, but my preference is to alter the posterior portal's location.

The exact location of the posterior portal varies with the clinical diagnosis. For rotator cuff repairs and arthroscopic subacromial decompressions, I make the posterior incision for the portal in a more superior and lateral position, approximately 1 cm inferior and 1 cm medial to the pos-

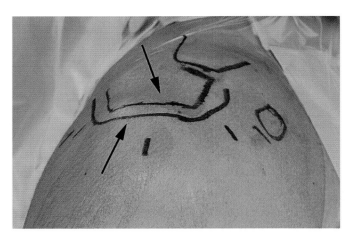

FIGURE 3–2. Superior and inferior bone edges.

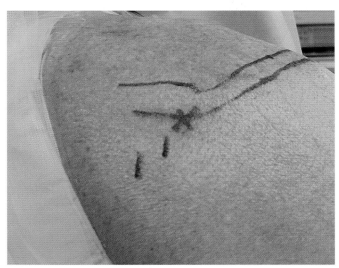

FIGURE 3–4. Soft spot—superolateral posterior portal for subacromial surgery.

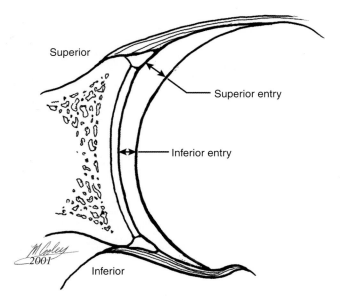

FIGURE 3–5. Glenohumeral joint space.

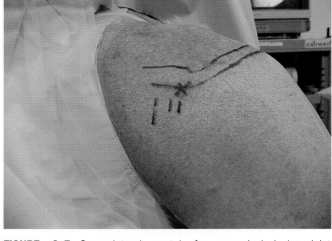

FIGURE 3–7. Superolateral portal for acromioclavicular joint resection.

require only a brief glenohumeral joint inspection (Fig. 3–6). If I am performing an acromioclavicular joint resection, I move the posterior incision 5 mm more laterally. This more lateral position affords me a better view of the distal clavicle (Fig. 3–7).

Lateral Portals

I do not routinely use a lateral subacromial portal during diagnostic glenohumeral joint arthroscopy. There are occasions when I wish to inspect the subacromial space, particularly to view the bursal rotator cuff surface to evaluate that structure for partial-thickness rotator cuff tear. More commonly, I use a lateral portal during arthroscopic subacromial decompression and rotator cuff repair, and discuss it in detail in Chapter 12. I mark the portal location with a skin marker 3 to 5 cm distal to the lateral acromial border and 1 to 3 cm posterior to the anterior acromion. I regard the mark as only an approximation. Once I have entered the subacromial space, I identify the lateral portal with a spinal needle before I incise the skin. I use two additional lateral portals during rotator cuff repair. Occasionally, I need an anterolateral or posterolateral portal to retrieve sutures during the repair of a massive rotator cuff repair. These portals are positioned midway between the anterior and lateral or posterior and lateral portals and again are identified with the use of a spinal needle (Figs. 3–8 and 3–9).

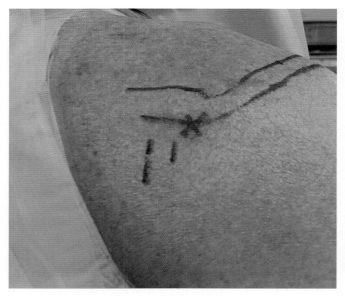

FIGURE 3–6. Superior medial portal for glenohumeral joint surgery.

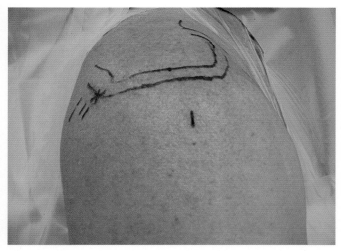

FIGURE 3–8. Midlateral portal for arthroscopic subacromial decompression.

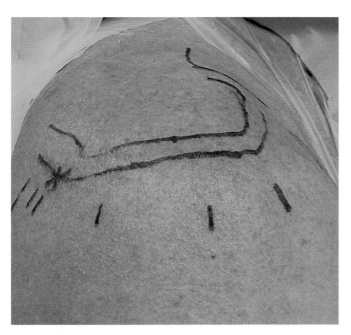

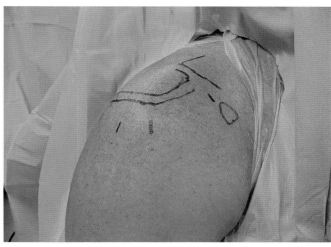

FIGURE 3–11. Anteromedial portal for acromioclavicular joint resection.

FIGURE 3–9. Anterior and posterior lateral portals.

Anterior Portals

The four basic anterior portals are anterior-inferior, anterior-superior, lateral, and medial (Figs. 3–10 and 3–11). The anterior-inferior and anterior-superior portals are used for glenohumeral reconstruction or SLAP lesion repair. I use the anterior-medial portal for acromioclavicular joint resection and the lateral portal during rotator cuff repair. I mark the anterior-inferior portal 5 mm lateral to the coracoid. I mark the location for the anterior-superior portal 1.5 cm lateral and 1 cm superior to the anterior-inferior portal. The lateral anterior portal is 2 to 3 cm distal to the anterior acromion and parallel to its lateral border. The medial portal is 1 to 3 cm distal to the acromioclavicular joint. Again, the marks are only approximations because the exact portal sites are identified during arthroscopy with a spinal needle. If I perform a glenohumeral reconstruction or a SLAP lesion repair, I will make the posterior portal 2 cm medial and 1 to 1.5 cm inferior to the posterior-lateral acromial border.

Because a patient's pain on physical examination may cause the surgeon to underestimate the range of motion or stability of the shoulder, I examine both shoulders for range of motion and stability after the induction of anesthesia. I record the range of motion in elevation, in external rotation with the arm adducted, and in external and internal rotation with the arm abducted 90 degrees. I then examine the shoulder for stability by applying anterior, posterior, and inferior force while changing the positions of abduction and rotation (Figs. 3–12 to 3–20).

I incise the skin only and avoid plunging the knife into the underlying structures because superficial skin nerves are susceptible to neuroma formation, and muscle bleeding unnecessarily complicates the procedure.

I do not insufflate the joint with a needle because I find I can better determine my entry point into the glenohumeral joint with the more rigid trocar than I can with a needle. I use only blunt-tipped trocars in shoulder arthroscopy and advise surgeons never to use a sharp trocar at any time.

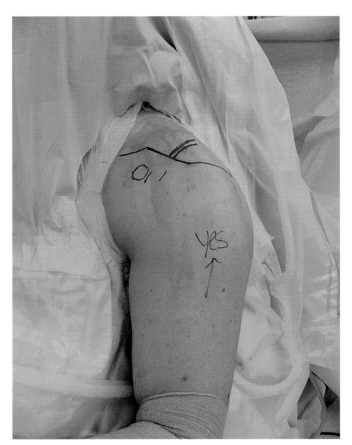

FIGURE 3–10. Anterior-inferior and anterior-superior portals for glenohumeral reconstruction.

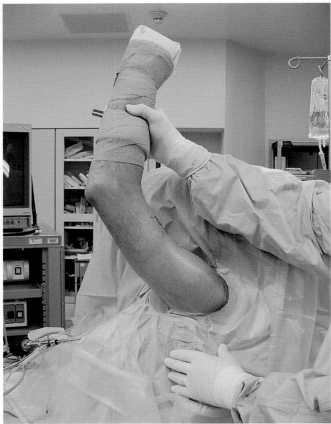

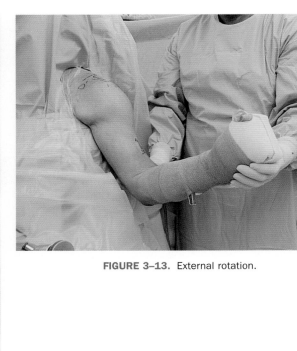

FIGURE 3–13. External rotation.

FIGURE 3–12. Elevation.

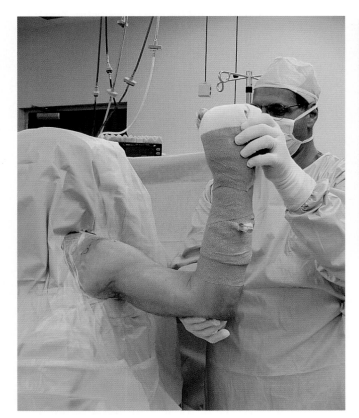

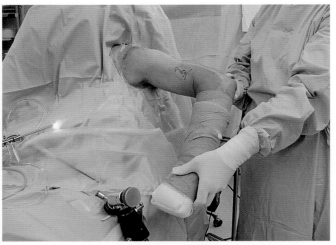

FIGURE 3–15. Internal rotation in abduction, coronal plane.

FIGURE 3–14. External rotation in abduction, anterior stress.

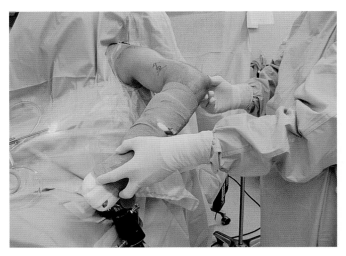

FIGURE 3–16. Internal rotation in abduction, scapular plane.

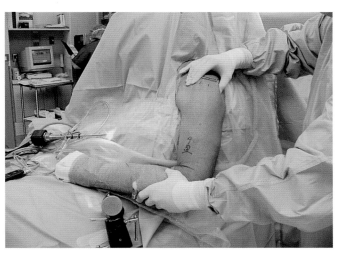

FIGURE 3–17. Sulcus test, internal rotation.

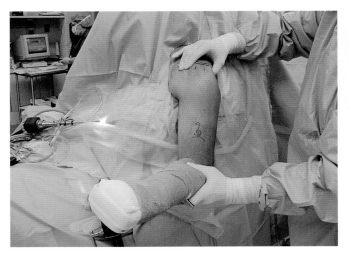

FIGURE 3–18. Sulcus test, external rotation.

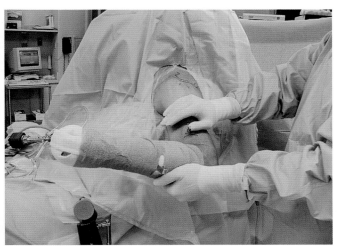

FIGURE 3–19. Inferior stress.

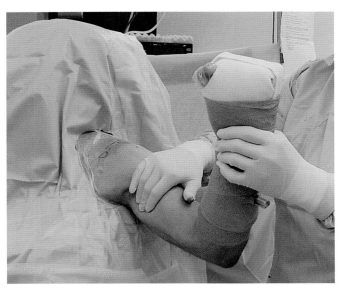

FIGURE 3–20. Posterior stress.

Insert the cannula and trocar through the skin incision, and gently advance it through the deltoid muscle until bone resistance is felt. With your opposite hand pushing the humeral head posteriorly against the trocar tip, you can palpate to determine whether the bone is the glenoid or the humeral head. You can also grasp the forearm and rotate the shoulder. If you feel the bone rotate, the trocar tip is resting against the humeral head, and you must direct the arthroscope medially to enter the joint. If no rotation is felt, the trocar is touching the glenoid, and you must direct it laterally to enter the joint. When the trocar tip is at the joint line, a slight lateral movement will allow you to palpate the head, and a slight medial movement will contact the glenoid. The posterior joint line is medial to the posterolateral acromion, and the direction of entry is generally oriented toward the tip of the coracoid. Angle the cannula slightly superiorly and advance it into the joint. Usually, a distinct "pop" is felt as the trocar enters the glenohumeral joint. Remove the trocar, insert the arthroscope through the cannula, and begin the diagnostic inspection. If you have not entered the joint, remove the cannula and trocar to check the bone landmarks drawn on the patient's skin (Fig. 3–21).

VIDEO

Diagnostic and Normal Anatomy

The diagnostic examination of the shoulder is systematic, to ensure that possible lesions are not overlooked. The plan described in Table 3–1 can serve as a guide.

TABLE 3–1. DIAGNOSTIC EXAMINATION OF THE SHOULDER

Anterior view: Arthroscope in posterior cannula

1. Biceps-labrum complex
2. Biceps tendon
3. Biceps exit from the joint
4. Anterior articular surface supraspinatus
5. Superior glenohumeral ligament
6. Rotator interval
7. Subscapularis tendon
8. Subscapularis recess
9. Middle glenohumeral ligament
10. Anterior labrum
11. Anterior-inferior glenohumeral ligament
12. Inferior labrum
13. Inferior capsule
14. Posterior-inferior glenohumeral ligament
15. Posterior labrum
16. Infraspinatus tendon
17. Posterolateral humeral head

Posterior view: Arthroscope in anterior cannula

1. Posterior glenoid labrum
2. Posterior capsule
3. Posterior rotator cuff (site of internal impingement)
4. Subscapularis recess
5. Middle glenohumeral ligament and its humeral attachment
6. Anterior-inferior glenohumeral ligament and its humeral attachment

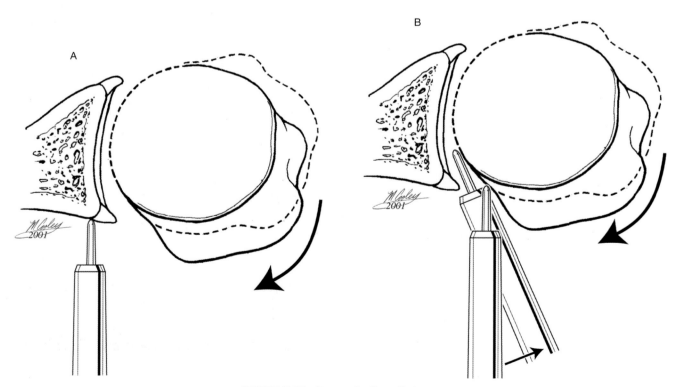

FIGURE 3–21. Bone palpation with trocar.

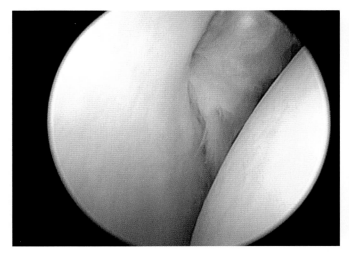

FIGURE 3–22. Glenohumeral joint, vertical orientation.

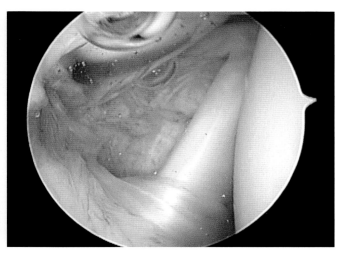

FIGURE 3–24. Rotator interval.

Once you have entered the glenohumeral joint, identify the biceps tendon-labrum complex and rotate the camera to orient the glenoid on the monitor screen. Some surgeons prefer the glenoid oriented vertically so that it is similar to its position if the patient were standing, seated in the beach-chair position, or on an anterior-posterior radiograph. Other surgeons prefer to orient the glenoid so that it appears parallel to the floor. I do not believe one technique is superior to the other but consider it a matter of surgeon preference (Figs. 3–22 and 3–23).

Advance the arthroscope into the joint and rotate it so that it appears to be at the 1 o'clock position relative to the glenoid surface. Inspect the rotator interval and superior glenohumeral ligament. Apply inferior distraction and observe the tension that develops. Distract the patient's arm with the shoulder externally rotated and internally rotated and note any difference. Perform this portion of the exami-

nation first because the anterior cannula will pass through the rotator interval and will alter the local anatomy. The rotator interval may appear normal in patients with subacromial impingement, contracted in patients with shoulder stiffness, and widened or lax in patients with glenohumeral instability (Figs. 3–24 to 3–30).

There are two basic techniques to establish an anterior portal: inside out and outside in. To establish the anterior portal with the inside-out technique, advance the arthroscope until it is in the middle of the triangular space bordered by the glenoid rim, the superior border of the subscapularis tendon, and the biceps tendon. Press the arthroscope against the rotator interval, and hold the cannula in position while you remove the arthroscope from the cannula. Insert a blunt-tipped (Wissinger) rod through the cannula and advance it through the capsule until it tents the skin anteriorly. Maintain pressure on the rod, and make

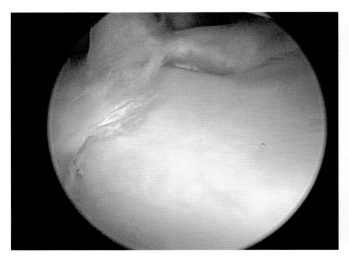

FIGURE 3–23. Glenohumeral joint, horizontal orientation.

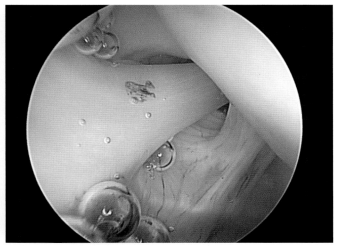

FIGURE 3–25. Rotator interval, normal superior glenohumeral ligament.

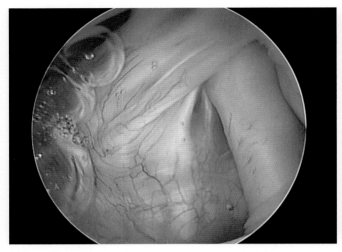

FIGURE 3–26. Rotator interval, prominent superior glenohumeral ligament.

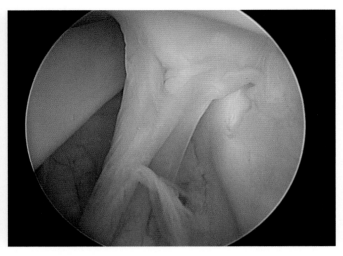

FIGURE 3–27. Partial tear, superior glenohumeral ligament.

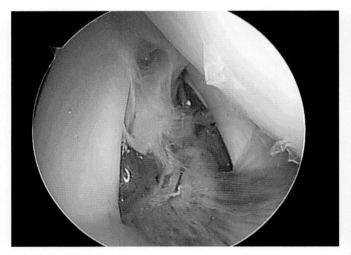

FIGURE 3–28. Contracted rotator interval.

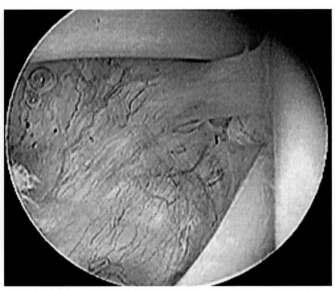

FIGURE 3–29. Widened rotator interval.

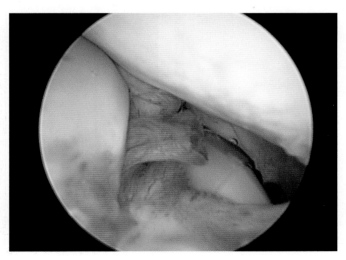

FIGURE 3–30. Rotator interval synovitis.

a skin incision directly over its tip. Advance the rod anteriorly so that it projects 5 to 10 cm. Slide a second cannula over the rod tip anteriorly, and advance this cannula into the joint until you can feel the two cannulas touch each other. Remove the rod, and reinsert the arthroscope into the posterior cannula. Adjust the anterior cannula until you can see 15 to 20 mm within the joint. Outflow may remain connected to the arthroscope cannula, or it may be moved to the anterior cannula as desired. I used this technique early in my arthroscopic experience because it enabled me to enter the glenohumeral joint reliably. As I began doing more reconstructive shoulder operations, I discovered some inadequacies with this approach. The inside-out approach allows for some variability in the precise entry spot for the anterior portal because, inevitably, there is some manipulation of the arthroscope with the necessary sequence of maneuvers. For glenohumeral joint reconstruction for instability, I need two anterior cannulas, and their positions are critical. If the inferior cannula is placed too superiorly, there will not be adequate space for the anterior-superior cannula. If the cannulas are placed too medially or too laterally, anchor insertion is complicated and suture placement is compromised. For these reasons, I now establish the anterior cannulas with an outside-in approach.

To establish the anterior portal with the outside-in technique, point the arthroscope at the rotator interval and use your index finger to push on the skin of the anterior shoulder lateral and superior to the coracoid process. Observe where your finger indents the anterior capsule, and move that location until the anterior capsule is indented in the middle of the rotator interval. Mark this location on the anterior shoulder with a marking pen, and then use a spinal needle to enter the joint at this point. I prefer to place the anterior cannula immediately superior to the superior border of the subscapularis tendon and 1 cm lateral to the glenoid surface. Note the angle that the needle makes with respect to the patient's anterior shoulder. Remove the spinal needle, make a small incision, and place the cannula and trocar into the joint. As noted earlier, outflow may remain connected to the arthroscope cannula, or it may be moved to the anterior cannula as desired (Figs. 3–31 to 3–33).

Rotate the arthroscope so that it is pointed at 1 o'clock for a right shoulder (or 11 o'clock for a left shoulder), advance it anteriorly, and inspect the subscapularis recess and the superior border of the subscapularis tendon. Rotate the arthroscope until it is pointed at 3 o'clock for a right shoulder (or 9 o'clock for a left shoulder), advance it anteriorly, and inspect the anterior labrum and the middle glenohumeral ligament. The opening of the foramen at the anterior-superior labrum is a normal structure and should not be confused with a Bankart lesion. Observe the anterior labrum for signs of glenohumeral instability such as fraying, tearing, or separation from the glenoid. Insert a probe through the anterior cannula, and test the anterior labrum's attachment to the glenoid. Use the probe to test the tension of the middle glenohumeral ligament. Translate the humeral head anteriorly, inferiorly, and posteriorly and observe the tension that develops in the ligament. Perform these maneuvers with the patient's arm internally and then externally rotated. The appearance of the middle glenohumeral ligament is variable, and it may be poorly defined, prominent, or cord-like (Figs. 3–34 to 3–45).

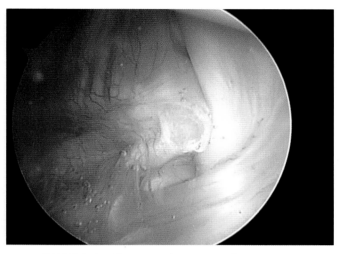

FIGURE 3–31. Entry point for anterior-inferior cannula.

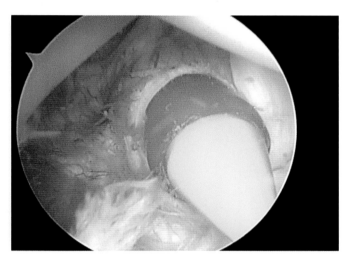

FIGURE 3–32. Cannula and trocar entry.

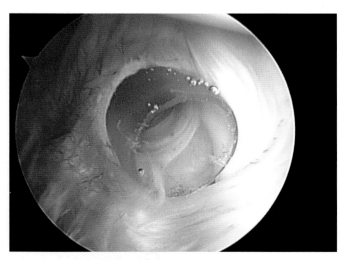

FIGURE 3–33. Trocar removed.

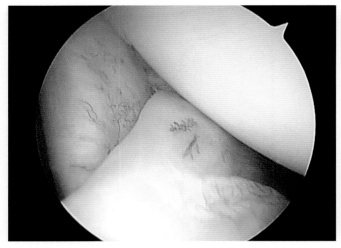

FIGURE 3–34. Middle glenohumeral ligament, thick.

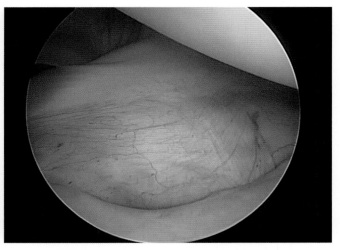

FIGURE 3–35. Middle glenohumeral ligament, broad.

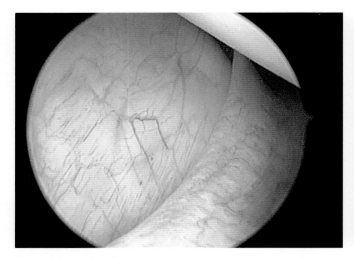

FIGURE 3–36. Middle glenohumeral ligament, subscapularis poorly defined.

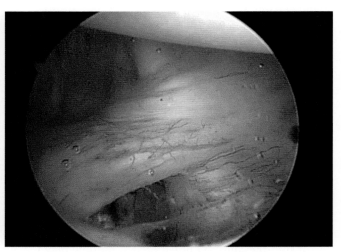

FIGURE 3–37. Middle glenohumeral ligament, partial tear.

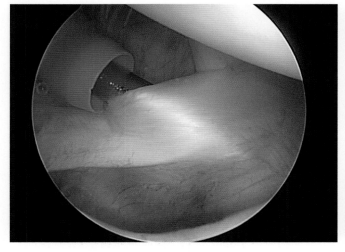

FIGURE 3–38. Middle glenohumeral ligament, cord.

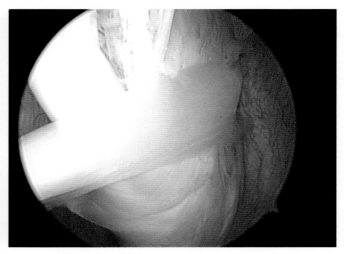

FIGURE 3–39. Middle glenohumeral ligament, cord.

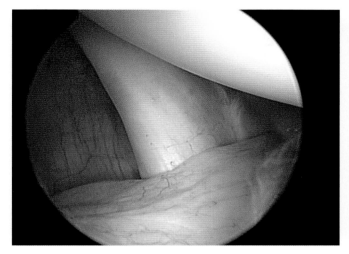

FIGURE 3–40. Subscapularis.

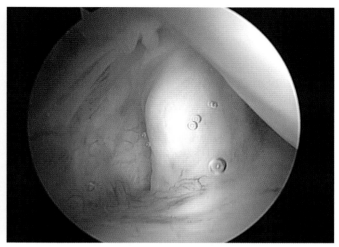

FIGURE 3–41. Subscapularis.

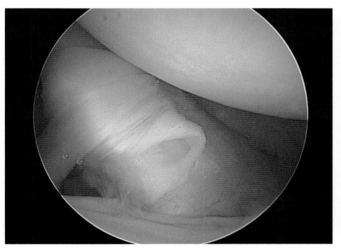

FIGURE 3–42. Subscapularis, synovial tear.

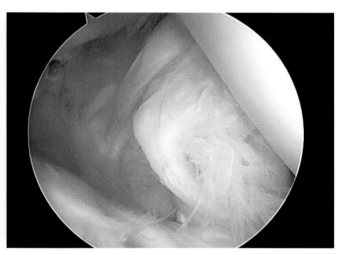

FIGURE 3–43. Subscapularis, partial tear superior border.

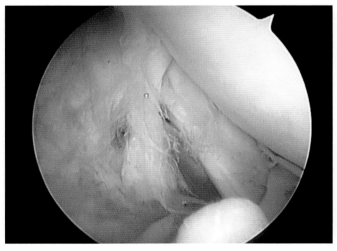

FIGURE 3–44. Subscapularis, partial tear superior border.

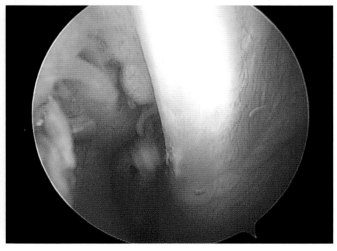

FIGURE 3–45. Subscapularis recess.

Rotate the arthroscope until it is pointed at 5 o'clock, and inspect the anterior-inferior labrum and glenohumeral ligament. Test their tension and insertion integrity as described earlier.

Move the arthroscope inferiorly, and note the presence or absence of a drive-through sign. This sign describes the ease with which the arthroscope passes between the humeral head and the glenoid surface at the 6-o'clock position. The drive-through sign is a measure of glenohumeral laxity or translation and is not an indication in and of itself of glenohumeral instability. Observe the laxity of the inferior capsule as the shoulder is distracted inferiorly and laterally and then is rotated. Determine whether there is an inferior labral lesion, and carefully inspect the humeral attachment of the inferior capsule for signs of trauma (Figs. 3–46 to 3–56).

Return the arthroscope to the biceps-labrum complex. To view the posterior labrum adequately from a posterior cannula, you must maximize the distance from the arthroscope

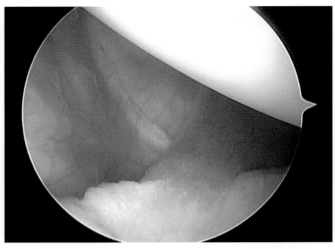

FIGURE 3–48. Anterior-inferior glenohumeral ligament less well defined.

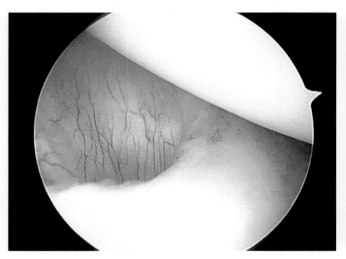

FIGURE 3–46. Rotate arthroscope.

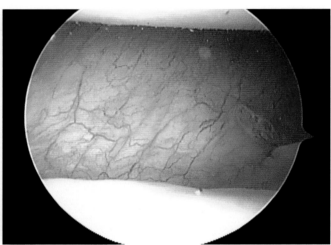

FIGURE 3–49. Anterior-inferior capsule.

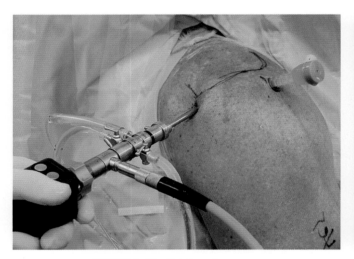

FIGURE 3–47. Anterior-inferior glenohumeral ligament.

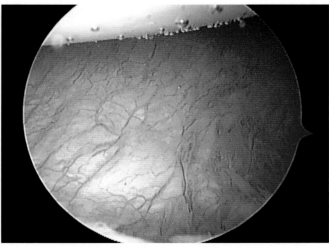

FIGURE 3–50. Axillary recess.

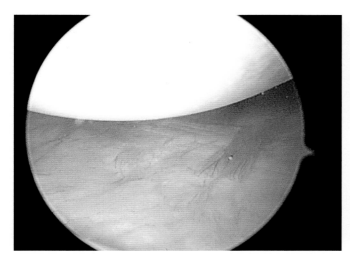

FIGURE 3–51. Inferior-posterior capsule.

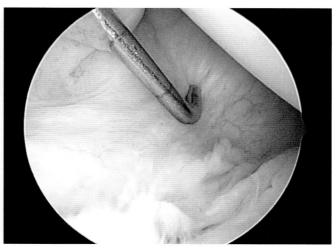

FIGURE 3–52. Palpate anterior-inferior glenohumeral ligament.

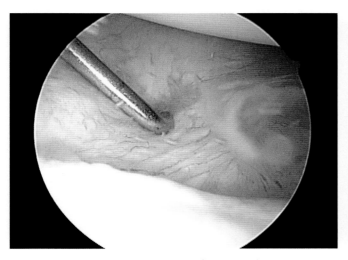

FIGURE 3–53. Palpate inferior capsule.

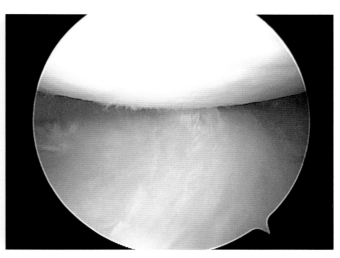

FIGURE 3–54. Inferior-posterior labrum.

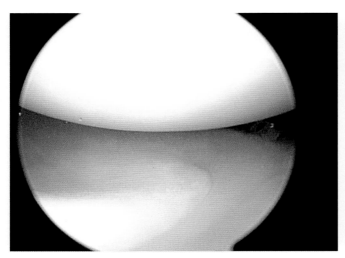

FIGURE 3–55. Posterior-inferior labrum.

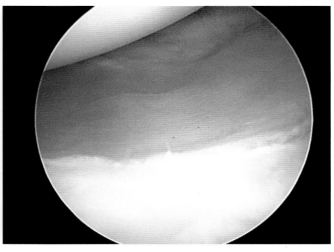

FIGURE 3–56. Posterior labrum, arthroscope posterior.

to the labrum. This requires that you withdraw the arthroscope until it is immediately anterior to the posterior capsule. My difficulty was that I would repeatedly pull the arthroscope completely out of the joint. My technique to minimize (but not eliminate) the problem is as follows. Pinch your index finger and thumb around the cannula where it exits the skin. This increased sensory feedback will help you to control the distance the cannula moves as well as giving you immediate control. Gently withdraw the arthroscope as posteriorly as possible. Rotate the objective lens of the arthroscope so that it is pointed to the 6-o'clock position. This will give you the best view of the biceps-labrum complex (Figs. 3–57 and 3–58).

Examine the biceps tendon, use an instrument to draw the intra-articular portion into the joint, and inspect it for inflammation or tearing. Follow the biceps tendon to its joint exit. Adhesions may exist between the biceps tendon and the supraspinatus tendon that may appear either congenital or post-traumatic (Figs. 3–59 to 3–78).

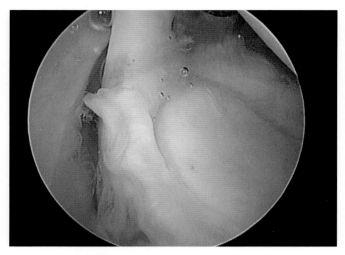

FIGURE 3–59. Biceps-labrum complex.

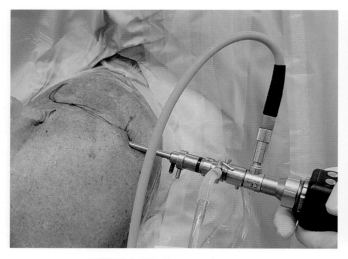

FIGURE 3–57. Pinch cannula and withdraw arthroscope.

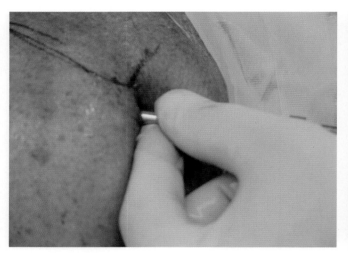

FIGURE 3–60. Biceps tendon synovitis.

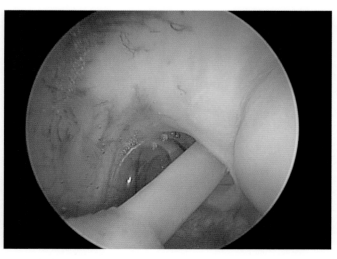

FIGURE 3–58. Rotate arthroscope.

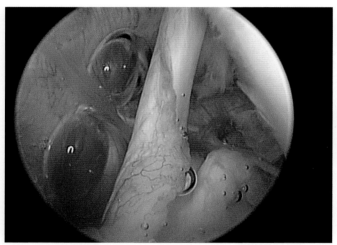

FIGURE 3–61. Biceps tendon exit from glenohumeral joint.

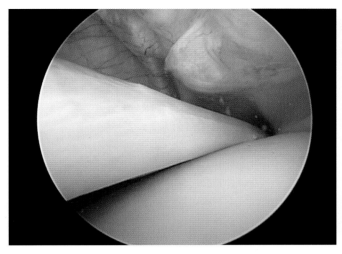

FIGURE 3–62. Biceps tendon entering bicipital groove.

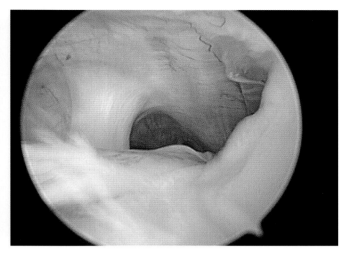

FIGURE 3–63. Bicipital groove.

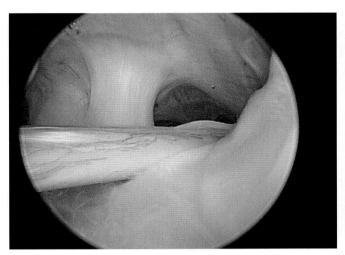

FIGURE 3–64. Bicipital groove.

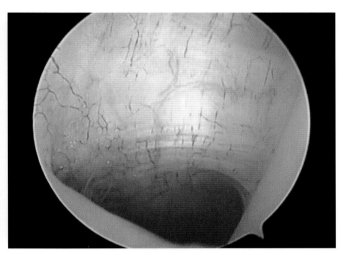

FIGURE 3–65. Bicipital groove, synovial lining.

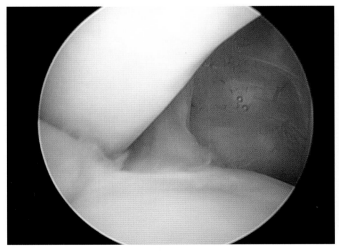

FIGURE 3–66. Bordering ligament.

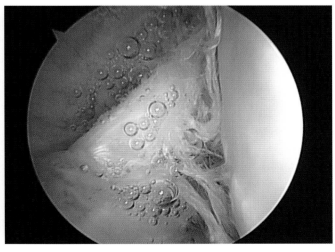

FIGURE 3–67. Partial biceps tendon tear.

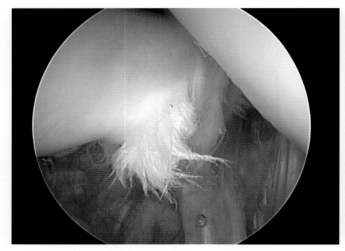

FIGURE 3–68. Partial biceps tendon tear.

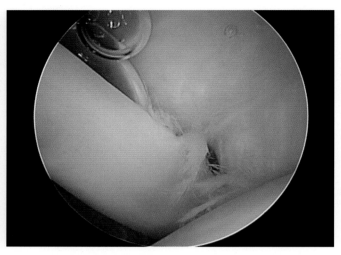

FIGURE 3–69. Partial biceps tendon tear.

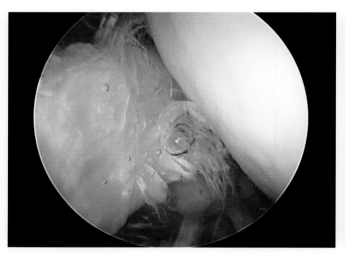

FIGURE 3–70. Partial biceps tendon tear.

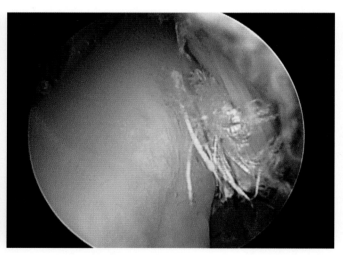

FIGURE 3–71. Partial biceps tendon tear.

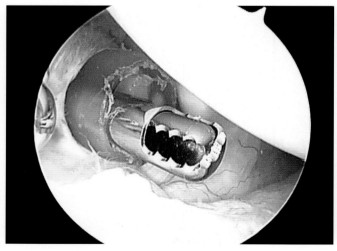

FIGURE 3–72. Introduce shaver.

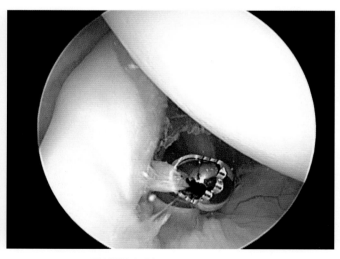

FIGURE 3–73. Lateral to biceps.

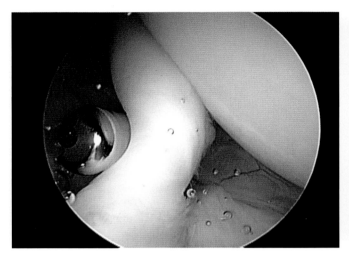

FIGURE 3–74. Medial to biceps.

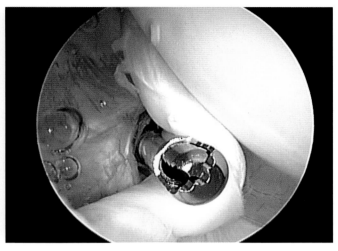

FIGURE 3–75. Pull extra-articular biceps tendon into glenohumeral joint.

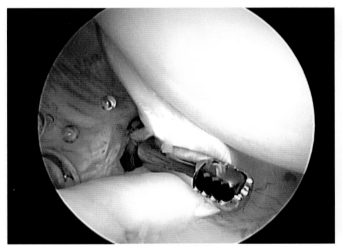

FIGURE 3–76. Pull extra-articular biceps tendon into glenohumeral joint.

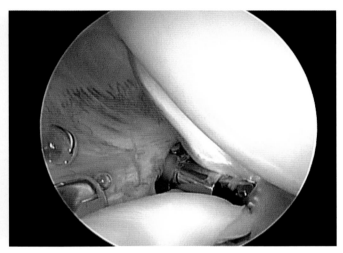

FIGURE 3–77. Pull extra-articular biceps tendon into glenohumeral joint.

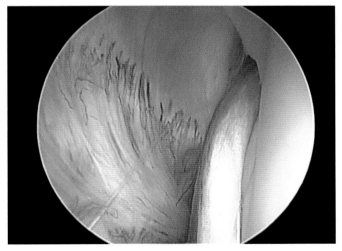

FIGURE 3–78. Extra-articular biceps tendon synovitis.

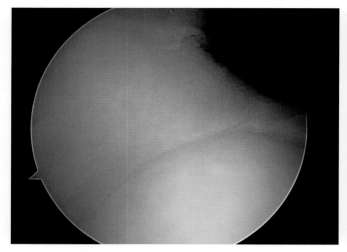

FIGURE 3–79. Normal superior labrum.

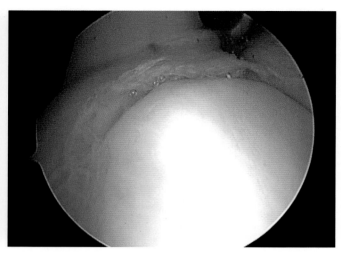

FIGURE 3–81. Minor separation.

Rotate the arthroscope so that it is pointed to 6 o'clock. Follow the posterior labrum from superior to inferior and note any labrum separation, fraying, or tears. Continue inferiorly until you can see the posterior-inferior glenohumeral ligament. Internally rotate the patient's arm, and observe the normal tightening of the posterior-inferior glenohumeral ligament.

Introduce a probe from the anterior portal, and evaluate the biceps-labrum complex. Often, a SLAP lesion is obvious, but sometimes probing is necessary. Abduct and externally rotate the patient's shoulder to see whether the superior labrum peels off the glenoid (Figs. 3–79 to 3–85). Adhesions may exist between the biceps tendon and the supraspinatus tendon that may appear either congenital or post-traumatic (Figs. 3–86 and 3–87).

Move your hand and the camera toward the floor to point the arthroscope superiorly and to view the rotator cuff tendons. Abduct and externally rotate the patient's shoulder until you see the anterior supraspinatus, which is marked anteriorly by the biceps tendon. Move your hand holding

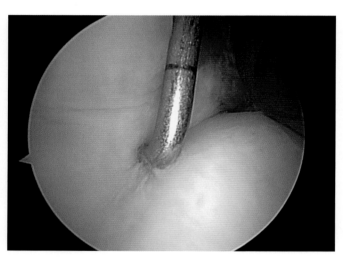

FIGURE 3–82. Probe for separation.

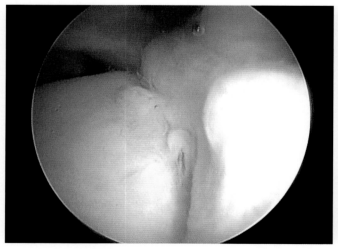

FIGURE 3–80. Minor fraying.

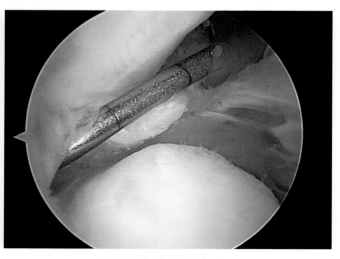

FIGURE 3–83. SLAP lesion.

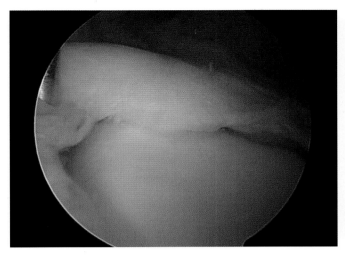

FIGURE 3–84. SLAP lesion continuing into anterior-superior labrum.

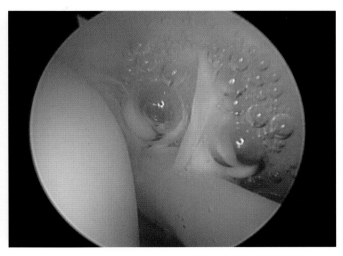

FIGURE 3–87. Biceps–rotator cuff adhesion.

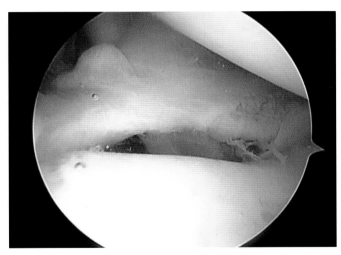

FIGURE 3–85. Normal anterior-superior labral foramen.

the camera medially and inferiorly (so that the arthroscope tip moves laterally and superiorly) and follow the cuff insertion from its anterior to posterior margins. At the same time, abduct and rotate the humeral head so that the arthroscope follows the cuff insertion from anterior to posterior. The small holes in the humeral head near the posterior cuff are normal vascular channels.

When you identify the posterior cuff insertion, tilt the arthroscope inferiorly, and continue to rotate the patient's shoulder externally. You can now see the posterolateral humeral head and can document the presence or absence of a Hill-Sachs lesion. Withdraw the arthroscope slightly so that the lens does not scrape against the humeral head, and allow it to return to the biceps tendon-labrum complex (Figs. 3–88 to 3–101).

Inspect the cartilage on the humeral head and glenoid for signs of osteoarthrosis such as eburnation and cobblestoning. Normally, the cartilage is thin in the central glenoid, and this should not be confused with osteoarthrosis (Figs. 3–102 to 3–107).

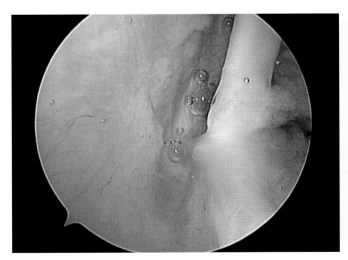

FIGURE 3–86. Biceps–rotator cuff adhesion.

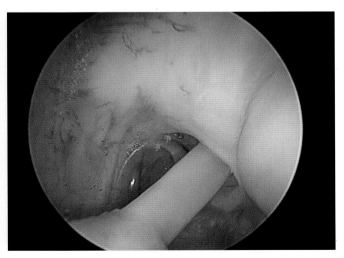

FIGURE 3–88. Anterior supraspinatus.

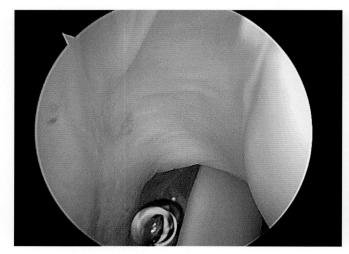

FIGURE 3–89. Anterior supraspinatus.

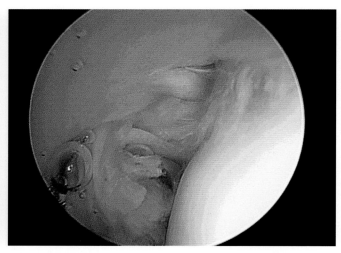

FIGURE 3–90. Articular surface partial-thickness rotator cuff tear, supraspinatus.

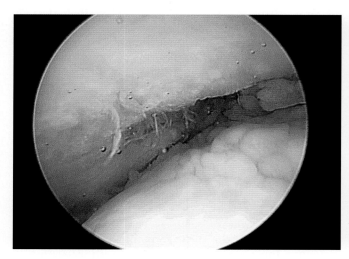

FIGURE 3–91. Full-thickness supraspinatus tear.

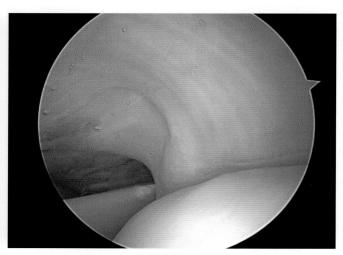

FIGURE 3–92. Midsupraspinatus.

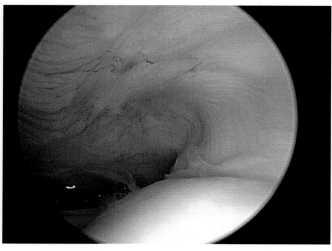

FIGURE 3–93. Midposterior supraspinatus.

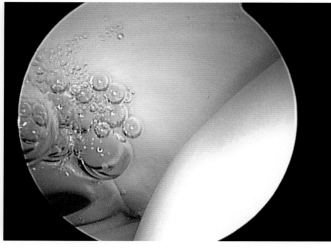

FIGURE 3–94. Posterior supraspinatus.

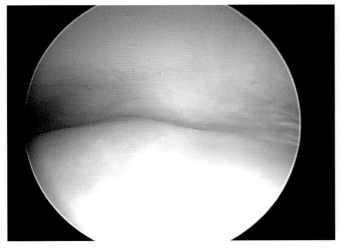

FIGURE 3–95. Posterior supraspinatus.

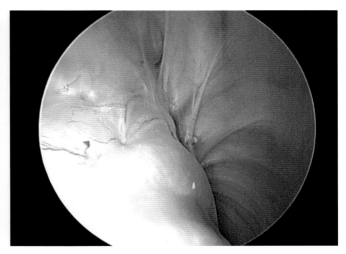

FIGURE 3–96. Infraspinatus.

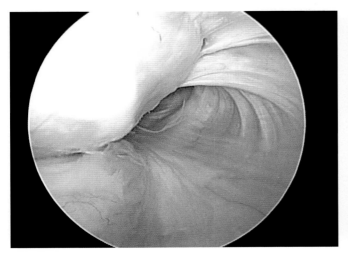

FIGURE 3–97. Capsular reflection.

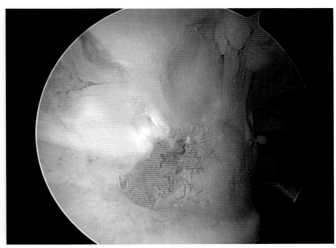

FIGURE 3–98. Bare area.

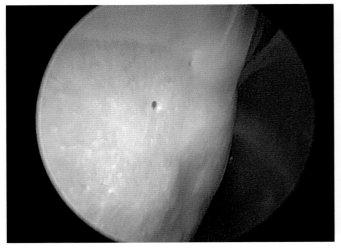

FIGURE 3–99. Vascular channels.

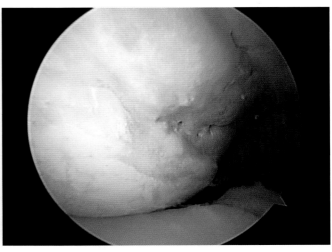

FIGURE 3–100. Bare area.

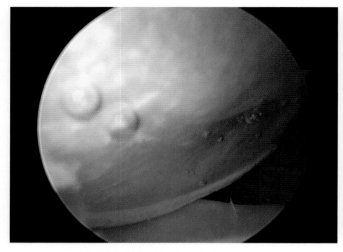

FIGURE 3–101. Shallow Hill-Sachs lesion.

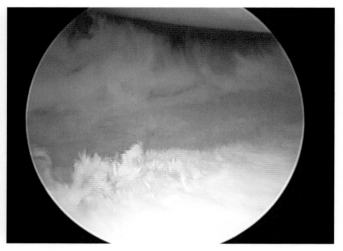

FIGURE 3–102. Anterior glenoid cartilage loss.

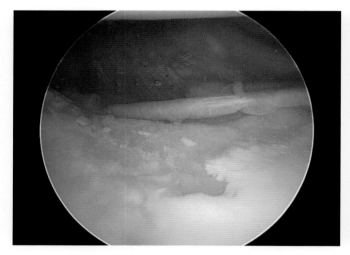

FIGURE 3–103. Anterior glenoid cartilage loss.

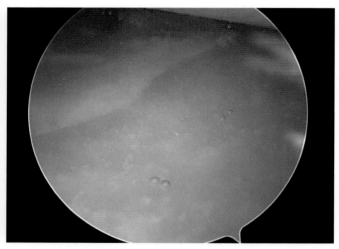

FIGURE 3–104. Osteoarthrosis, glenoid.

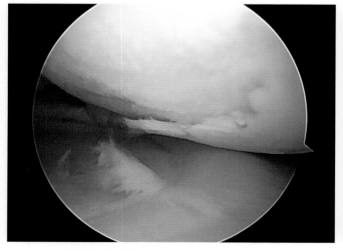

FIGURE 3–105. Humeral head cartilage tear.

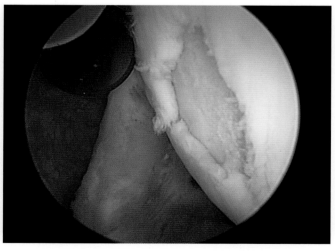

FIGURE 3–106. Full-thickness cartilage loss.

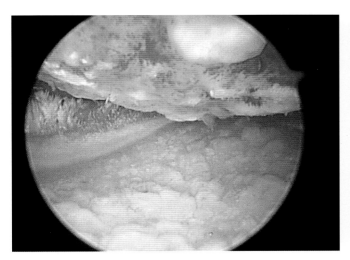

FIGURE 3–107. Osteoarthrosis, humeral head.

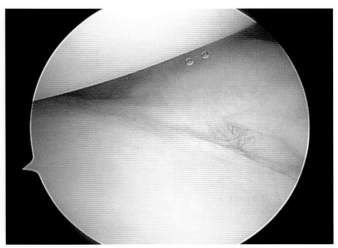

FIGURE 3–110. Inferior-posterior labrum.

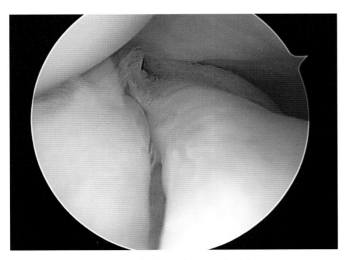

FIGURE 3–108. Posterior-superior labrum.

Remove the arthroscope from the posterior cannula, reinsert in into the anterior cannula, and again inspect the posterior labrum, capsule, and posterior rotator cuff. Move the patient's arm into abduction and external rotation, and evaluate the shoulder for internal impingement between the posterior superior labrum and the posterior cuff and capsule (Figs. 3–108 to 3–111). This completes a routine inspection of the glenohumeral joint. Withdraw both cannulas, and proceed to the subacromial space.

Diagnostic Subacromial Space Anatomy

The diagnostic examination of the subacromial space is systematic, to ensure that you do not overlook any possible lesions. The plan described in Table 3–2 ensures that you can accomplish this goal.

The subacromial space is a pseudoarticulation that permits gliding between the proximal humerus and the coracoacromial arch. Arthroscopic experience has led us to

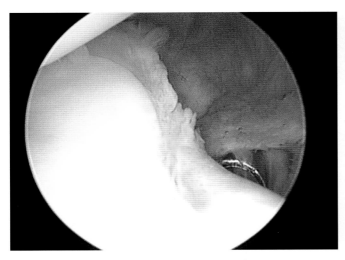

FIGURE 3–109. Posterior labrum and gutter.

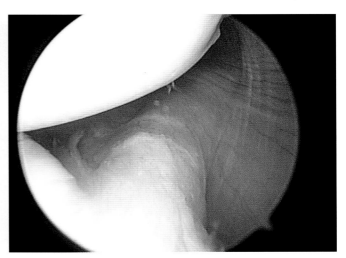

FIGURE 3–111. Posterior-inferior glenohumeral ligament.

TABLE 3–2. DIAGNOSTIC EXAMINATION OF THE SUBACROMIAL SPACE

View from posterior portal
1. Acromial undersurface
2. Coracoacromial ligament
3. Anterior bursa
4. Supraspinatus insertion into greater tuberosity
5. Subdeltoid adhesions
6. Acromioclavicular joint

View from lateral portal
1. Posterior rotator cuff
2. Posterior bursa
3. Rotator interval

surgeon penetrate a veil or curtain of bursal tissue that separates the anterior from the posterior space. Anterior, posterior, and lateral gutters can be defined (Fig. 3–112). The medial confines are below the acromioclavicular joint, and exposure of the lateral clavicle requires resection of thick fibrofatty and vascular tissue. The lateral wall lies beyond the greater tuberosity, and the anterior margin is the anterior acromial border.

It is often difficult to visualize the subacromial space because of reactive bursitis and fibrosis. It is helpful to position the arthroscope anteriorly in the subacromial space to minimize the effect of the bursal tissue that is posteriorly located within the space.

Use the same posterior skin incision to enter the subacromial space. Place the trocar and cannula through the skin incision, and palpate the posterior edge of the acromion. Slide immediately beneath the bone, and advance the trocar and cannula anteriorly. With your other hand, palpate the anterior acromion and advance the trocar beyond the anterior acromion; you can feel the trocar tip. Withdraw the trocar until it is just posterior to the anterior acromion. Usually, you can palpate the coracoacromial ligament. Remove the trocar while you maintain the cannula

define the subacromial space that reveals well-defined borders when it is cleared of the hypertrophic bursal tissue associated with chronic subacromial impingement. The arthroscopic subacromial space begins halfway back from the anterior acromion, and posterior entry requires that the

FIGURE 3–112. Bursa anatomy.

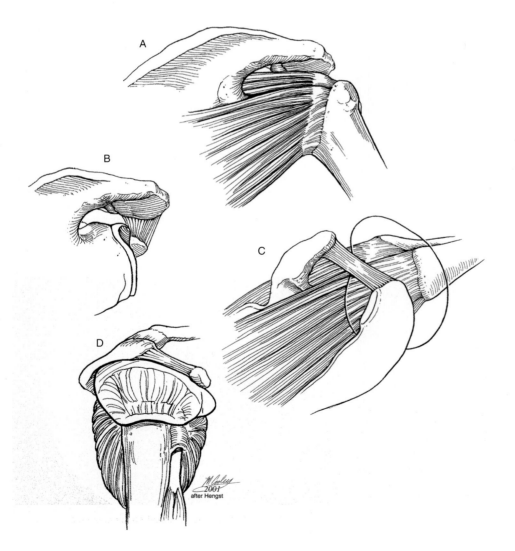

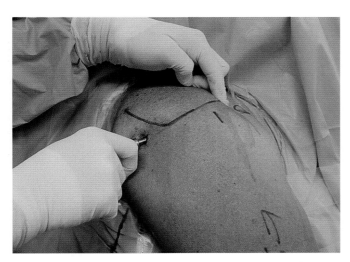

FIGURE 3–113. Palpate anterior acromion and trocar tip.

the inferior surface of the acromion. The distance the incision is located distal to the lateral acromial border will vary depending on the patient's size, but in general place the lateral portal 2 to 3 cm distal to the lateral acromial border.

If you cannot see well, advance the arthroscope anteriorly to free it of any surrounding bursal tissue, and then withdraw it posteriorly until the acromion is visualized. If visualization at this point remains poor, I have found triangulation technique helpful.

Insert the cannula and trocar as described earlier. Create a lateral portal by incising the skin 1 to 2 cm posterior to the anterolateral acromial border. The distance the incision is located distal to the lateral acromial border will vary depending on the patient's size, but in general place the lateral portal 2 to 3 cm distal to the lateral acromial border. You want the lateral cannula to enter the subacromial space parallel to and immediately beneath the inferior surface of the acromion. Insert a cannula and trocar through the lateral portal, and, with one hand holding each cannula and trocar, position them so they touch one another. Often, you can sense bursal tissue interposed between the two cannulas. Rub them together to remove the bursal tissue until you feel the two cannulas making direct contact. Advance the lateral cannula medially until it is past the tip of the posterior trocar. Push the posterior trocar until it is in direct contact with the lateral cannula. Hold both cannulas pressed together, remove the trocar from the posterior cannula, and insert the arthroscope. You should now be looking directly at the lateral cannula.

Remove the lateral trocar, and insert a motorized soft tissue resector. Palpate the acromion above and the rotator cuff below with the resector tip to help with orientation. Use the resector to remove enough bursal tissue until you can see clearly. Direct the shave blade superiorly if the shaver is on the rotator cuff so as not to damage it. Direct the shaver blade inferiorly when you are working near the acromion. Be careful not to contact the cuff or the acromion with the resector, because this will alter the subacromial space anatomy (Figs. 3–115 to 3–120).

position, and insert the arthroscope. Rotate the arthroscope so that it is directed toward the acromion, and determine whether there are any alterations in the coracoacromial ligament or the acromion (Figs. 3–113 and 3–114).

Now orient the arthroscope lens so that it is pointing directly down at the rotator cuff. If you maneuver the patient's shoulder through a range of motion and rotate the arthroscope, you will obtain a view of the superior portion of the subscapularis, the supraspinatus, and the superior portion of the infraspinatus. If you desire a better view of the posterior rotator cuff or if you cannot see clearly, establish a lateral portal. Identify the precise location of the lateral portal with a spinal needle. Introduce the needle percutaneously until the needle is 1 to 2 cm posterior to the anterior acromion and located midway between the acromion and the rotator cuff. This will allow the lateral cannula (because of its increased size) to enter the subacromial space parallel to and immediately beneath

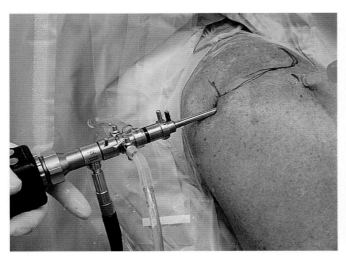

FIGURE 3–114. Lateral cannula location.

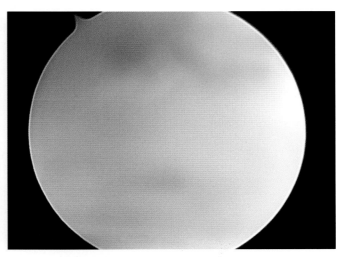

FIGURE 3–115. Subacromial space obscured.

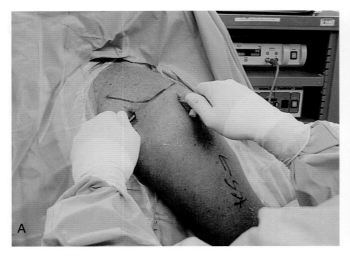

FIGURE 3–116. *A,* Palpate lateral cannula with trocar tip. *B,* Visualize lateral cannula.

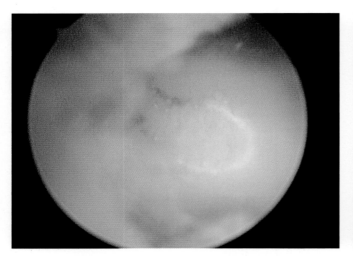

FIGURE 3–117. Withdraw arthroscope slightly.

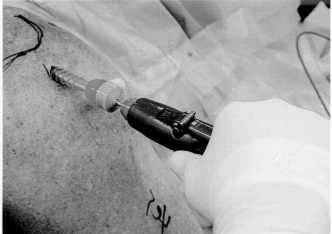

FIGURE 3–118. Introduce shaver.

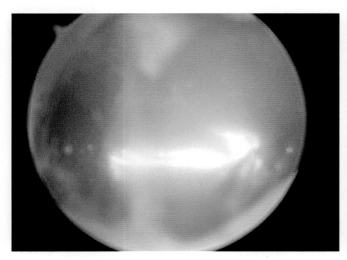

FIGURE 3–119. Visualize shaver within lateral cannula.

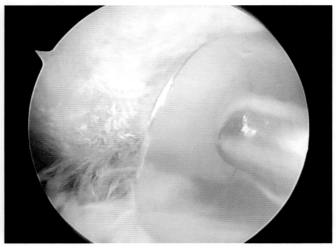

FIGURE 3–120. Withdraw lateral cannula.

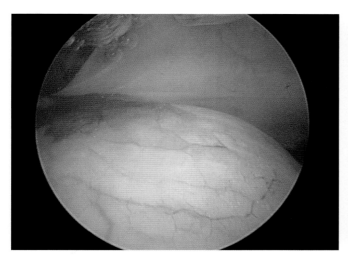

FIGURE 3–121. Rotator cuff.

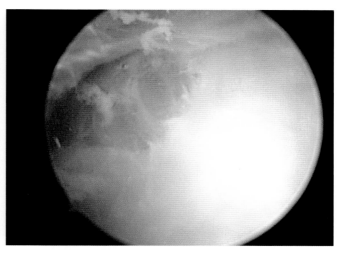

FIGURE 3–124. Musculotendinous junction.

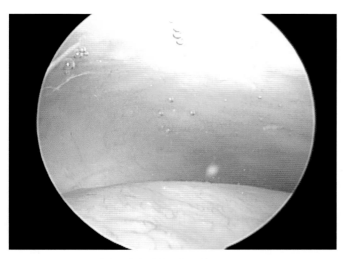

FIGURE 3–122. Anterior gutter.

Once you can see clearly, perform a diagnostic inspection of the subacromial space. Observe the acromion and coracoacromial ligament for signs of impingement such as fraying or erythema. Rotate the arthroscope so that it looks directly at the rotator cuff, and at the same time move the arthroscope tip superiorly so that the distance between the arthroscope and the rotator cuff is maximized. This will improve your perception of the extent of any disease. Signs of impingement include fraying, fibrillation, and partial tearing of the rotator cuff bursal surface.

Advance the arthroscope anteriorly to view the anterior gutter. Rotate the arthroscope to observe the lateral gutter. Move the arthroscope to the lateral portal. This will allow a better view of the subscapularis tendon and posterior rotator cuff. If bursa is covering the rotator cuff tendons, resect it until you can see the tendon fibers. This completes the diagnostic examination of the glenohumeral joint and subacromial space (Figs. 3–121 to 3–142).

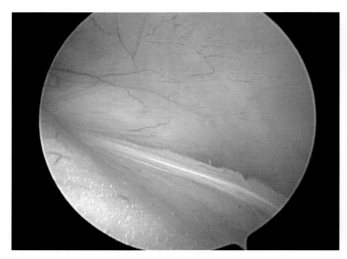

FIGURE 3–123. Anterolateral gutter.

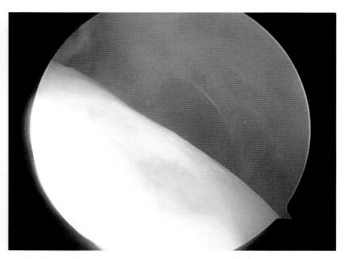

FIGURE 3–125. Lateral gutter.

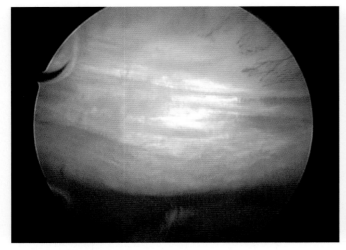

FIGURE 3–126. Coracoacromial ligament.

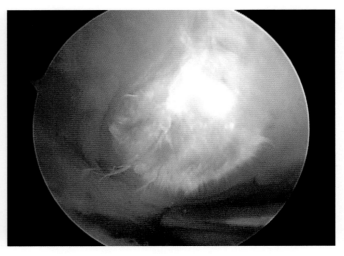

FIGURE 3–127. Coracoacromial ligament fraying.

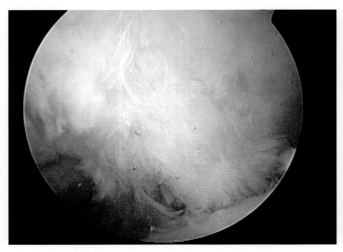

FIGURE 3–128. Coracoacromial ligament fraying.

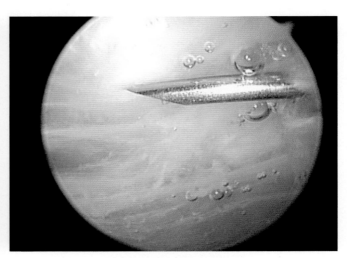

FIGURE 3–129. Spinal needle.

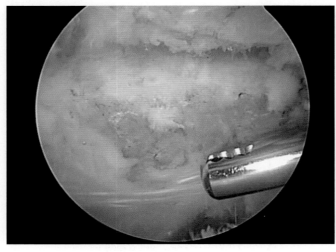

FIGURE 3–130. Os acromiale.

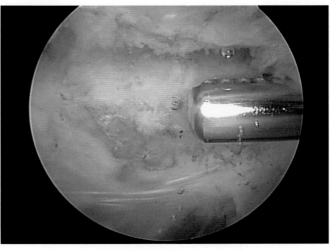

FIGURE 3–131. Os acromiale.

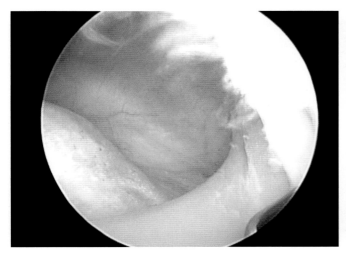

FIGURE 3–132. Lateral subacromial adhesion.

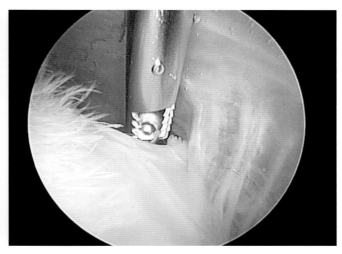

FIGURE 3–133. Resect adhesion.

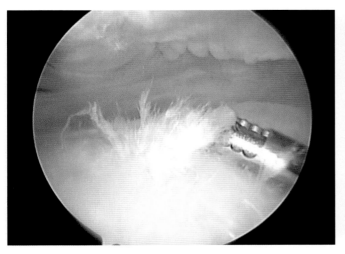

FIGURE 3–134. Partial-thickness rotator cuff tear, bursal surface.

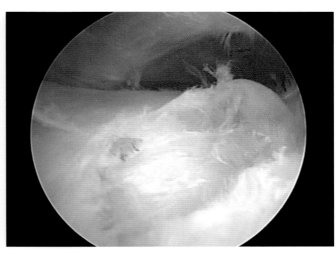

FIGURE 3–135. Partial-thickness rotator cuff tear, bursal surface.

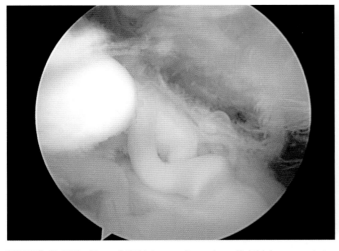

FIGURE 3–136. Near full-thickness bursal partial-thickness rotator cuff tear.

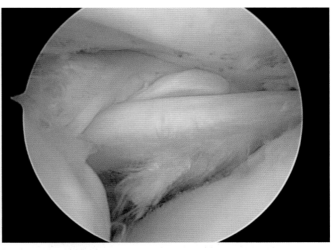

FIGURE 3–137. Full-thickness rotator cuff repair.

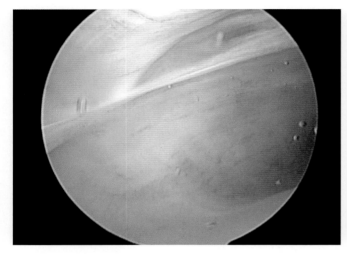

FIGURE 3–138. Coracoacromial ligament, arthroscope in lateral cannula.

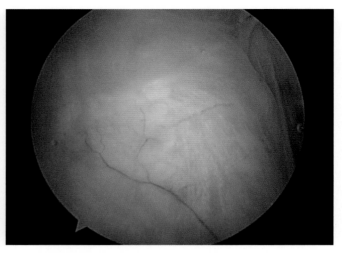

FIGURE 3–139. Rotator cuff, arthroscope in lateral cannula.

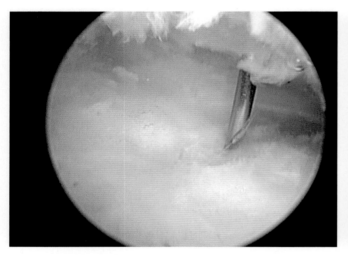

FIGURE 3–140. Rotator interval, arthroscope in lateral cannula. Needle probes anterior supraspinatus.

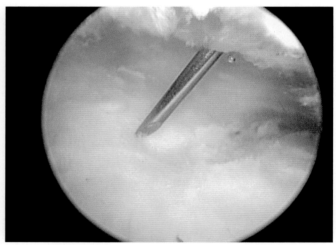

FIGURE 3–141. Rotator interval, arthroscope in lateral cannula. Needle probes superior subscapularis.

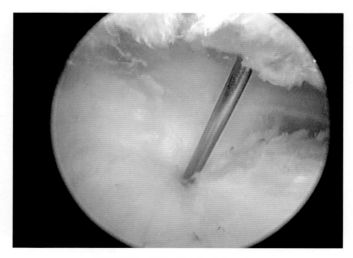

FIGURE 3–142. Rotator interval.

GLENOHUMERAL JOINT SURGERY

Glenohumeral Instability

Introduction

The fundamental desire on the part of orthopedic surgeons to search for a simple solution to glenohumeral instability has dictated various operative approaches. Initially, surgeons observed that the shoulder dislocates anteriorly in abduction and external rotation, and early operations sought to limit motion by limiting external rotation. Subsequently, the Bankart lesion rose in importance and became regarded as the essential lesion, so that labrum repair predominated. This change was also motivated by the eventual failure of many overtightening procedures. Although labrum repair operations were successful in some, but not all, patients, the underlying rationale could not provide an intellectual framework to explain or address dislocations that occurred without a Bankart lesion. Consequently, patients with recurrent anterior dislocations without labral detachment were treated with an anterior capsular tightening procedure. Again, many patients benefited, but others continued to dislocate or subluxate their shoulders. With the understanding that some shoulders were unstable in multiple directions, interest shifted to global capsular tightening. The capsular shift, as described by Neer, provided and continues to provide a solution to this challenging condition.

More recently, the desire to control glenohumeral instability while retaining patient function in overhead sports has motivated the search for newer techniques involving arthroscopy. The advantages of arthroscopic stabilization include the following: smaller skin incisions, more complete glenohumeral joint inspection, ability to treat all intra-articular lesions, access to all areas of the glenohumeral joint for repair, less soft tissue dissection, and maximal preservation of external rotation. Arthroscopy has provided a tremendous advantage by enabling surgeons to inspect the entire glenohumeral joint clearly and to observe lesions that exist in the unstable shoulder. Concurrently, clinical and basic science investigations have increased our understanding of the pathophysiology of glenohumeral instability. We now have the background, knowledge, and requisite technical skill to solve the problems of glenohumeral instability, and I believe the coming decade will bring both exciting advances and improved patient outcomes. Because my current treatment is linked directly to our recent past, I would like to summarize how I interpret the intellectual history of arthroscopic shoulder stabilization.

Literature Review

Early arthroscopic repairs used a staple to advance the Bankart lesion superiorly and *medially* and were associated with failure rates of up to 30%. When immobilization was extended, the failure rate approached 10% to 15%. Because of potential complications from staples within the glenohumeral joint, other surgeons employed techniques that used a transglenoid suture repair of the Bankart lesion. The essential element of these techniques is passage of sutures through the avulsed labrum and then through drill holes in the scapular neck. The sutures were tied posteriorly over soft tissue or bone. Early publications reported initial success rates up to 100%, but these results deteriorated with longer follow-up.

Later research and outcomes documented two flaws with these two approaches: the medial location of the repaired labrum and the failure to address capsular laxity. T. Neviaser first identified the ALPSA lesion (anterior labroligamentous periosteal sleeve avulsion) in shoulders with anterior inferior glenohumeral instability. The detached labrum-ligament complex had healed medially on the scapular neck, and this allowed excessive humeral translation. It was apparent that the staple and transglenoid suture techniques described earlier repaired the labrum medially to create an ALPSA lesion. Savoie and colleagues arthroscopically examined shoulders that had dislocated after arthroscopic stabilization. These investigators found that the labrum had been repaired 5 mm medial to the glenoid rim and were the first to point out that the attachment site of the repaired ligaments was critical. Savoie and associates subsequently modified their technique by moving the entry position of the anchor from the medial scapular neck to the glenoid articular surface and reported improved results with the newer technique.

The advent of bone suture anchors enabled repair of the detached labrum directly to the glenoid rim. This approach was pioneered by Wolf and colleagues for arthroscopic repair of instability and was later popularized by others. Improved outcomes occurred as surgeons learned to position the glenoid labrum onto the glenoid rim correctly. Harryman, Sidles, Harris, and Matsen introduced the term *concavity-compression* to explain the important role of the labrum in glenohumeral instability. However, further investigation raised two questions. Was the Bankart lesion the only labrum lesion responsible for anterior inferior instability? Could *any* labrum lesion or combination of labrum lesions produce glenohumeral instability without any other lesion?

Rodosky and associates described the role of the biceps-labrum complex in anterior inferior instability. Detachments of the superior labrum (superior labrum from anterior to posterior, or SLAP lesion) performed in the laboratory allowed increased anterior humeral head translation. Speer also used a cadaver model to determine that although a Bankart lesion allowed increased humeral head translation, it alone did not cause the humeral head to dislocate. Capsular stretch or elongation, in addition to the Bankart lesion, was necessary for dislocation. McMahon and colleagues emphasized that the rate of capsular stretch was an important variable because the rate of speed of the injury may determine where the capsular ligament is damaged. In a laboratory study, Bigliani and colleagues demonstrated predominantly ligament injury at faster strain rates, whereas testing at a slower strain rate demonstrated a higher percentage of failures at the ligament insertion site. Bigliani and associates also studied the tensile properties of the shoulder capsule of patients with an acute dislocation and found that capsular damage was almost always present to some extent even with a Bankart lesion. Baker arthroscopically inspected the shoulders of 45 patients within 10 days of an acute dislocation and found that the capsule had been stretched or torn in all patients with or without an associated Bankart lesion. We are all indebted to Michael Gross, who elegantly summarized much of this information.

Most descriptions of arthroscopic technique have also omitted treatment of the rotator interval. This area of the glenohumeral joint capsule is the soft tissue between the superior border of the subscapularis tendon and the anterior edge of the supraspinatus tendon, and it includes the superior glenohumeral ligament and a portion of the coracohumeral ligament. Neer and Foster and Rowe and Zarins described the role of the rotator interval in open repair of shoulder instability. Rowe and Zarins inspected the superior aspect of the rotator cuff and found that 20 of 37 patients undergoing operation had a large opening in the capsule between the supraspinatus and subscapularis. The laboratory studies of Harryman and colleagues advanced our understanding of the rotator interval. These investigators found that opening the rotator interval increased inferior posterior translation.

Perhaps the most subjective (and therefore difficult) area of instability treatment is capsular tensioning. Thermal treatment represents the latest therapeutic modality and was received by the orthopedic community with great interest. Thermal treatment is a technique by which the surgeon can alter the soft tissue tension easily and can observe the effects directly. However, clinical application outpaced basic science investigation. It is only recently that we have gained some appreciation of thermal technique's complexity, appropriate role, limitations, and complications.

I believe that the high failure rates previously reported for arthroscopic repairs are the result of technical factors, such as a medial repair of the anterior labrum, as well as the failure to treat other lesions, such as those of the capsule or rotator interval, that contribute to glenohumeral instability. My colleagues and I recently reported my early results. Our work emphasized several concepts, as follows:

1. Glenohumeral instability occurs in several directions.
2. These directions are classified as anterior, posterior, bidirectional (anterior inferior or posterior inferior), or multidirectional (inferior, anterior, and posterior).
3. The classification of direction is somewhat arbitrary.
4. The primary direction of instability is determined through a combination of patient history, physical examination, radiographic analysis, examination while the patient is under anesthesia, and evaluation of the glenohumeral joint at the time of arthroscopic surgery.
5. The lesions observed are usually multiple.
6. Instability in any direction may be the result of various combinations of lesions.
7. A combination of lesions may produce instability in a certain direction in one patient, whereas in another patient the same lesions may produce instability in another direction.
8. Instability correction requires the surgeon to identify all the lesions and repair them.
9. It may be necessary to operate on areas of the glenohumeral joint on the side opposite the primary instability to balance the shoulder and to prevent iatrogenic instability.
10. Glenohumeral instability should probably be considered a single entity defined as symptomatic excessive humeral head translation. The clinical expression of this translation is variable in each individual patient.

Orthopedic surgeons diagnose this clinical expression of glenohumeral instability on the basis of patient history, physical examination, radiographic analysis, and operative findings. Unidirectional instabilities are well appreciated and are generally categorized as anterior or posterior. Patients with multidirectional instability have symptoms on physical examination of pain and apprehension when the shoulder is stressed in anterior, posterior, *and* inferior directions. Neer's pioneering concepts were twofold: glenohumeral instability can occur in multiple directions, *and* correction of all three *symptomatic* directions was necessary. My experience was that there was an additional group of patients who were symptomatic in only two directions. There is little in the literature concerning bidirectional glenohumeral instability, that is, inferior instability with *either* an anterior or a posterior component. This entity is separate from multidirectional instability and unidirectional anterior or posterior instability. Neer and Foster discussed instability in two directions in their article on multidirectional instability. Altchek and colleagues described their results with operation for multidirectional instability of the anterior and inferior types. Bigliani and associates specifically used the term *bidirectional* in their article on recurrent posterior shoulder instability. In a search for a unifying approach to the many forms of glenohumeral instability, I found the analysis by Bigliani and colleagues most helpful. In their article on anterior inferior shoulder instability, Bigliani and associates discussed the complexities of instability classification and stressed the need to address *all* components of glenohumeral *laxity* to balance the shoulder. Previous articles had focused on correcting the laxity in the direction of the instability, but Bigliani and colleagues were the first to report that an area of *asymptomatic* laxity must be treated to correct symptomatic instability in another direction.

The clinical expression of glenohumeral joint laxity is termed *instability*, and my own philosophy is that the direction(s) of instability are the result of laxity in various areas of the glenohumeral capsule and insertion tears of the labrum. Successful arthroscopic treatment requires that the surgeon identify the direction and degree of clinical instability on preoperative evaluation, identify the areas responsible for excessive translation on arthroscopic evaluation, and then correct all necessary areas of the glenohumeral joint. A prime example of this approach is the patient with recurrent posterior glenohumeral subluxation. That patient likely will have excessive laxity in the posterior inferior capsule, but correction of that area alone will not control excessive humeral head translation. Although the patient is not symptomatic in the direction of the rotator interval or the anterior inferior glenohumeral ligament, tightening of both these areas is usually required.

There are many similarities between arthroscopic rotator cuff repair and arthroscopic glenohumeral reconstruction, but I believe that these procedures have important fundamental differences. Arthroscopic rotator cuff repair has certain advantages over the traditional open approach, as described in Chapter 12. However, fundamentally the primary goal of both the arthroscopic operation and the open procedure is identical: to reattach the torn edge of the rotator cuff tendon to its normal point of anatomic insertion. Although operations within the glenohumeral joint are technically less demanding than those within the tight confines of the subacromial space, few would argue that an arthroscopic glenohumeral reconstruction is a simple operation. It is true that the glenohumeral joint is better visualized and has greater space for the surgeon to manipulate instruments than within the tight confines of the subacromial space. However, the less demanding technical aspects are offset by a greater deficit in knowledge. For example,

there are no objective standards by which to judge ligament or capsular tension, so the surgeon can only estimate the tightening that is needed.

Diagnosis

Patient History

I collect sufficient data to rate patients according to the American Shoulder and Elbow Surgeons' Shoulder Index, the Constant scoring system, the scoring system of Rowe, and the University of California at Los Angeles Shoulder Scale. Recently, my colleagues and I developed our own shoulder scoring system that allows us to compare patients with high as well as low levels of shoulder function without an excessive response burden. Before operation, all patients complete self-assessment questionnaires to document their levels of shoulder pain, satisfaction, and function.

To increase diagnostic precision, I classify each shoulder in regard to chronicity, degree, and traumatic onset. I document (according to the patient's description) whether the instability is chronic or acute (less than 6 weeks' duration), and I also classify the instability as a recurrent dislocation, a recurrent subluxation after a single dislocation, or a recurrent subluxation without prior dislocation. I record whether or not patients developed instability after a traumatic event of a magnitude sufficient to damage the glenohumeral ligaments (traumatic or atraumatic) and use guidelines similar to those described by Wirth and associates. A traumatic cause is supported by an injury with the arm forcefully abducted, externally rotated and extended, sudden sharp pain, the need for manipulative reduction, and residual aching in the shoulder for several weeks. Atraumatic instability is characterized by an insidious onset or that developing after minor trauma, and it is associated with mild pain and spontaneous reduction. All patients are questioned about arm position or activity that reproduces their symptoms.

Additionally, I record sports participation, if any, of each patient. To define the sports category accurately, I classify sports according to the method described by Allain and colleagues. Type 1 sports are nonimpact activities and consist of breaststroke swimming, rowing, running, or sailing. Type 2 sports are high-impact activities and include bicycle riding, snow-skiing, soccer, or water-skiing. Type 3 sports require overhead use of the arm with hitting movements, such as crawl-stroke swimming, golf, tennis, throwing, and weightlifting. Type 4 sports involve overhead hitting movements and sudden stops such as basketball, football, handball, ice hockey, judo, karate, kayaking, lacrosse, polo, rodeo, volleyball, windsurfing, and wrestling. I also record which shoulder is dominant.

Physical Examination

I measure active ranges according to the Constant rating system that includes forward flexion, abduction, external rotation in abduction, and behind-the-back internal rotation. Passive elevation and external rotation (with the arm adducted), as well as external rotation and internal rotation with the arm abducted 90 degrees, are measured. I measure internal rotation at 90 degrees of abduction in the coronal

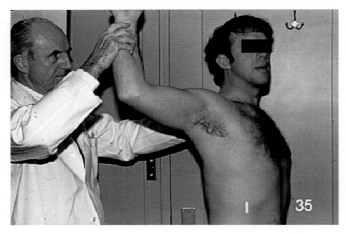

FIGURE 4–1. Dr. Rowe examining a patient for anterior instability.

The stability examination is performed on both shoulders. I compress (load) the humeral head into the glenoid during all maneuvers. I assess glenohumeral translation in eight directions: anterior superior, anterior, anterior inferior, inferior anterior, inferior, inferior posterior, posterior inferior, and posterior. An essential element of the instability examination is patient relaxation because an effective examination cannot be performed with voluntary resistance on the part of the patient. If the patient is comfortable, I perform the examination with the patient standing, but if relaxation is not adequate, I examine the patient while he or she is seated or supine. I assess anterior superior translation with the patient's arm externally rotated in 90 degrees of abduction while I grasp the humeral head and move it anterior superiorly. Anterior translation is assessed with an anterior force applied to the shoulder with the arm in 90 degrees of abduction, and anterior inferior translation is tested in the same arm position but with the direction of force changed anterior inferiorly (Fig. 4–1). I also perform the relocation test (Fig. 4–2). Dr. Rowe instructed me in the performance and importance of a particularly useful maneuver, and I use the Rowe test to assess inferior anterior translation. To perform this examination, the patient stands

plane as well as in the scapular plane. Elevation strength is measured using a dynamometer with the arm elevated in the scapular plane 90 degrees and internally rotated, with the result recorded in pounds.

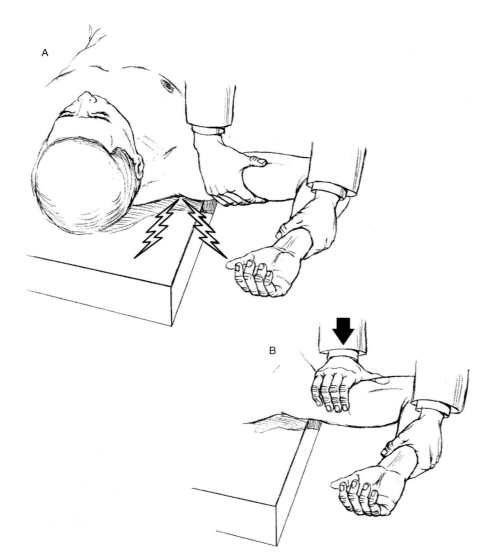

FIGURE 4–2. *A* and *B*, Relocation test.

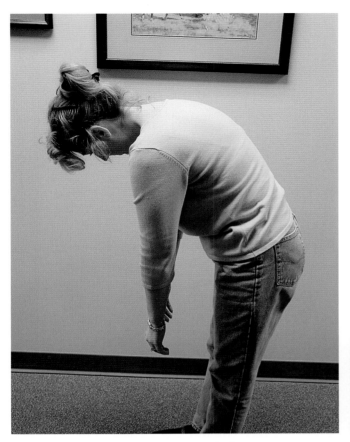

FIGURE 4–3. Patient position for Rowe test.

and flexes the trunk from the hips approximately 30 degrees. I instruct the patient to relax the arms and let them hang from the shoulder toward the floor. In this relaxed position, the shoulders are effectively elevated 30 degrees, and the examiner applies a distraction force (Fig. 4–3). Inferior translation is assessed with an inferior force applied with the shoulder at 0 degrees of abduction (sulcus test). If the translation force is applied in an inferior posterior direction, the surgeon will gain additional information. Posterior translations are examined with the arm elevated 90 degrees, adducted slightly, and rotated internally approximately 30 degrees. I translate the shoulder in a posterior inferior direction and record the result. I then apply a posterior force and assess the translation. Typically, the posterior translation produces minimal complaints, but as the shoulder is extended and reduces, the patient expresses pain.

I record the presence or absence of pain and apprehension for each instability maneuver and grade the amount of humeral head translation on the glenoid surface as 0 (stable or trace laxity), 1 (up to 50%), 2 (more than 50% but not dislocatable), and 3 (dislocatable). The grading of instability is subjective, because I have only recently made an attempt to measure the degree of translation with fluoroscopic observation. I record the presence of laxity in the contralateral shoulder and the elbows and the patient's ability to bring the thumb to the forearm, but I do not use any formal grading system for the degree of generalized ligament laxity. Ligament laxity is categorized as present or

absent on the basis of this examination. I exclude other sources of shoulder pain (rotator cuff lesions, acromioclavicular joint arthritis, thoracic outlet syndrome, brachial plexus lesions, and glenohumeral arthritis) through patient history, physical examination, and radiographic analysis.

Radiographs

Routine radiographs include anterior posterior glenoid, axillary, and supraspinatus outlet views. Other radiographic imaging (magnetic resonance imaging, computed tomography, arthrography) is not routinely obtained. Direct radiographic evidence of glenohumeral instability consists of radiographs that demonstrate humeral head dislocation. Indirect plain radiographic signs of instability include calcification adjacent to the anterior glenoid, a bone Bankart lesion, or a Hill-Sachs lesion. Magnetic resonance imaging and computed tomographic evidence of instability include not only the foregoing but also detachment of the glenoid labrum from the glenoid bone, capsular stripping from the glenoid, and ligament insufficiency (Figs. 4–4 to 4–13).

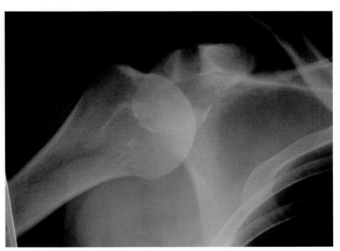

FIGURE 4–4. Anterior inferior dislocation.

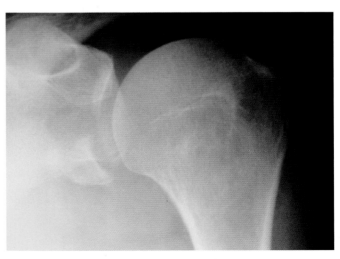

FIGURE 4–5. Glenoid rim fracture.

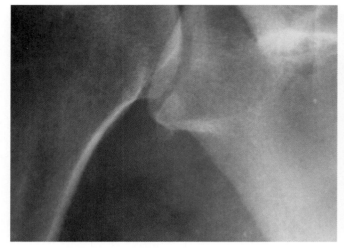

FIGURE 4–6. Bone Bankart lesion.

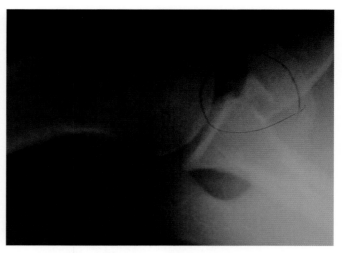

FIGURE 4–7. Bone Bankart lesion *(circled)*, axillary view.

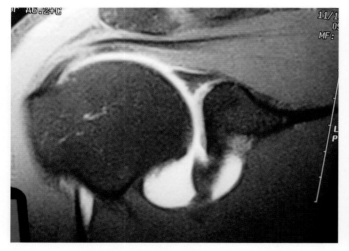

FIGURE 4–8. SLAP lesion.

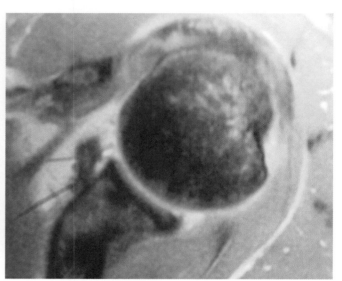

FIGURE 4–9. Bankart lesion.

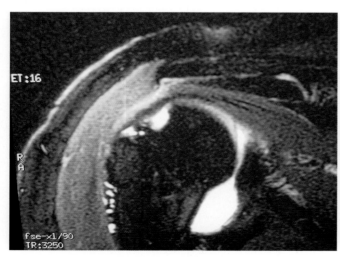

FIGURE 4–10. Hill-Sachs lesion.

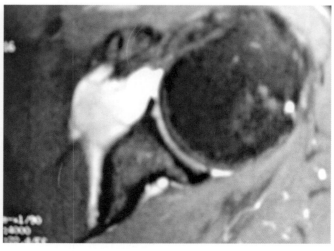

FIGURE 4–11. Anterior capsular stripping.

If the diagnosis is in doubt, an arthroscopic examination or examination with the patient under anesthesia is helpful. I observe humeral head movement under direct arthroscopic visualization and also find intra-articular lesions helpful in determining the predominant direction of instability. These lesions are located in the humeral head and glenoid (chondral or osteochondral defects), labrum (fraying or separation from the glenoid), and capsular ligaments (tear or laxity).

Nonoperative Treatment

Nonoperative treatment consists of avoidance of painful activities, nonsteroidal anti-inflammatory medication, and a home physical therapy program designed to eliminate contracture and to maintain or improve shoulder girdle strength and neuromuscular coordination. My goal is to improve the strength of those muscles responsible for glenohumeral stability. Therefore, patients perform resistive exercises of the deltoid, internal rotators, external rotators, biceps, triceps, and scapular muscles with surgical tubing and light weights (maximum, 5 pounds). Patients are instructed in exercises to improve neuromuscular coordination and proprioception. Areas of contracture are identified and are corrected with specific stretching. Posterior contracture commonly occurs in patients with anterior inferior glenohumeral instability (Figs. 4–14 and 4–15).

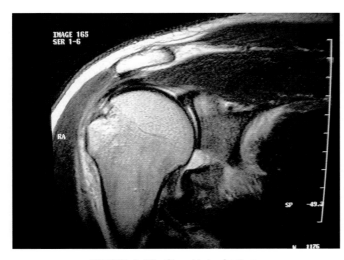

FIGURE 4–12. Glenoid rim fracture.

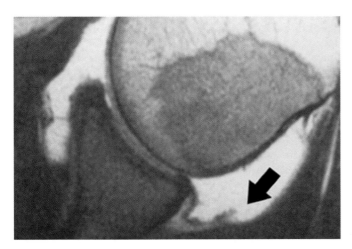

FIGURE 4–13. Posterior humeral glenohumeral ligament tear (*arrow*).

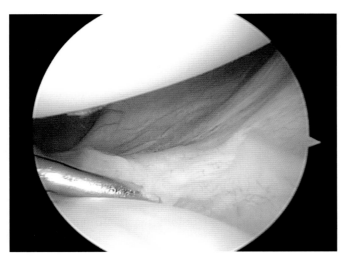

FIGURE 4–14. Contracted posterior inferior capsule.

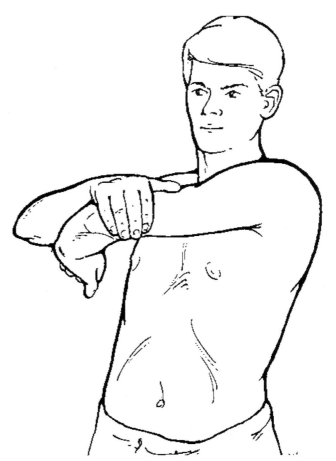

FIGURE 4–15. Adduction stretch.

Indications for Surgery

The primary indication for operation is persistent shoulder pain resulting from glenohumeral instability that has not responded to a minimum 6-month nonoperative program, as described earlier. The only exceptions are patients who desire operative repair acutely (within 6 weeks of an initial traumatic dislocation).

When a patient sustains an initial dislocation that occurs with sufficient energy that I can classify it as traumatic, I believe that surgical repair is an option. I consider nine factors: patient age, amount of trauma involved in the dislocation, reduction method, arm dominance, present activity level, desired activity level, the patient's sensation of instability, radiographic findings, and timing during a sports season. Fundamentally, I believe that the decision for operation is the patient's choice, and I present the natural history of initial shoulder dislocation in the context of the patient's particular situation.

Factors influencing the decision for acute repair include age younger than 30 years, traumatic cause (as opposed to dislocations that occur with minimal force), reduction required (as opposed to spontaneous reduction), dominant arm, high present activity level, a desire to continue that activity level, or a sensation of instability while the arm is in the sling or with movement during sling removal or dressing. A displaced bone fragment indicates that the labrum does not lie in its anatomic location and will heal with the attached soft tissue in a medial position. If the patient is currently participating in team sports and the season is less than 2 months from completion, then we discuss the patient's desire to return to that sport or another seasonal sport. For example a high school junior with an interest in football may elect to have the shoulder repaired to return for the senior season, whereas a patient who also participates in a spring sport may not wish to take a chance on missing baseball, particularly if that is the patient's area of concentration. I explain the percentages of recurrent instability in light of the patient's particular situation and let the patient and family decide on operative or nonoperative care.

I think historians will find our past treatment of the patient with a traumatic dislocation curious. Essentially, we have a patient with a 30% to 90% recurrence rate and a treatment with a 90% to 95% success rate, yet this treatment is performed uncommonly. Orthopedic surgeons operate on acute ligament injuries of the knee and ankle but rarely on the shoulder. I believe that as our technique and equipment continue to improve, the patient with an acute shoulder dislocation will have more access to surgical care.

Contraindications for Surgery

Absolute contraindications include patients who demonstrate glenohumeral instability with selective voluntary muscle contractions and those with questionable emotional stability. Relative contraindications include failed prior operations for instability and those with large bone defects of the glenoid or humeral head. Itoi and colleagues demonstrated in a cadaver experiment that anterior glenoid defects greater than 4 mm result in glenoid insufficiency

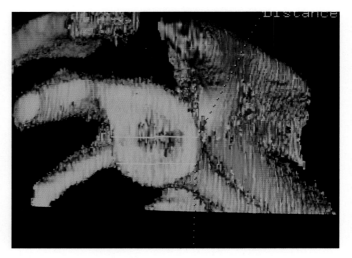

FIGURE 4–16. Three-dimensional computed tomographic reconstruction.

that the surgeon cannot correct with soft tissue repair. I use 4 mm only as a guideline because Itoi's laboratory experiment does not take into account the variability of capsular advancement that can be achieved in a particular patient. I have found three-dimensional computed tomographic reconstruction to be the most helpful radiographic aid but rely most on my inspection of the glenoid shape at the time of arthroscopic examination (Fig. 4–16).

Most Hill-Sachs lesions do not affect the operative result because with restoration of soft tissue tension, the Hill-Sachs lesion does not engage the anterior glenoid. However, when the humeral head defect is large enough, there is insufficient surface area to allow adequate external rotation. Prior operations dealt with this issue by purposefully restricting external rotation, but such an approach restricts function and may lead to asymmetric loading and arthrosis. I have found that arthroscopy is the most effective means of evaluating whether the Hill-Sachs lesion is large enough to require open procedures such as humeral head allograft or rotational osteotomy.

Operative Approach

I would like to describe why I choose to repair various structures within the glenohumeral joint (operative rationale), then describe when I repair the lesions (intraoperative decision making and indications), and finally how I repair the lesions (operative technique). As discussed earlier, I consider glenohumeral instability to be a single entity with variable clinical expression. Therefore, I do not present separate sections on the treatment of each instability direction.

Operative Rationale

The underlying principle of my arthroscopic repair is to identify and repair all lesions that contribute to glenohumeral instability. These include débridement, repair of ligament and labrum tears, capsular tensioning, and, if needed, repair of the rotator interval.

My approach to a patient with glenohumeral instability is to first determine the directions of instability by a thorough history, physical examination, examination with the patient under anesthesia, and examination during glenohumeral arthroscopy. I then evaluate all the structures within the glenohumeral joint and decide which of these structures requires operation. A patient with unidirectional anterior instability may require an anterior labrum repair, but if capsular stretching has occurred, the patient may also require an anterior capsular imbrication. Another patient with the same direction and degree of translation may not be stabilized with these two maneuvers but could also require a superior labrum repair. A patient with posterior inferior instability may not be stabilized after posterior labrum or posterior capsular repair but may require tightening of the inferior capsule and anterior inferior glenohumeral ligament. A rotator interval repair may be necessary. Decision making is complex, but I believe it accurately reflects the complexity of the clinical situation (Figs. 4–17 to 4–21).

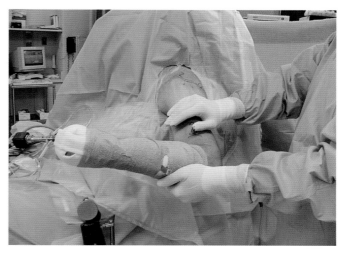

FIGURE 4–19. Inferior translation in abduction.

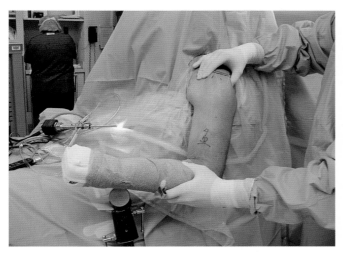

FIGURE 4–17. Inferior translation, shoulder internally rotated.

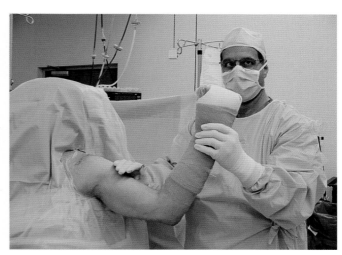

FIGURE 4–20. Anterior translation.

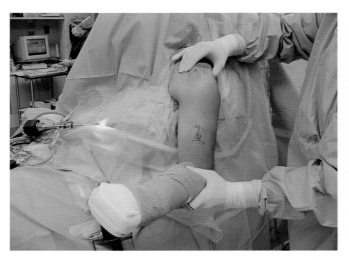

FIGURE 4–18. Inferior translation, shoulder externally rotated.

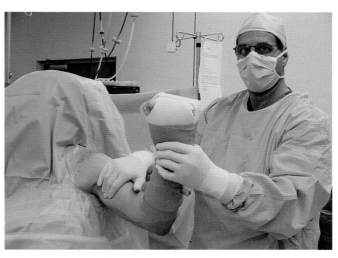

FIGURE 4–21. Posterior translation.

The goal of débridement is to remove sources of mechanical irritation or functional instability. Only minor labrum flap tears (less than 50% of the labrum thickness) are removed, and every attempt is made to repair the lesions.

The purpose of ligament and labrum reattachment to bone is twofold. Adequate capsular tension is impossible to achieve unless labrum and ligament are securely attached to the glenoid. Therefore, I repair all traumatic tears of the superior, anterior, and inferior labra because I believe that all lesions contribute to glenohumeral instability. Second, anatomic repair of the ligament and labrum restores concavity-compression to the glenohumeral joint. Lippitt and colleagues demonstrated that compression of the humeral head into the glenoid by muscular force is an effective stabilizer to humeral translation, and resection of the labrum decreases the stability by 20%.

However, reattachment of the anterior inferior ligament-labrum complex to the glenoid may not restore sufficient stability to the glenohumeral joint. Speer and associates demonstrated only a small increase in humeral translation with a simulated Bankart lesion and believed that capsular stretching or elongation is necessary to produce glenohumeral instability. Therefore, the final portion of the operation is to restore capsular tension.

I classify capsular elongation as primary or secondary. I use the term *primary elongation* to refer to permanent deformation of the capsular fibers resulting from a single traumatic event or multiple instability episodes. Secondary elongation occurs when there is a tear at the insertion site, thereby decreasing capsular tension. This may occur within the anterior inferior capsule after a Bankart lesion, but it may also result from a superior labrum tear. The biceps-labrum complex contributes to anterior inferior translation, and its detachment results in increased humeral translation. Based on these data, I repair all *traumatic* superior labrum detachments. Rotator interval and superior glenohumeral ligament tears also affect glenohumeral stability. I have observed, at the time of operation, that repair of the rotator interval decreases inferior and posterior translation of the humeral head. If the repair also incorporates the superior portion of the middle glenohumeral ligament, anterior capsular tension is increased. Thus, the surgeon can restore capsular tension by two methods: primary capsular elongation requires operation directly on the capsule, and secondary elongation responds to repair of insertion site tears.

I correct primary capsular elongation by four techniques, used singly or in combination: (1) advancement of the capsule to the labrum, (2) advancement of the capsule to the glenoid with suture anchors, (3) capsular imbrication, and (4) thermal capsulorrhaphy.

The goals of this portion of the procedure are to restore ligament and capsule tension and to eliminate excessive humeral head translation, which I define as greater than 25%. To estimate the percentage of translation, I visually divide the humeral head into four segments and observe how much of the humeral head translates with relation to the glenoid. Any or all of the following areas may require tightening: middle glenohumeral ligament, anterior inferior glenohumeral ligament, inferior capsule, posterior inferior glenohumeral ligament, and posterior capsule.

My preference is to advance the capsule to the intact or repaired labrum with monofilament or braided sutures.

Only if the labrum is small or absent is the capsule repaired to the glenoid rim with bone suture anchors. Drill holes for the suture anchors are placed through the glenoid articular surface approximately 1 to 2 mm from the peripheral glenoid rim. The detached labrum is sutured so that it contacts the scapular neck and extends onto the glenoid articular surface. This reestablishes the labrum "bumper" 'and recreates an optimal surface for concavity-compression. I estimate the amount of tightening based on both the degree and direction of translation and use guidelines similar to those described by Warner and associates for open operations. A soft tissue grasper is used to apply traction to the various portions of the capsule while the patient's arm is positioned in varying degrees of abduction and external rotation and while I apply translation forces. I try to establish tension in different parts of the capsule according to their role in glenohumeral stability. I estimate appropriate capsular tension of the inferior capsule with the patient's arm in 60 degrees of abduction and 60 degrees of external rotation, the middle glenohumeral ligament with the arm in 30 degrees of abduction and external rotation, and the rotator interval with the arm in 0 degrees of abduction and 30 degrees of external rotation. Because I am technically unable to perform the repair with the patient's arm in complete abduction or external rotation, I estimate the appropriate amount of tension, return the arm to 20 degrees of abduction and 30 degrees of external rotation, and then complete the arthroscopic repair.

If areas of the capsule do not advance adequately after suture repair, I use thermal application to contract the capsule and ligaments further. I believe that it is not appropriate to perform thermal capsulorrhaphy initially in ligaments that require suture repair. First, because the ligaments shorten with thermal capsulorrhaphy, they are more difficult to repair to the glenoid rim. Second, I believe it is more difficult to determine the appropriate amount of ligament advancement after thermal application is applied. The indication for thermal shrinkage is limited to those shoulders in which capsular suture tightening fails to restore adequate soft tissue tension to all areas of the capsule. This is a common finding, and although thermal application is not used as the primary operative technique, it is used as needed to supplement the primary technique of suture repair. I believe that one reason for the high failure rates experienced by other surgeons is their failure to address the quality of the ligaments. Although suture tightening can increase ligament tension, in certain patients it may serve only to tighten attenuated soft tissue and may fail to address plastic deformation at a cellular level. This is particularly true when the surgeon operates on the posterior capsule, as demonstrated by Tibone's laboratory analysis. In my experience, the effectiveness of thermal application is variable because some areas of the capsule respond, whereas others do not. Although the long-term effectiveness of thermal application remains to be described, I believe there is enough evidence in laboratory studies to justify its use.

With the greater visualization afforded by the arthroscope, the surgeon can now selectively repair the damaged portions of the capsule. This is an advantage over open reconstructions for anterior instability. With the increased selectivity of arthroscopic repairs comes the promise of improved patient outcomes, but also a new set of required decisions. This is less of a problem with tears of the labrum insertion because the goal of returning the labrum to its anatomic location is relatively well understood. More difficult are decisions regarding ligament or capsule tightening because the surgeon now has to decide *what portions* of the capsule should be tightened, *how much* tightening is necessary, and *by which technique* tightening should occur.

Intraoperative Decision Making and Indications

Débridement

I débride only minor flap tears of the labrum. Flap tears of greater than 50% are repaired with absorbable monofilament sutures. I find that labrum palpation with a probe is necessary to determine adequately the presence of minor flap tears, cleavage tears that exist within the labrum substance, and minor separations of the labrum from the glenoid. Loose bodies are removed with surgical forceps.

Labrum Repair

The labrum normally is attached securely to the glenoid bone anteriorly, inferiorly, and posteriorly below the glenoid equator, and I consider separations in these areas as lesions. The anterior superior labrum is usually not well attached to the glenoid (sublabral foramen), and separation in this area is considered normal. The superior labrum attachment is variable, and a mobile superior labrum without evidence of trauma is not classified as a tear of the superior labrum from anterior to posterior (SLAP lesion). When the superior labrum separation is a normal variant, the superior glenoid is covered with smooth cartilage, and the labrum shows no evidence of trauma. Signs of traumatic separation include tears within the substance of the superior labrum, cartilage loss with exposed bone at the site of labrum attachment, and an increase in superior labrum separation with abduction and external rotation of the arm. I repair the superior labrum anatomically and make no attempt to shift the superior labrum anteriorly or posteriorly. In contrast, during repair of the anterior, inferior, or posterior labrum, I will, if necessary, shift the labrum laterally so that it projects onto the glenoid surface to reestablish the labrum as a bumper and to aid in concavity-compression.

Capsular Tensioning

I estimate the location of the ligament repair site (and therefore the ligament tension) by grasping the ligament and placing it at different locations on the glenoid. Humeral head translation is performed with the torn ligament positioned at possible repair sites until humeral head translation is less than 25% of the glenoid's diameter. Typically, one requires 5 to 15 mm of lateral and superior ligament advancement. Arm position will affect ligament and capsule tension, so I routinely maintain the patient's shoulder in 20 degrees of abduction and 30 degrees of external rotation during this portion of the operation. I alter the patient's arm position when I perform the operation on the dominant

arm of a competitive, throwing athlete. In these patients, I determine the ligament repair site after I position the arm in 60 degrees of external rotation.

Rotator Interval

After I perform débridement, labrum repair, and capsular tensioning, if the shoulder demonstrates persistent excessive translation, I turn my attention to the rotator interval. If the direction of translation is inferior or inferior posterior, I place a monofilament suture through the soft tissue immediately adjacent to the anterior border of the supraspinatus and then through the soft tissue superior to the subscapularis tendon. I place the suture as far laterally as possible so as not to interfere with postoperative external rotation. Traction on this suture is applied, and I again assess humeral head translation. If the correction is adequate, the suture is tied. If the correction is inadequate, the suture is removed and is placed in a more medial position until excessive translation is corrected. If the direction of persistent translation is inferior anterior, the inferior limb of the suture is passed through the superior portion of the middle glenohumeral ligament to increase tension in that portion of the capsule.

Thermal Capsulorrhaphy

If persistent translation is not corrected after labrum and capsular suture repair and tension on the rotator interval suture, I perform a thermal capsulorrhaphy. I use the thermal probe to contract areas of the capsule that correspond to the direction of excessive humeral head movement.

Operative Technique

Before induction of general anesthesia, all patients receive an interscalene block to diminish postoperative pain. The anesthesiologist administers 1 g of cephalosporin intravenously. I place patients in the sitting position and examine both shoulders as described earlier.

The shoulder joint is entered with a cannula and blunt trocar through a posterior skin incision placed 1.5 cm inferior and 2 cm medial to the posterolateral border of the acromion. I place the posterior portal in a more superior location than the soft spot. This allows me more access if I must introduce a second, inferior posterior portal later during the procedure. I perform a brief inspection and evaluate the rotator interval for evidence of trauma or laxity. Because the anterior portals will pass through the rotator interval and will alter its appearance, this assessment must be done first. An anterior portal is identified with a spinal needle so that the cannula enters the shoulder joint immediately superior to the subscapularis tendon and 1 cm lateral to the glenoid. The more laterally the surgeon places the anterior inferior cannula, the easier it is to place anchors perpendicular to the glenoid surface but the more difficult it is to reach the inferior aspects of the glenohumeral joint. If the anterior inferior cannula is placed more medially, it is easier to reach the inferior glenohumeral joint but more difficult to place suture anchors.

I then inspect the glenohumeral joint completely. I reexamine the shoulder for translation while viewing it through the arthroscope, and I use a probe to examine the labrum for tears and palpate the capsule to evaluate ligament tension (Figs. 4–22 to 4–36). I then establish the anterior superior portal with a spinal needle. The anterior superior cannula is 1 cm superior and 5 mm lateral to the anterior inferior cannula (Figs. 4–37 to 4–40). The arthroscope is removed and is inserted through the anterior superior cannula to inspect the posterior glenohumeral joint more completely (Figs. 4–41 to 4–44).

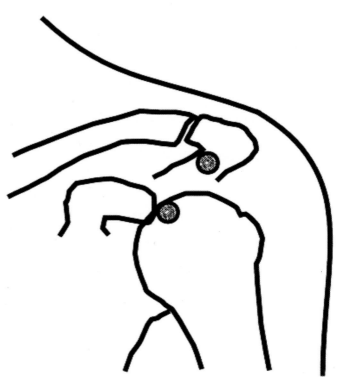

FIGURE 4–24. Anterior portals.

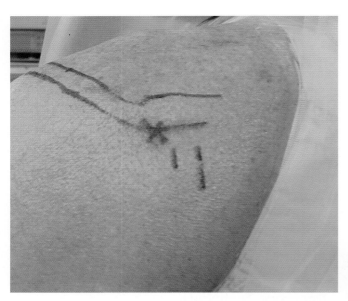

FIGURE 4–22. Portal for arthroscopic subacromial decompression, glenohumeral reconstruction, traditional soft spot.

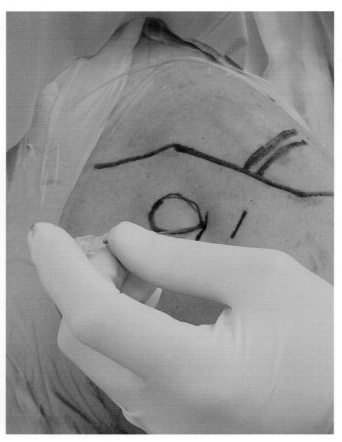

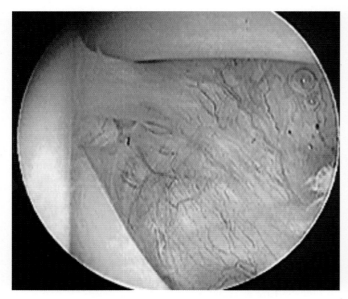

FIGURE 4–23. Widened, thin rotator interval.

FIGURE 4–25. Anterior inferior portal.

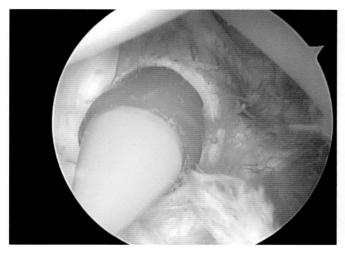

FIGURE 4–26. Cannula in anterior inferior portal.

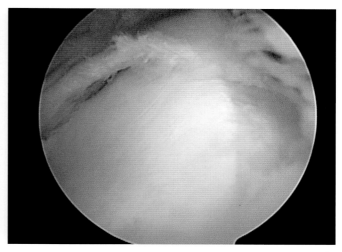

FIGURE 4–27. Superior labrum tear.

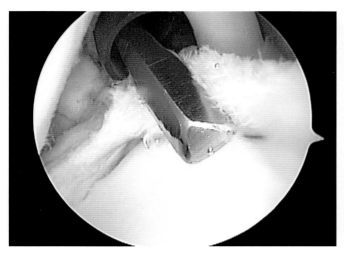

FIGURE 4–28. Palpating for superior labrum tear.

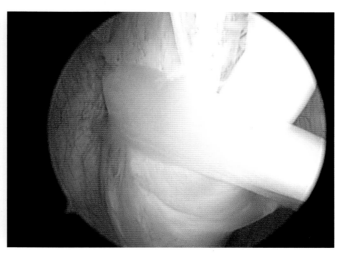

FIGURE 4–29. Poorly defined middle glenohumeral ligament.

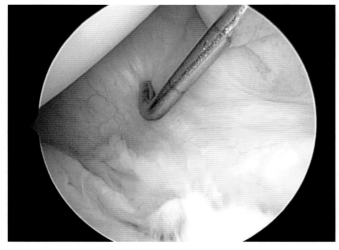

FIGURE 4–30. Palpation of anterior inferior glenohumeral ligament.

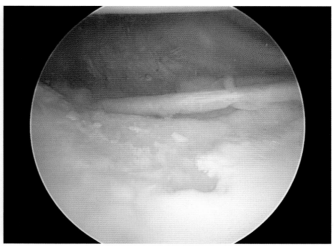

FIGURE 4–31. Anterior cartilage loss.

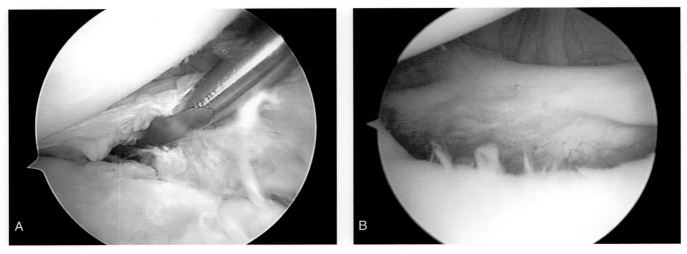

FIGURE 4–32. *A*, Chisel exposing small Bankart lesion. *B*, Bankart lesion.

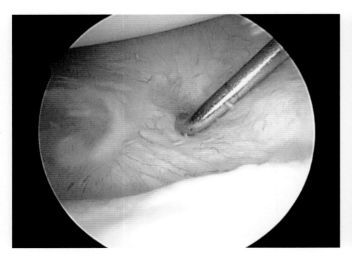

FIGURE 4–33. Palpation of inferior capsule.

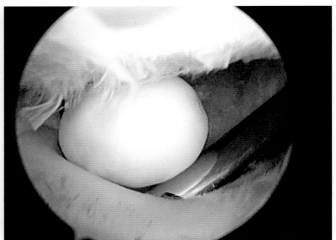

FIGURE 4–34. Loose body removal.

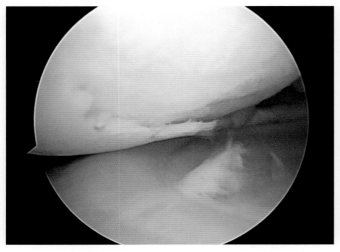

FIGURE 4–35. Humeral head cartilage lesion.

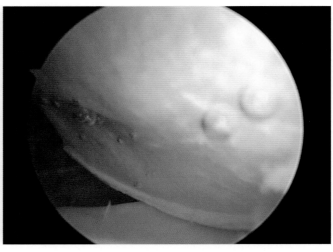

FIGURE 4–36. Shallow Hill-Sachs lesion.

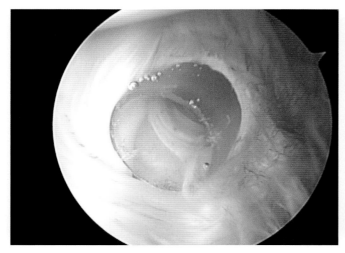

FIGURE 4–37. Anterior inferior cannula.

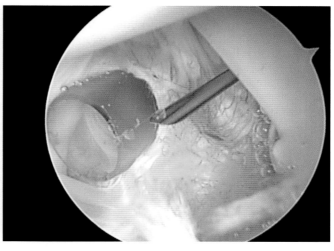

FIGURE 4–38. Needle identifies anterior superior portal location.

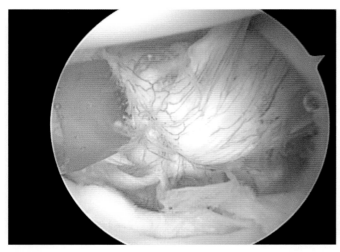

FIGURE 4–39. Introduce anterior superior cannula and palpate rotator interval.

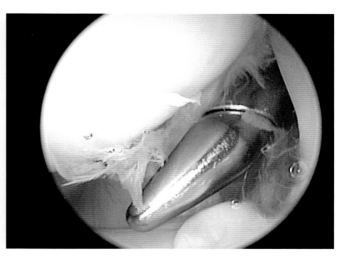

FIGURE 4–40. Metal cannula, arthroscope moving to anterior superior portal.

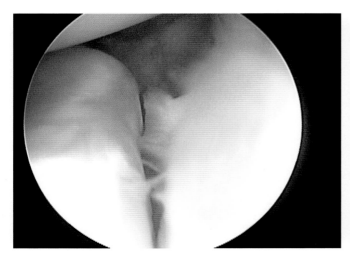

FIGURE 4–41. Anterior Bankart lesion seen from anterior superior cannula.

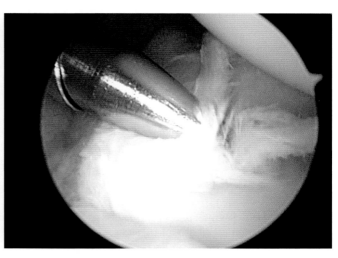

FIGURE 4–42. Posterior labrum fraying.

I then return the arthroscope to the posterior cannula. All structures within the glenohumeral joint are examined systematically, and all lesions consistent with instability are recorded. Such lesions are variable and include tears of the rotator cuff (partial and complete), rotator interval, glenoid labrum, glenohumeral ligaments, and biceps tendon. I have noted, as have other surgeons, that the glenohumeral ligaments may tear at either the glenoid or the humeral head insertion. To evaluate the glenohumeral ligaments for midsubstance tear or plastic deformation, I also assess them for laxity by directly observing and palpating them (with an arthroscopic probe) and applying translation stresses as I rotate the shoulder. I document the location on the glenoid and the extent (superior to inferior and medial to lateral) of labrum detachment. Labra that are frayed or have midsubstance tears are noted. The presence or absence of loose bodies is recorded.

The cartilage is inspected for damage to the glenoid and humeral head (Hill-Sachs lesion). I believe the surgeon can gain additional information by evaluating the cartilage lesions carefully. I closely examine the glenoid. I use an arthroscopic probe inserted through the anterior inferior cannula to measure the glenoid width. The inferior portion below the glenoid equator should have a greater anterior posterior width than the glenoid superior to the equator. If it does not, bone loss from the anterior inferior glenoid is sufficient that a bone graft will be necessary to restore glenoid width. I perform this operation with open technique.

I then examine the Hill-Sachs lesion and record its location, dimensions, and orientation. A posterolateral location indicates anterior instability, and an anteromedial location is consistent with posterior instability. I note the lesion's dimensions of length, width, and depth and maneuver the shoulder until I can determine what amount of external rotation allows the Hill-Sachs lesion to engage the glenoid rim. I center the humeral head by compressing it against the glenoid while performing the foregoing maneuver. Usually, the Hill-Sachs lesion will not engage the glenoid rim without anterior translation. If the Hill-Sachs lesion engages the glenoid rim with the humeral head centered and the amount of external rotation is 40 degrees or less, I stop the arthroscopic procedure and perform an open reconstruction and bone graft of the humeral head defect. This rarely occurs. If the external rotation is greater than 40 degrees, I proceed with arthroscopic stabilization. I then examine the orientation of the Hill-Sachs lesion. I position the patient's arm so that the Hill-Sachs lesion is parallel to the anterior glenoid rim and observe the amount of abduction and external rotation. This is the position of the arm during the moment of dislocation and indicates which areas of the capsule were damaged. As a general rule, the greater the amount of abduction needed to align the Hill-Sachs with the anterior glenoid rim, the more inferior capsule damage exists. A smaller amount of abduction indicates more anterior capsule (middle glenohumeral ligament) damage (Figs. 4–45 to 4–46). If a posterior repair is necessary, I perform this before superior, anterior, or inferior capsular repair because repair in any of these areas dramatically limits access to the posterior and, especially, the posterior inferior glenohumeral joint (Figs. 4–47 to 4–59).

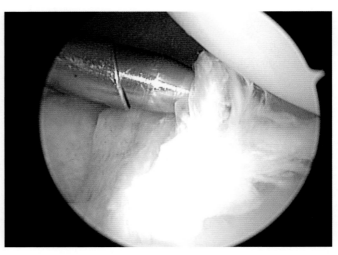

FIGURE 4–43. Posterior labrum split.

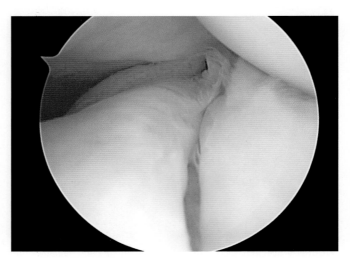

FIGURE 4–44. Posterior Bankart lesion.

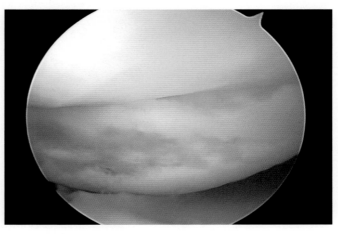

FIGURE 4–45. Hill-Sachs lesion, arm resting at side.

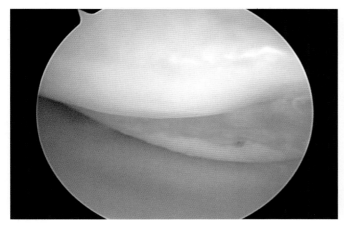

FIGURE 4–46. Hill-Sachs lesion, arm positioned until lesion is parallel to anterior glenoid rim.

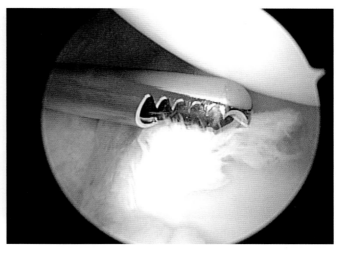

FIGURE 4–47. Débride posterior labrum.

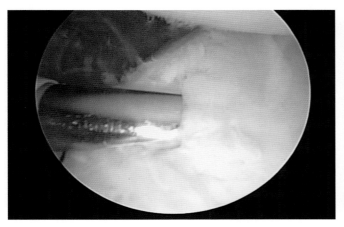

FIGURE 4–48. Abrade posterior glenoid with round bur.

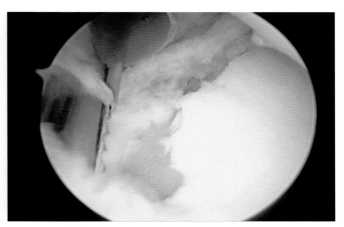

FIGURE 4–49. Posterior glenoid prepared.

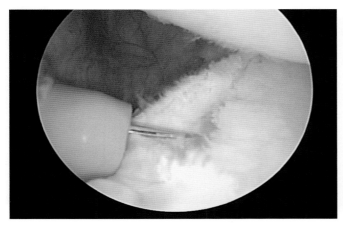

FIGURE 4–50. Drill inferior anchor hole.

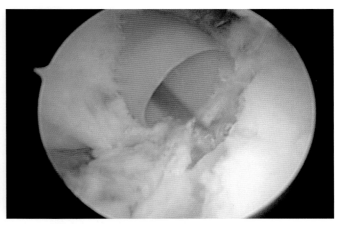

FIGURE 4–51. Drill superior anchor hole.

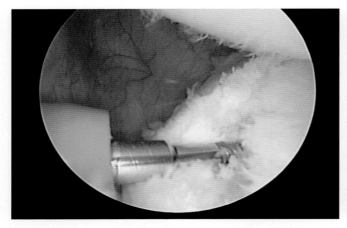

FIGURE 4–52. Insert anchor.

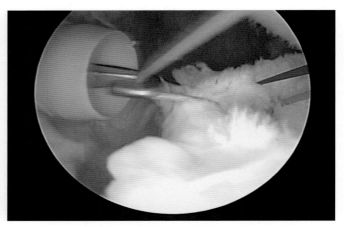

FIGURE 4–53. Retrieve braided suture.

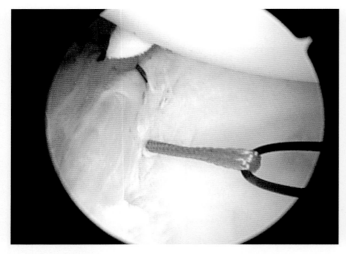

FIGURE 4–54. Pass through labrum and retrieve with nylon loop through anterior-inferior cannula.

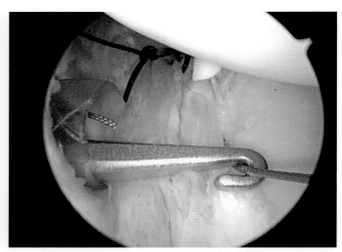

FIGURE 4–55. Retrieve braided suture from anterior inferior cannula to posterior cannula.

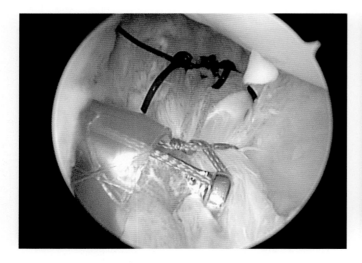

FIGURE 4–56. Tie knots.

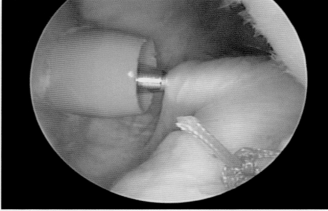

FIGURE 4–57. Tighten inferior posterior capsule.

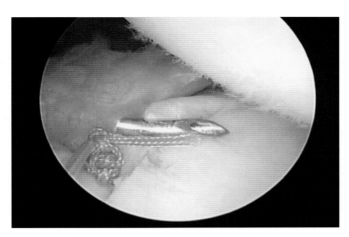

FIGURE 4–58. Repair to now-intact labrum.

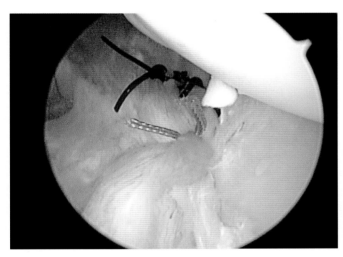

FIGURE 4–59. Completed repair.

Posterior Repair

 — Posterior Bankart

 — Posterior Revision

The principles of posterior repair are similar to those of anterior and inferior repair, but there are certain specific distinctions, and I want to discuss them in a separate section. Because posterior repair is performed less frequently than anterior repair, the surgeon is not as familiar with the hand maneuvers needed to position instruments within the glenohumeral joint. I understand that my movements will be slower and less fluid than when I operate anteriorly, and I mentally give myself some leeway during this operation.

Portal Placement

To establish the posterior portal I move the arthroscope to the anterior superior cannula. I leave the anterior inferior cannula in place to provide outflow and through which I can insert the crochet hook to retrieve sutures. While I view the posterior capsule through the arthroscope, I remove the posterior metal cannula and instrument a larger diameter plastic cannula through the same skin incision. I advance it until the tip tents the capsule. I then move the tip inferiorly and advance it external to the capsule until it reaches the appropriate entry point. This point is located near the inferior glenoid for inferior posterior capsular tensioning or may be at the glenoid equator if a labrum is the only damaged structure.

Scapular Neck Preparation

I use the 4-mm round bur. Because of the portal location, the bur enters the glenohumeral joint parallel to the glenoid surface, and I advance it into the joint and move it superiorly and inferiorly over the desired distance. It helps to advance the arthroscope as far into the joint as possible and to rotate it so that you have the best view of the posterior glenoid.

Drill Holes

There are two basic approaches. You can move the arthroscope back to the posterior portal and insert the drill through the anterior superior cannula. This is effective for anchors at the level of the glenoid equator or superiorly, but it is not effective for posterior inferior anchors. I prefer to leave the arthroscope in the anterior superior cannula and insert the drill posteriorly. I place the posterior drill holes on the posterior scapular neck. This is different from when I perform the procedure anteriorly, in which the drill holes are positioned on the glenoid articular surface. One reason is technical, in that I cannot maneuver the posteriorly located drill to penetrate the articular cartilage at an appropriate angle. Second, because in most posterior repairs I also incorporate posterior capsule, I incorporate enough capsule with the labrum that I can recreate the labrum bumper even with anchors located in this position. The posterior labrum bumper is smaller than the one I create anteriorly, but this corresponds to the normal labrum anatomy. I locate the drill holes 2 to 3 mm medial to the articular surface. The angle is parallel to the surface or slightly posterior to it. I insert the anchors and repair the labrum and capsule from inferior to superior.

Suture Passing

I use the Spectrum crescent hook and pierce the posterior inferior capsule and advance it superiorly. The instrument tip penetrates the capsule and is visible. I then advance the soft tissue superiorly, pierce the labrum, and advance the two free ends of the 2-0 nylon suture into the glenohumeral joint. Dr. Hammerman inserts a crochet hook through the anterior inferior cannula and retrieves the sutures and applies a hemostat. I remove the crescent hook from the joint. The anchor sutures exit the joint through the posterior cannula. We then reverse the loop with another monofilament suture so that the loop end is out the anterior inferior cannula and the two free ends exit the posterior cannula. I insert a crescent hook through the anterior inferior cannula and retrieve one of the anchor suture strands. I place it through the looped end of the monofilament suture and pull it through the labrum and the posterior cannula until it exits posteriorly. I tie the knot through the posterior cannula. I repeat this sequence until the posterior repair is complete and then proceed to capsular tensioning. If no posterior repair is needed, I return the arthroscope to the posterior cannula and proceed with the glenohumeral reconstruction.

Anterior Inferior Repair

 — Bankart Standard Repair

 — Bankart Repair with Complications

The repair sequence varies and depends on the specific combination of lesions identified. In general, I follow a pattern of débridement, ligament or labrum reattachment, and capsular tensioning.

Débridement

Débridement is performed to smooth frayed or remove torn labrum fragments. Débridement is performed if necessary to identify the depth of partial-thickness rotator cuff tears. Loose bodies are removed. Loose body removal is almost always frustrating because the inflow blows the pieces around the joint. I find it helpful to attach suction to the outflow cannula to let the flow of fluid bring the loose body to the mouth of the cannula, and then to grasp the loose body with forceps.

Insertion Tears

I then treat labrum and ligament insertion site tears. The labrum tear is then repaired beginning with the posterior labrum, if needed, and proceeding as necessary to the inferior, anterior, and superior labrum. Technical considerations dictate the order of labrum repair. As the labrum (and attached ligaments) is repaired, the ability to displace the humeral head and to insert bone and soft tissue suture anchors or sutures is compromised. I repair the posterior labrum first, because access to this lesion becomes difficult after superior or anterior labrum repair. Posterior, inferior, and superior labral tears are usually easily identified and are minimally displaced. This is not the situation for anterior labrum tears. I classify the following three types of anterior labrum detachment: (1) the labrum is separated from the glenoid bone, but it remains at the level of the glenoid articular surface (type A); (2) the labrum is separated and retracted medially (type B); and (3) the labrum is retracted and has healed medially on the glenoid (type C, equivalent to an ALPSA lesion) (Figs. 4–60 to 4–62).

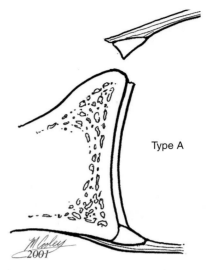

FIGURE 4–60. Type A lesion.

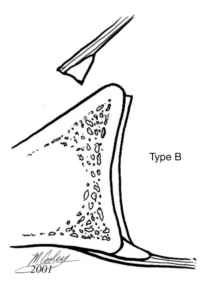

FIGURE 4–61. Type B lesion.

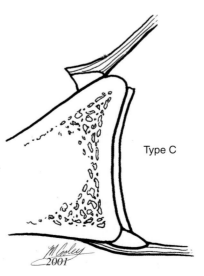

FIGURE 4–62. Type C lesion.

Type B and C lesions require that the surgeon dissect the labrum from the glenoid and place it laterally on the glenoid articular surface. I perform this with a combination of a thermal probe, a power bur, scissors, and blunt dissection.

If the anterior inferior and middle glenohumeral ligaments are retracted and adherent to the subscapularis, I then release the ligaments before insertion site repair. I make an incision with scissors along the superior border of the middle glenohumeral ligament. I then insert a blunt instrument (posterior to the capsule and anterior to the subscapularis tendon) to separate the two structures. If the labrum and capsule have healed medially, I insert the sharp chisel dissector along the scapular neck to peel these structures from the bone. I advance the arthroscope (located in the posterior cannula) as far anteriorly as possible and rotate it so that I have the best anterior view. If the view is not satisfactory, I transfer the arthroscope to the anterior superior cannula. Once the capsule and labrum have been separated from the bone, I try to advance them laterally. If further mobilization is necessary, I insert arthroscopic scissors through the anterior inferior cannula and divide the soft tissue attachment that is present in the base of the letter "V" formed by the scapular neck posteriorly and the capsule anteriorly. I continue to divide the soft tissue until I can see the muscular fibers of the subscapularis (Figs. 4–63 to 4–66).

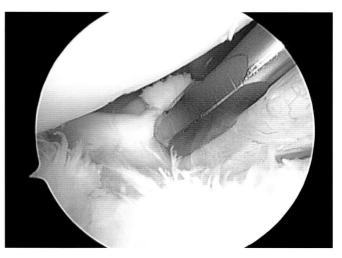

FIGURE 4–64. Chisel to dissect labrum from glenoid.

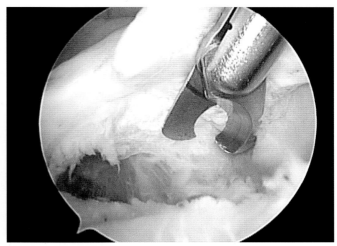

FIGURE 4–65. Scissors to mobilize labrum and capsule.

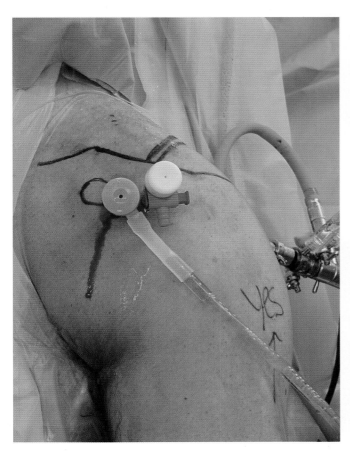

FIGURE 4–63. Location of two anterior cannulas for anterior repair.

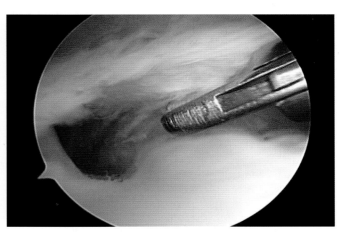

FIGURE 4–66. Muscular fibers of subscapularis.

Bone Bankart Fragment

— Acute Dislocation

Patients with traumatic unidirectional instability often have a piece of bone attached to the anterior labrum that has avulsed from the glenoid during a dislocation. Often, these fragments are so small they are not seen on radiographs but are easily seen and palpated during arthroscopy. I try to retain these fragments and incorporate them in the labrum repair because they add to the bulk of the labrum-capsule repair. The tip of the suture passer must pass underneath the fragment so that it is lifted by the suture and reduced laterally. Larger bony Bankart lesions are more critical and must be retained. If the fragment is excised, the glenoid width decreases. Studies have shown that glenoid narrowing as small as 4 mm significantly compromises containment of the humeral head by the glenoid. Second, if the fragment is excised, the glenohumeral ligaments will not have sufficient length. I believe that the labrum and ligaments should be repaired with the shoulder in external rotation. If there is insufficient ligament length, the surgeon is forced to make the repair with the patient's shoulder internally rotated, and this makes it if very difficult for the patient to regain adequate external rotation.

Anterior Scapular Neck Preparation

After I complete labrum and ligament mobilization, the scapular neck is abraded to a depth of 1 mm. The abraded area begins at the level of the glenoid cartilage and extends 2 cm medially on the scapula. It is important not to abrade too deeply and to risk compromising glenoid width and creating the problems discussed earlier. This may be done with the arthroscope in the posterior portal and the bur in the anterior inferior cannula, or the arthroscope may be moved to the anterior superior cannula (Figs. 4–67 to 4–69).

Drill Holes

Drill holes for the suture anchors are placed through the glenoid articular surface approximately 1 to 2 mm from the lateral glenoid margin. I space the drill hole sites (typically, three are used) proportionally along the anterior glenoid. I use the round bur to remove a small area of cartilage and mark the drill hole site for five reasons, as follows:

1. The cartilage in these patients is usually thick, and because the length of the drill is fixed, the greater the amount of cartilage, the smaller the amount of screw will be in the bone.
2. If the drill hole is made in cartilage, the drill hole can be hard to identify.
3. I want to recess the screw as far as possible.
4. I can create a small shelf in the bone to decrease the acuity of the approach angle.
5. I want to maximize the area of labrum bone contact because I believe that labrum will heal more securely to bone than it will to cartilage.

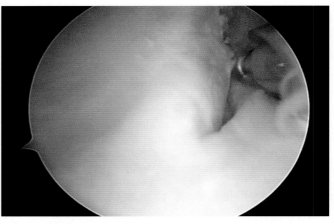

FIGURE 4–67. Abrade anterior scapular neck.

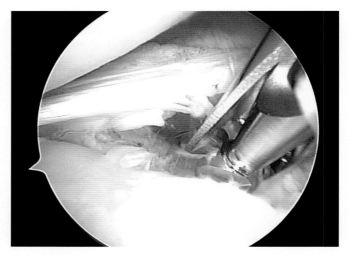

FIGURE 4–68. Anterior view.

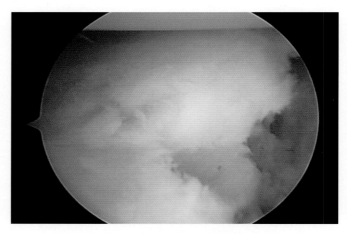

FIGURE 4–69. Completed abrasion.

Drill holes are created in the anterior and inferior glenoid with a power drill inserted through the anterior superior cannula. To reach the most inferior portion of the glenoid, I ask the assistant to distract the humeral head laterally and posteriorly.

Distraction occurs during three segments: placing the drill hole, passing the suture passer through the inferior capsule or labrum, and suture tying. During the remaining portions of the procedure, the arm rests in the arm holder without any distraction force.

I place the drill holes through the anterior superior cannula for two reasons: the angle of approach to the glenoid is easier, and I minimize the number of times I must transfer sutures from the anterior inferior to the anterior superior cannula. The anterior superior cannula is located slightly more superior and posterior to the anterior inferior cannula and presents a less tangential approach to the articular glenoid surface. It is also easier to insert the anchors through the same cannula as I used for the drill because the anchors enter the glenoid at the same angle as the drill. If I place the drill holes (and anchors) through the anterior inferior cannula, I must transfer the sutures to the anterior superior cannula before inserting the suture passer because the suture passer barely fits in the larger anterior inferior cannula. I avoid sutures in this cannula and thereby eliminate the possibility that the sharp tip of the suture passer may cut one of the sutures. In addition, the suture passer must be inserted through the larger anterior inferior cannula because the anterior inferior aspect of the glenoid

cannot be reached from the anterior superior cannula. Because of the approach angle made by the drill, it is easier to insert the anchors through the same cannula used for the drill.

Anchor Insertion

I prefer to insert an anchor, pass the suture and tie it, and then go on to the next anchor, as opposed to inserting all the anchors at one time. This method minimizes the number of suture strands within the glenohumeral joint. I place the anchors inferiorly to superiorly. The first suture anchor is inserted through the anterior superior cannula into the most inferior glenoid drill hole. The number of suture anchors varies and depends on the size of labrum detachment, but I typically use three anchors. As Dr. Hammerman inserts each anchor, I distract the humeral head to allow him easier access to the drill hole. The anchor inserter has two vertical lines that mark the eyelet orientation. As he seats the anchor, he checks to see that the vertical lines (and eyelet) are oriented anterior posteriorly rather than superior inferiorly. This method minimizes suture strand twisting and allows the suture to slide freely in the anchor during knot tying (Figs. 4–70 to 4–73).

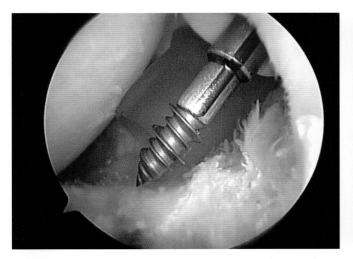

FIGURE 4–70. Insert anchor through anterior superior cannula.

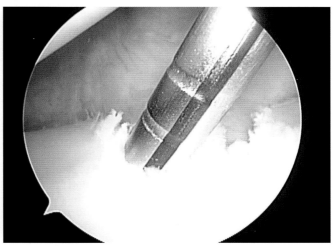

FIGURE 4–72. Inserter orientation lines.

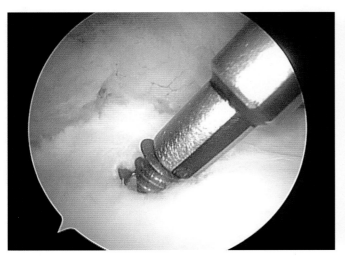

FIGURE 4–71. Anchor inserted on glenoid surface.

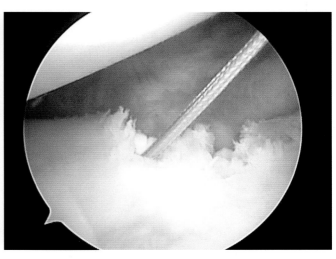

FIGURE 4–73. Anchor and suture in glenoid.

Suture Passing

The most difficult suture to place is the most inferior because access to the glenohumeral joint is generally quite limited. Suture passing is less difficult in patients with multidirectional instability because the inferior capsular laxity that accompanies that condition allows the surgeon greater access. The first decision I make is whether to repair only the detached labrum or to incorporate the inferior capsule with the repair, to perform capsular imbrication. If capsular imbrication is not necessary and I want to repair the labrum alone, I use the suture passer to pierce the labrum at a point that will bring the labrum to its normal anatomic insertion site on the glenoid. The torn labrum is usually displaced medially and inferiorly. Therefore, I must pierce the labrum with the suture passer so that when the knot is tied, the labrum is translated superiorly and laterally. This will bring the labrum above the glenoid articular surface so that I reestablish the labrum as a bumper, and concavity-compression is restored (Fig. 4–74).

I often take the suture passer without a suture and grasp the labrum at various points and bring it to the glenoid until I am satisfied that the appropriate entry point has been established. Only then do I load the suture passer with the nylon passing suture for the final repair.

I prefer to use the angled Spectrum suture passer for this portion of the procedure. I use a right-angled instrument for right shoulders and a left-angled instrument for left shoulders. I normally incorporate some amount of capsule along with the labrum to correct capsular laxity. I find it easier to choose the correct spot in the capsule with the tip of the instrument before I insert the suture passer through the labrum. If the right-angled instrument is used in a left shoulder, the surgeon must pass it from labrum to capsule, and once the instrument has pierced the labrum, it is hard to manipulate and find the appropriate area of capsule. (Figs. 4–75 and 4–76) In addition, the left-angled instrument allows me to pierce the capsule and to advance it so that I can clearly see where the tip of the instrument exits the soft tissue near the glenoid. When I advance the nylon passing suture, it comes to lie on the glenoid within reach of the crochet hook. Once the nylon suture is in the joint, I distract the humeral head, and Dr. Hammerman inserts a crochet hook through the anterior superior cannula, retrieves the suture strands, and places a hemostat on the two free ends. I then remove the suture instrument from the anterior inferior cannula. The loop end now exits from the anterior inferior cannula, and the two free ends exit from the anterior superior cannula. (Figs. 4–77 to 4–81) The foregoing description is reversed for a right shoulder.

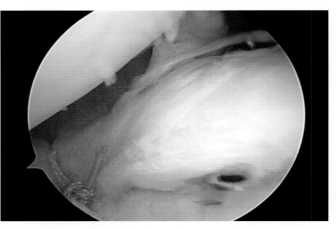

FIGURE 4–74. Advance labrum onto glenoid articular surface.

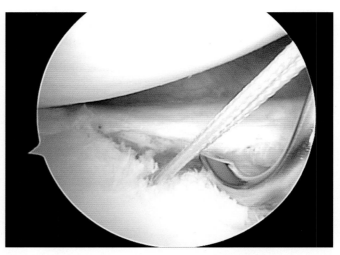

FIGURE 4–75. Right-angled instrument in left shoulder.

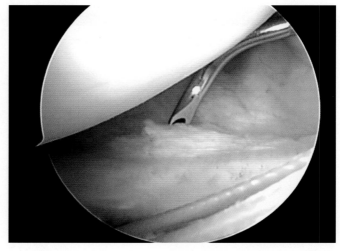

FIGURE 4–76. Left-angled instrument in left shoulder.

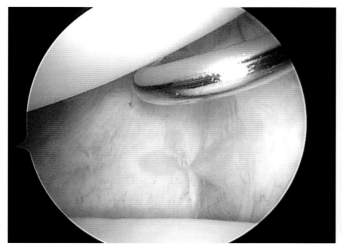

FIGURE 4–77. Piercing capsule.

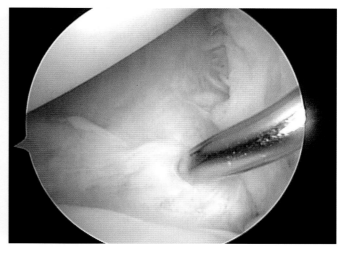

FIGURE 4–78. Advance capsule to labrum.

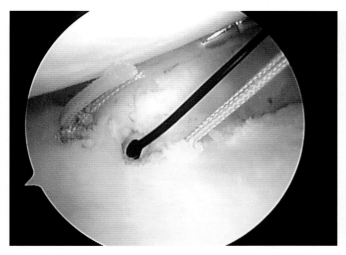

FIGURE 4–79. Puncture labrum and advance nylon suture.

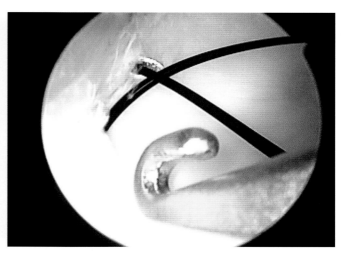

FIGURE 4–80. Access to nylon suture for crochet hook.

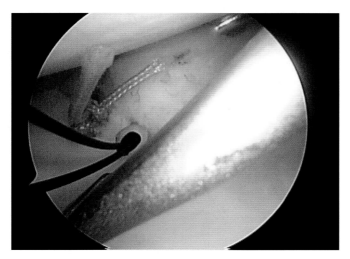

FIGURE 4–81. Retrieve suture through anterior-superior cannula.

Loop Reversal

Because I have passed the suture in this manner, if I place an anchor suture in the loop end, it will pass through the labrum in the wrong direction. The anchor suture will pass from the anterior position to the posterior position. This loop around the labrum inhibits suture sliding and therefore the security of the knot. I want the anchor suture to pass from the anchor through the labrum from posterior to anterior. Therefore, I use a monofilament suture to reverse the loop. The two free ends of the monofilament suture are placed through the loop of the nylon. By pulling on the two free nylon ends, the loop of monofilament is brought into the anterior inferior cannula, through the labrum and capsule, and out the anterior superior cannula. The loop of monofilament suture is now in the same anterior superior cannula that contains the suture anchor sutures (Fig. 4–82).

Obviously, these steps could be avoided by initially passing the suture passer in the opposite direction. However, loop reversal takes about 10 seconds to accomplish, and the advantages of piercing the labrum from anterior to posterior as described earlier far outweigh this extra step.

An exception to this technique occurs during the repair of a shoulder with a large bone Bankart fragment. Because of the size of the bone, I am unable to pass the suture from the labrum and capsule toward the glenoid (from lateral to medial). In this situation, I use a right-angled suture passer (for a left shoulder), place the instrument tip under the bone fragment, and rotate the instrument so that I obtain an adequate amount of soft tissue. No loop reversal is needed.

— Acute Dislocation

Passing the Anchor Suture

I insert a crochet hook through the anterior inferior cannula and grab one of the suture anchor limbs. I remove the most posterior anchor suture limb out the anterior inferior cannula. The anterior suture anchor limb and the monofilament loop are now in the anterior superior cannula. Dr. Hammerman places 8 cm of the suture anchor limb through the loop. He then pulls the hemostat clamped to the two free ends of the monofilament suture in the anterior inferior cannula and, while I provide humeral head distraction, pulls the suture from the anterior superior cannula into the joint, through the labrum and capsule, and out the anterior inferior cannula. He then removes the monofilament suture. Both suture anchor limbs are now out the anterior inferior cannula, and I tie the knot (Figs. 4–83 and 4–84).

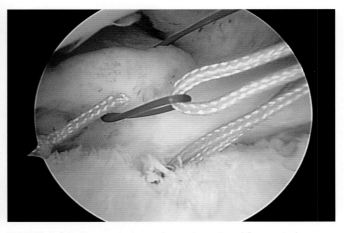

FIGURE 4–83. Retrieve posterior anchor suture strand out anterior inferior cannula.

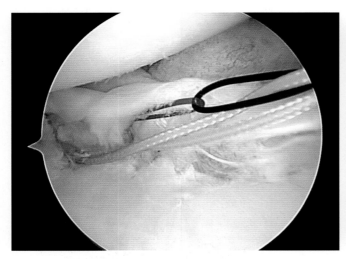

FIGURE 4–82. Reverse loop direction with Prolene (blue) suture.

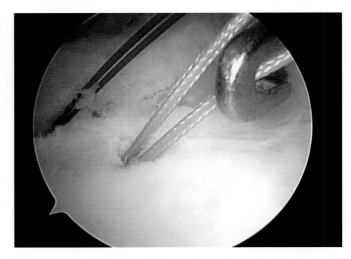

FIGURE 4–84. Pass anterior anchor suture strand from anterior superior cannula through labrum and capsule to anterior inferior cannula.

Knot Tying

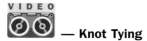 — **Knot Tying**

I first apply traction to both suture ends to eliminate any twists in the sutures. I then pass the loop suture grasper into the joint and encircle the suture that does not pass through the labrum. I select this suture because I want this strand to be the post. This allows me to slide the knots and to gain better knot security. I then place a half-hitch throw and use the knot pusher to push the throw into the joint and to bring the labrum to the glenoid. I then throw another half hitch in the same direction and push it into the joint. I then pull on the post strand while releasing any tension from the other suture anchor strand and slip the knot and labrum until the labrum is in its desired location and the knot is tied firmly. Next I throw a half hitch in the opposite direction and tighten it. I then reverse the post and tie another half hitch. Finally, I reverse the post again and tie another half hitch. This results in a secure knot (Figs. 4–85 and 4–86).

Superior Labrum Repair

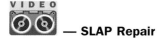 — **SLAP Repair**

 — **Bankart and SLAP Variations**

After the inferior and anterior labra are repaired, any tear of the labrum from the superior glenoid bone is identified. The superior glenoid bone is abraded with a power bur, and two suture bone anchors are inserted. The location of the suture anchors varies and depends on the anatomy of the lesion, but in general I place one suture anchor one third of the tear length from the posterior margin and a second anchor one third of the tear length from the anterior margin of the tear. I prefer nonabsorbable No. 2 braided suture and currently employ a metallic screw-in anchor exclusively. The details of this portion of the procedure are described in the discussion of SLAP repair in Chapter 5 (Fig. 4–87).

Capsular Repair

The superior view obtained with arthroscopic inspection (when compared with open surgery) has allowed me to become increasingly selective in my capsular repair. I can identify and repair lesions restricted to only one of the glenohumeral ligaments without tightening the undamaged portions of the capsule. A typical example is a tear of the middle glenohumeral ligament. Once I identify the tear, I use monofilament sutures to repair it to the intact labrum. I insert the suture passer through the anterior inferior cannula, piece the torn capsule, and puncture the labrum at the

site of desired repair. I then advance the suture and use a crochet hook to retrieve it out the anterior superior cannula. I then retrieve the suture limb and tie the strands through the large anterior inferior cannula. These steps are repeated as needed (Figs. 4–88 to 4–100).

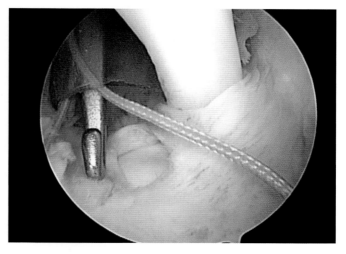

FIGURE 4–85. Retrieve both limbs of anchor suture.

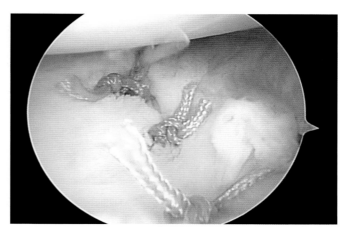

FIGURE 4–86. Final repair.

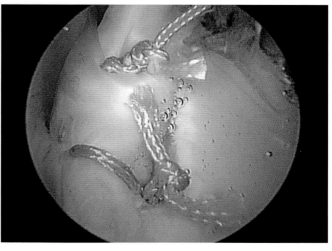

FIGURE 4–87. SLAP repair.

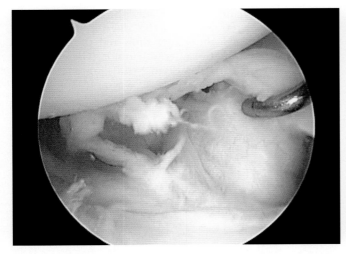

FIGURE 4–88. Middle glenohumeral ligament tear.

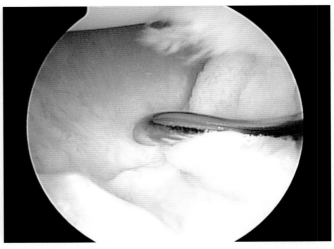

FIGURE 4–89. Spectrum pierces middle glenohumeral ligament inferior to tear.

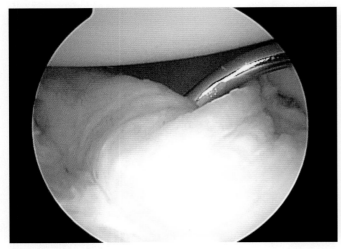

FIGURE 4–90. Advance intact middle glenohumeral ligament superiorly.

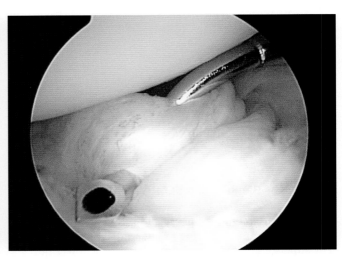

FIGURE 4–91. Pierce capsule.

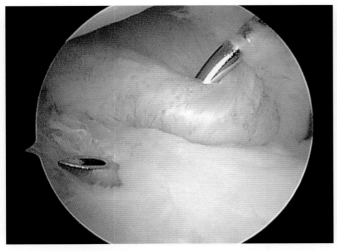

FIGURE 4–92. Pierce labrum.

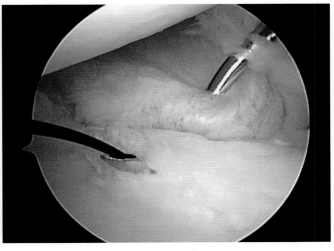

FIGURE 4–93. Advance nylon suture.

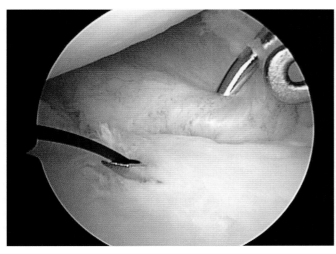

FIGURE 4–94. Retrieve suture limb out anterior superior cannula.

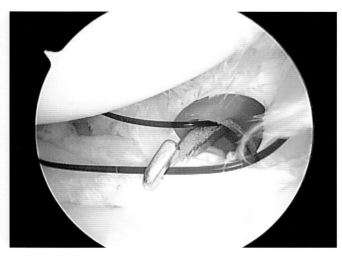

FIGURE 4–95. Remove Spectrum and withdraw suture limb out anterior inferior cannula.

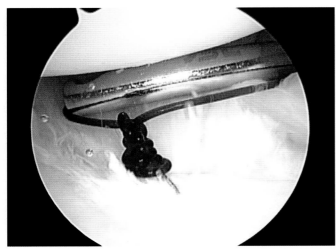

FIGURE 4–96. Both suture limbs exit anterior inferior cannula.

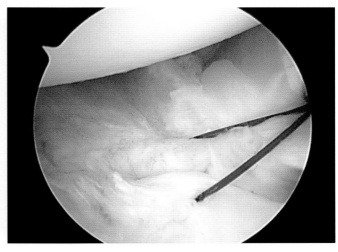

FIGURE 4–97. Test tension in repaired middle glenohumeral ligament.

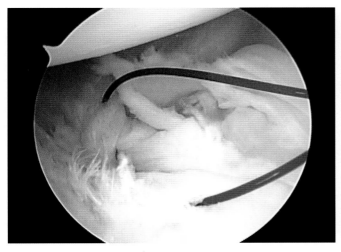

FIGURE 4–98. Tie knots.

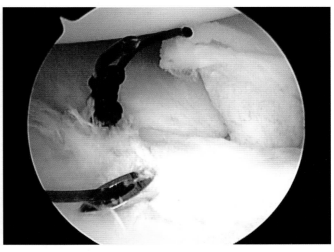

FIGURE 4–99. Repeat as needed.

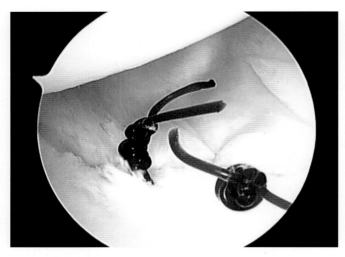

FIGURE 4–100. Final middle glenohumeral ligament repair.

Determining Capsular Tension

I have experimented with various techniques for determining the appropriate amount of capsular tension. I have attempted to measure the amount of translation in centimeters and have tried to measure capsular tension with various types of strain gauges, but I have not been successful. My current technique is to tighten the capsule maximally while varying the position of the shoulder. As in an open capsular shift procedure, it is possible to tighten different areas of the capsule selectively. I position the patient's shoulder in elevation and internal rotation. I grasp the posterior capsule with forceps and determine its maximum superior advancement on the glenoid. I then suture it in this position. I tighten the inferior capsule in 0 degrees of abduction and neutral rotation. I tighten the anterior capsule in 45 degrees of abduction and 45 degrees of external rotation.

If persistent inferior or inferior posterior translation remains, I proceed to a rotator interval repair. I tension the sutures, and if further anterior or anterior inferior tightening is required, I proceed to thermal capsulorrhaphy. Therefore, the repair sequence is to place the rotator interval sutures, test the capsular tension, perform thermal capsulorrhaphy if necessary, and then tie the rotator interval sutures.

Capsular Tensioning

If capsular tightening is necessary, there are two options. First, you can repair the labrum to its anatomic location and then with a second suture advance the capsule to the now-repaired labrum. A second option is to repair the labrum and tighten the capsule in one step. There are advantages and disadvantages to each approach. If the surgeon chooses to repair the capsule and labrum with two separate sutures, then two suture-passing steps are required. If the surgeon chooses to repair the capsule and labrum in with one suture, then the decision making needed is more complex and the amount of tightening possible is more limited. The surgeon must choose precisely where the suture passer enters both the capsule and the labrum to advance the capsule superiorly and laterally as well as repair the labrum. Once the suture passer enters the capsule, the ability of the surgeon to maneuver the needle tip and pierce the labrum is limited. It is also difficult to obtain more than 1 cm of capsular tightening with this technique. This may be sufficient for most cases of traumatic unidirectional instability, but more capsular tightening may be necessary for bidirectional and multidirectional instability. I also débride the capsule lightly with a whisker shaver to aid capsular healing (Fig 4–101). I modify the repair technique when the labrum is intact but the glenohumeral ligament is torn from the labrum. If the labrum is of sufficient size to allow suture placement within its substance, the ligament is repaired directly to the labrum with monofilament suture. If the labrum is absent, the capsule is advanced onto the glenoid articular cartilage surface and is repaired with suture anchors (as described earlier) to create a labrum bumper.

If the labrum-ligament complex is attached to the glenoid but the ligament lacks sufficient tension to contain the humeral head, I operate directly on the capsule using the methods described earlier. The goals of this portion of the procedure are to restore ligament and capsule tension and to eliminate excessive humeral head translation. The capsule can be tightened by advancing it radially and suturing it to the labrum, or it can be translated superiorly 1 to 2 cm and then sutured. I load a monofilament suture into a Spectrum suture passer and through the anterior inferior cannula and pierce the capsule at the point where I want to advance to the glenoid. For sutures in the inferior labrum or capsule, the assistant provides distraction to the humerus as I reach down to grab the capsule. After the instrument has pierced the capsule, I advance the tip of the suture passer to the labrum and penetrate it. I advance the monofilament suture into the joint. I maintain the distraction while Dr. Hammerman reaches into the joint with a crochet hook and retrieves the suture out the anterior superior cannula. Next I insert the crochet hook through the anterior inferior cannula and retrieve the other suture limb. I then tie the knot. These steps are repeated as necessary. Finally, I examine the shoulder for translation. If I have established adequate tension, the operation is concluded.

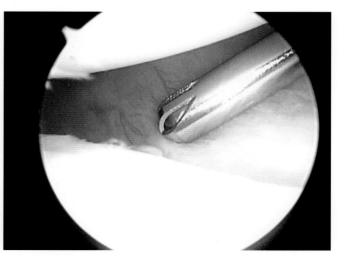

FIGURE 4–101. Whisker shaver to abrade capsule lightly.

Capsular Shift

 — Bankart Capsular Shift

The capsule of patients with multidirectional instability or bidirectional instability may not tighten adequately with simple advancement or with 1 to 2 cm of superior translation. If further capsular movement is necessary, I perform a capsular shift. To shift the anterior capsule superiorly, I divide the attachment of the middle glenohumeral ligament to the subscapularis. I use scissors to incise along the superior border of the middle glenohumeral ligament from a point overlying the subscapularis to the glenoid. I then use a blunt dissector to separate these two structures. I divide the capsular attachment to the glenoid with scissors. I start anteriorly and continue until I reach the 6-o'clock position. I then incise the capsule radially approximately 2 cm. I use the blunt dissector to free the anterior and inferior capsule from the underlying subscapularis muscle. The capsule is now mobilized sufficiently to allow significant advancement superiorly and is sutured as described earlier. If a posterior capsular shift is necessary, I transfer to arthroscope to the anterior superior cannula and divide the posterior capsule from the glenoid.

Rotator Interval Repair

 — Interval Repair

Rotator interval repair is the last step performed within the glenohumeral joint, because cannulas cannot be inserted anteriorly once this repair is completed. Through the anterior inferior cannula, a suture passer is used to place a monofilament suture through the capsule superior to the subscapularis tendon. I advance the suture into the joint and withdraw it through the anterior superior cannula. I then load a doubled 2-0 nylon suture into the suture passer, insert it through the anterior superior cannula, and position it in the joint. I withdraw the anterior superior cannula until it is external to the capsule. I then withdraw the suture passer external to the capsule and pierce the superior capsule. I advance this suture into the joint and withdraw the two free ends out the anterior inferior cannula. The monofilament suture through the anterior superior cannula is placed in the nylon loop. Traction of the two free ends of the nylon (exiting the anterior inferior cannula) draws the suture through the superior capsule and out the anterior inferior cannula. The knot is then tied, and an additional suture is placed if necessary. If a greater degree of tightening is required, the superior capsular tissue is sutured to the middle glenohumeral ligament (Figs. 4–102 to 4–108).

Thermal Capsulorrhaphy

 — Thermal Technique

 — The Throwing Athlete

If excessive translation remains after I apply traction to the rotator interval suture, I do not tie the suture. I perform a thermal capsulorrhaphy and then tie the rotator interval suture at the conclusion of the procedure. I insert the thermal probe and identify those areas of the capsule that correspond to the direction of excessive translation (usually inferior or inferior anterior). Heat is applied over a very limited area of the capsule until the capsule contracts.

I consider the following 13 variables when I perform a thermal capsulorrhaphy:

1. Which areas of the capsule to treat
2. The amount of capsule treated
3. The pattern of capsulorrhaphy
4. The direction of shrinkage
5. The degree of shrinkage

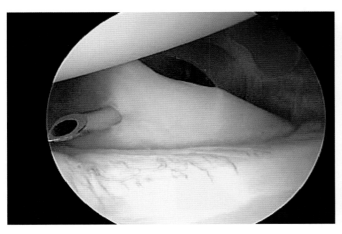

FIGURE 4–102. Pierce middle glenohumeral ligament with suture passer.

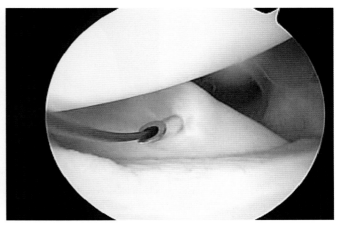

FIGURE 4–103. Advance monofilament suture.

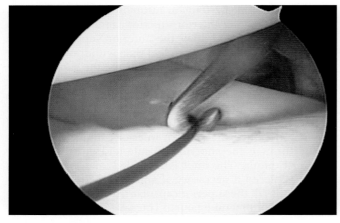

FIGURE 4–104. Insert crochet hook through anterior superior cannula.

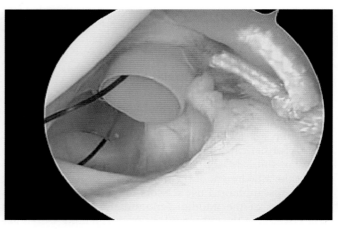

FIGURE 4–105. Retrieve suture out anterior superior cannula.

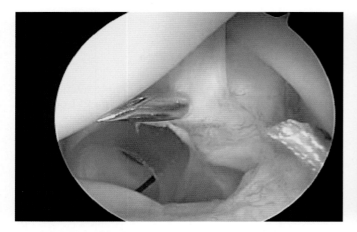

FIGURE 4–106. Puncture superior glenohumeral ligament.

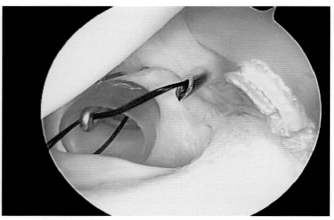

FIGURE 4–107. Advance nylon suture and withdraw out anterior inferior cannula.

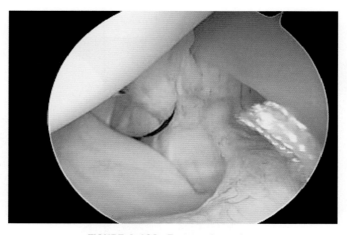

FIGURE 4–108. Test repair tension.

6. The sequence in which the different areas of the capsule are treated
7. Probe temperature
8. Probe pressure or depth
9. Probe angle of approach
10. The rate of probe movement across the capsule
11. The distance from any sutures used in the repair
12. Fluid temperature
13. Patient age

The physiology of heat and tissue response has been investigated. A temperature range of 65 to 70°C is critical for tissue shrinkage. There is an unwinding of the collagen triple helix and a renewed formation of bonds in the new contracted position. The depth of tissue reaction is related to the degree of applied energy. The altered structural property is one of decreased tissue stiffness, as with any healing and remodeling of collagenous tissue. Experimental studies suggest that tissue may stretch if it is exposed to physiologic loads too early, and immobilization for 4 weeks reduces eventual stretching of thermally modified tissue but does not eliminate it. Some data indicate that the return of treated tissue to normal mechanical properties may take as long as 12 weeks.

The initial approach to thermal capsulorrhaphy was that because heat produces visible shrinkage, we should apply more heat to obtain greater degrees of increased capsular contracture. More recent research by Arnoczky suggests that this is not the case. He believes that greater amounts of heat result in greater areas of tissue necrosis. Rather than produce a larger amount of capsular contracture, the tissue death results in decreased tissue stiffness and greater laxity. The ultimate role of thermal energy may be as a low-level stimulant for inducing a biologic repair response, rather than as a highly aggressive mechanism for primary tissue shrinkage. Therefore, it is my practice to use heat sparingly.

1. Which areas of the capsule to treat. I treat those areas of the capsule that either are lax in the clinical direction of instability or require correction to control that direction of instability. For example, I may apply heat to the posterior capsule for a patient with posterior instability but also apply heat to the anterior inferior glenohumeral ligament if tightening that structure is needed to correct the excessive posterior translation.
2. The amount of capsule treated. The amount or area of treated capsule is variable and is proportional to the degree of ligament laxity. A patient with traumatic unidirectional instability may require thermal application only to the prominent superior band of the anterior inferior glenohumeral ligament, whereas a patient with multidirectional instability may require treatment to the entire middle glenohumeral ligament, anterior inferior glenohumeral ligament, inferior capsule, posterior inferior glenohumeral ligament, and posterior capsule.
3. The pattern of capsulorrhaphy. The pattern of thermal capsulorrhaphy is relatively constant. I always leave normal capsule between any two areas of thermal probe application to avoid thermal necrosis. The pattern that results consists of thin bands of treated capsule separated by 5-mm bands of untreated tissue.
4. The direction of shrinkage. The direction of capsulorrhaphy is from the humeral attachment to the glenoid attachment in a radial pattern.
5. The degree of shrinkage. The degree of shrinkage varies from patient to patient and among the different areas of the capsule. Generally, 1 to 2 cm of tightening can be obtained. The anterior inferior glenohumeral ligament responds best to thermal capsulorrhaphy, followed, in order of decreasing response, by the middle glenohumeral ligament, inferior capsule, posterior inferior glenohumeral ligament, and posterior capsule.
6. The sequence in which the different areas of the capsule are treated. The sequence with which I apply heat to the capsule varies by the predominant clinical direction of instability. For a patient with anterior instability who has persistent excessive anterior translation after repair of labrum detachment and suture capsular tightening, I first perform a thermal capsulorrhaphy to the anterior inferior glenohumeral ligament. I then reexamine the shoulder, and if further correction is necessary, I apply heat to the inferior capsule and then the posterior inferior glenohumeral ligament. If the patient has a clinical diagnosis of multidirectional instability, I apply heat to the inferior capsule, followed by the anterior inferior glenohumeral ligament and then the posterior inferior glenohumeral ligament if needed. If the patient has posterior instability and persistent, excessive posterior translation, I apply heat to the posterior capsule and examine the shoulder. The next areas to be treated are the anterior inferior glenohumeral ligament and then the inferior capsule or axillary pouch.
7. Probe temperature. The probe temperature is set before the operation and is controlled by the electrical unit. I prefer to use a temperature of 65°C. I believe that a critical issue is the cell temperature and that temperature is not related to the type of heat delivery system. Holmium laser and bipolar and monopolar systems are available. I prefer the monopolar system because the temperature control is more precise.
8. Probe pressure or depth. Probe pressure should be light, with just enough pressure to indent the capsule. Approximately 30% of the probe tip is below the capsule surface.
9. Probe angle of approach. I prefer to have the probe approach the capsule perpendicularly. This usually requires that I bend the probe tip before I insert it through the cannula. No bend is necessary for the middle glenohumeral ligament or the anterior inferior glenohumeral ligament. A small bend is sufficient for the inferior capsule. To reach the inferior posterior capsule through an anterior portal, the probe must be bent in two directions. Practice is required to gain sufficient bend in the probe so that it still fits through the straight cannula without breaking the plastic coating.
10. The rate of probe movement across the capsule. I position the probe against the capsule and wait until

there is a visible response. Once the capsule begins to shrink, I move it toward the glenoid at a rate of 1.5 to 2 cm per second. It is important not to allow the probe to contact the capsule without any movement because thermal capsular necrosis or axillary nerve damage is a possibility.

11. The distance from any sutures used in the repair. I try to perform any thermal application as far a possible from my repair sutures. The thermal treatment initially results in capsular weakness, and there is a danger that the sutures will pull out of any thermally treated tissue. I attempt to have 2 cm between any sutures and thermally treated tissue.

12. Fluid temperature. The temperature of the irrigating fluid within the glenohumeral joint has a marked effect on the soft tissue response. Cold fluid results in a sluggish response, and warmer fluid causes a brisk reaction. Another advantage of the warmer fluid is that the probe is in contact with the tissue for a shorter time, whereas the disadvantage is that the warmer fluid increases the conductivity to the surrounding tissues and increases the risk of thermal damage. I believe the advantages outweigh the disadvantages, and I have the circulating nurse take bags of fluid that were placed in the blanket-warming drawer and hang those during this portion of the procedure.

13. Patient age. Older patients' tissues respond less well to thermal energy because there is a higher degree of collagen cross-linking and the tissue is more thermally stable. I tend to use little or no thermal technique in patients older than 40 years and prefer to use sutures exclusively.

If persistent excessive translation remains after thermal capsulorrhaphy, I tie the rotator interval repair suture (Figs. 4–109 to 4–115).

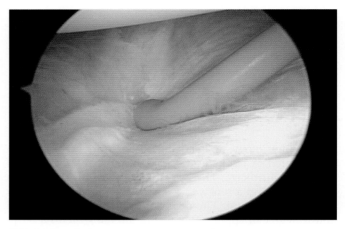

FIGURE 4–110. Thermal capsulorrhaphy of inferior posterior capsule.

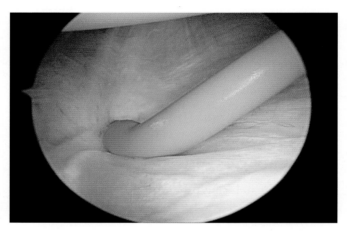

FIGURE 4–111. Thermal capsulorrhaphy of inferior capsule.

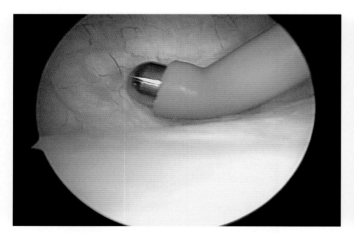

FIGURE 4–109. Test capsular tension.

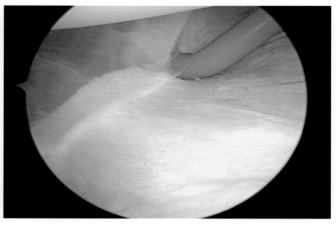

FIGURE 4–112. Thermal capsulorrhaphy of inferior anterior capsule.

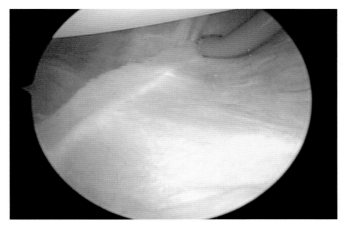

FIGURE 4–113. Thermal capsulorrhaphy of inferior capsule.

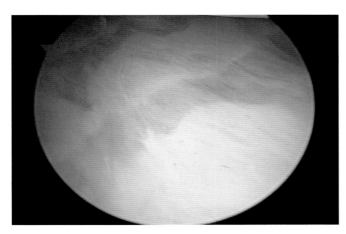

FIGURE 4–114. Capsular striping.

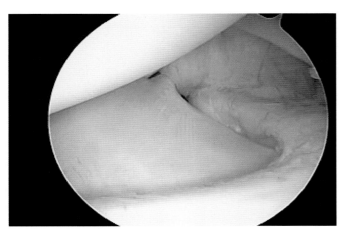

FIGURE 4–115. Completed interval repair.

Rotator Cuff Lesions

Overhead-throwing athletes may have rotator cuff lesions that range from minor fraying to full-thickness rotator cuff tears. When these tears are grade 3 or full-thickness tears, I repair them after I complete the glenohumeral joint reconstruction. I mark the area of tear with a spinal needle or monofilament suture and reinsert the arthroscope into the subacromial space. Anterior lesions are usually small tears and are easily repaired. Posterior lesions are repaired with the arthroscope in the lateral portal, and instruments are passed through the anterior and posterior portals.

VIDEO — **Posterior Bankart with Posterior Rotator Cuff Repair**

Postoperative Management

Postoperative management is similar for all patients. A soft pillow sling supports the arm in 15 degrees of abduction. If the primary direction of instability repair is anterior, I position the elbow anterior to the coronal plane of the shoulder with the arm internally rotated. I position the elbow posterior to the coronal plane with the arm in 10 degrees of external rotation if the primary direction is posterior. I place the elbow of a patient with multidirectional instability in neutral rotation and 25 degrees of abduction. An ice pack wrap decreases postoperative shoulder swelling and pain. I administer 1 g of a cephalosporin 8 hours postoperatively. Patients go home the morning after operation. Active range-of-motion exercises of the fingers, wrist, and elbow as well as deltoid muscle isometric exercises are started the morning after the operation and continue at home for 2 weeks. At 2 weeks, I obtain an anterior posterior radiograph to document the position of any metallic suture anchors.

Patients are allowed to remove their sling for active elevation and external rotation exercises twice daily, but they wear the sling at all other times. If the patient has had an anterior repair, I allow active elevation as tolerated. I instruct patients to limit external rotation to 20 degrees at week 2, 40 degrees at week 4, and 60 degrees at week 6. If the patient has had a posterior repair (either as the only operation or if it is performed along with an anterior or inferior repair), I restrict active elevation to 90 degrees and internal rotation to neutral, but I allow unlimited external rotation. If the patient has had a multidirectional instability operation, I instruct the patient to limit shoulder motion as much as possible. Generally, these patients have some degree of ligament laxity, and achieving full range of motion is not a problem. The sling is worn for 6 weeks, at which time it is removed, and the patient begins active range-of-motion (without restrictions) and strengthening exercises. Patients continue range-of-motion and strengthening exercises for 1 year.

TABLE 4–1. PREOPERATIVE PHYSICAL EXAMINATION FINDINGS: BIDIRECTIONAL

	0+	1+	2+	3+	Pain	Apprehension
Abd/ER (IA)	6	26	4	0	31	14
Abd/ER (IP)	2	12	2	0	14	7
Abd/Down (IA)	3	19	14	0	25	12
Abd/Down(IP)	0	7	9	0	9	6
Sulcus (IA)	0	13	23	0	36	23
Suclus (IP)	0	9	7	0	16	9
Rowe (IA)	2	10	24	0	32	22
Rowe (IP)	0	8	8	0	16	10
Posterior (IA)	24	11	1	0	2	0
Posterior (IP)	6	6	1	3	4	4

Abd/Down, abduction and downward force; Abd/ER, abduction and external rotation; IA, interior anterior; IP, interior posterior.

Results

Operative Repair

The lesions repaired at operation are variable, and most patients have more than a single lesion. I have summarized my experiences in Tables 4–1 to Tables 4–3. These early reports are consistent with my findings in the last 1000 operations. The average number of bone and soft tissue anchors used was 2.4 (range, 0 to 5). After ligament or labrum suture repair and suture imbrication or advancement to correct midsubstance laxity, I examine the shoulder for translation, and if further tightening is necessary, I use the thermal probe sparingly to increase ligament or capsular tension. I have not found any patients in whom I believed thermal capsulorrhaphy without ligament or labrum suture repair was adequate to restore soft tissue tension.

TABLE 4–3. FINAL RESULTS*

	ASES		Constant		Rowe		UCLA	
Unidirectional Instability								
	Pre	Post	Pre	Post	Pre	Post	Pre	Post
Score	45.5	91.7	56.4	91.8	11.3	91.9	17.6	32.0
SD	18.6	13.7	13.3	11.3	5.7	20.8	4.8	4.7
Bidirectional Instability								
	Pre	Post	Pre	Post	Pre	Post	Pre	Post
n = 54	45.5	94.0	57.0	92.4	20.3	92.1	18.6	32.7
SD	16.2	9.3	12.9	10.4	13.3	19.5	4.4	3.7
Multidirectional Instability								
	Pre	Post	Pre	Post	Pre	Post	Pre	Post
Score	45.4	94.7	60	91.7	14.2	93.7	17.4	33.1
SD	18.8	9.3	11.5	8.5	13	13.2	4.5	2.9

*All postoperative scores significant ($P = .0001$).
ASES, American Shoulder and Elbow Surgeons Shoulder Index; Post, postoperative; Pre, preoperative; SD, standard deviation; UCLA, University of California at Los Angeles.

Postoperative Scores and Shoulder Rating Systems

The four rating systems reflect an improvement in shoulder status. Comparing the scores before the surgical procedure with those at final follow-up, paired t-tests revealed significant increases in the total and subscales scores for the American Shoulder and Elbow Surgeons' Shoulder Index and the shoulder scores of the Constant, Rowe, and University of California at Los Angeles systems ($P=.0001$). Neither the Constant system nor the American Shoulder

TABLE 4–2. OPERATIVE FINDINGS

	Unidirectional (n = 53)	Bidirectional (n = 33)		Multidirectional (n = 47)
		Inferior Anterior	*Inferior Posterior*	
Labrum repair				
Superior	31	16	7	10
Anterior	48	9	0	10
Type A	25	—	—	—
Type B	15	—	—	—
Type C	8	—	—	—
Inferior	2	2	0	2
Posterior	0	0	2	6
Ligament suture imbrication				
Anterior	46	25	5	47
Middle	41	33	11	47
Inferior	31	19	7	47
Posterior	0	0	9	47
Thermal tightening				
Anterior	48	7	1	—
Middle	5	5	2	—
Inferior	11	17	9	—
Posterior	0	0	7	—
Rotator interval repair	14	22	1	28

and Elbow Surgeons' scoring system provides guidelines on what scores may be considered excellent or poor. Ellman and I categorized University of California at Los Angeles shoulder scores of 29 to 35 as good to excellent results and those less than 29 as fair to poor results. Rowe rated scores of 90 to 100 as excellent and 75 to 89 as good. My experience with all three types of glenohumeral instability, that is, traumatic unidirectional anterior, bidirectional, and multidirectional instability, are good and excellent results in about 90% of shoulders according to both the Rowe score and the University of California at Los Angeles shoulder score. The details of these results are summarized in the following sections.

Range of Motion

No patient lost more than 5 degrees of forward elevation. External rotation at 90 degrees of abduction averaged 88 degrees, compared with 83 degrees preoperatively. The gain in movement reflects the preoperative loss of external rotation that is typical in patients with traumatic anterior instability caused by medial healing of the Bankart lesion (ALPSA). Patients without an ALPSA have a similar loss of external rotation because they tend to limit that motion to avoid pain or instability.

Return to Sports Participation

I studied patients with unidirectional traumatic anterior glenohumeral instability. Forty-three patients participated actively in sports before the onset of their shoulder problem: no patients participated in type 1, 5 in type 2, 30 in type 3, and 8 in type 4 sports. When stratified by sports level of participation, 17 patients participated at level 1 (high school team sports), 1 at level 2 (college school team sports), and 35 at level 3 (recreational athletes). At final follow-up evaluation, 5 patients did not participate in sports because of issues unrelated to their shoulders. Reasons most commonly cited were work or family commitments, graduation from high school or college (and the associated lack of team sports), or injuries to the knee or lumbar spine. The remaining 38 patients participated in sports: 1 in type 1, 6 in type 2, 26 in type 3, and 5 in type 4 sports. The distribution of sports level of participation at final follow-up was 3 at level 1, none at level at 2, and 35 at level 3. Four patients with persistent shoulder instability had decreased their level of participation at final follow-up.

Ligament Laxity

The final Rowe score was stratified according to the presence or absence of generalized ligament laxity. Patients without evidence of ligament laxity ($n = 47$) had a final mean Rowe score of 94, and those with ligament laxity ($n = 6$) had a final score of 74. The difference is statistically significant ($P = .02$). The inferior results in patients with generalized ligament laxity may stem from a technically inadequate repair or may suggest that patients with anterior inferior instability and generalized ligament laxity require an open capsular reconstruction to achieve adequate soft tissue tension.

Complications

No major intraoperative or perioperative complications (permanent nerve injuries, wound infections) occurred. Two patients noted paresthesias in the musculocutaneous nerve distribution. All resolved by the 6-week postoperative visit. One patient noted minor wound drainage that resolved within 1 week without the use of antibiotics. I did not observe any complications from suture anchors.

Discussion

The many different treated lesions, patient populations, operative techniques, length of follow-up, and use of multiple scoring systems complicate comparison of arthroscopic technique with the results of open operations. However, the level of improvement of the various parameters described in multiple investigations allows me to conclude that arthroscopic repair of glenohumeral instability using the techniques I have described can produce outcomes that are improved over prior arthroscopic treatments and are equivalent to open repair.

The spectrum of operative findings does not support the concept of any "essential lesion." On the contrary, it appears that the etiology of glenohumeral instability is multifactorial, and successful treatment requires that any operative approach possess sufficient flexibility to deal with the variety of lesions found. The arthroscopic approach allows the surgeon to identify and treat all the lesions of shoulder instability. I believe that the success of arthroscopic treatment is the result of our ability to perform an anatomic repair of anterior, superior, and inferior labrum tears, to correct capsular elongation and, if necessary, to repair the rotator interval.

Currently, my operative treatment of glenohumeral instability is arthroscopic. No open operations are performed, except in the rare case of a large bony humeral head or glenoid defect requiring bone grafting. With arthroscopic technique, I inspect the entire glenohumeral joint and avoid soft tissue dissection. No division of the subscapularis is required. Although I am unable to document my impression statistically, I believe that arthroscopic repair provides improved cosmesis, decreased postoperative pain, and more rapid gains in motion when compared with open operative treatment of patients with similar lesions.

These techniques can be recommended only to the experienced orthopedic surgeon familiar with the normal and abnormal anatomy seen during both open and arthroscopic shoulder operations. A thorough understanding of the various conditions that produce pain in the shoulder is needed. The orthopedic surgeon who infrequently performs open glenohumeral instability repair should not undertake the arthroscopic procedure. The arthroscopic operation requires advanced arthroscopic techniques and is still in the developmental stage.

Bibliography

Allain J, Goutalliler D, Glorion C: Long-term results of the Latarjet procedure for the treatment of anterior instability of the shoulder. J Bone Joint Surg Am 80:841–852, 1998.

Altchek DW, Warren RF, Skyhar MJ, Ortiz G: T-plasty modification of the Bankart procedure for multidirectional instability of the anterior and inferior types. J Bone Joint Surg Am 73A:105–112, 1991.

Arnoczky SP, Aksan A: Thermal modification of connective tissues: Basic science considerations and clinical implications. Instr Course Lect 50:3–11, 2001.

Baker CL, Uribe JW, Whitman C: Arthroscopic evaluation of acute initial anterior shoulder dislocations. Am J Sports Med 18:25–28, 1990.

Bigliani LU, Kurziil PR, Schwartzbach, CC, et al: Inferior capsular shift procedure for anterior-inferior shoulder instability in athletes. Am J Sports Med 22:578–584, 1994.

Bigliani LU, Pollock RG, Soslowsky, LJ, et al: Tensile properties of the inferior glenohumeral ligament. J Orthop Res 10:187–97, 1992.

Blasier RB, Soslowsky LJ, Palmer, ML: Posterior glenohumeral subluxation: Active and passive stabilization in a biomechanical model. J Bone Joint Surg Am 79:433–440, 1997.

Burkhart SS, Morgan CD: The peel-back mechanism: Its role in producing and extending posterior type II SLAP lesions and its effect on SLAP repair rehabilitation. Arthroscopy 14:637–640, 1998.

Burkhead WZ Jr, Rockwood CA Jr: Treatment of instability of the shoulder with an exercise program. J Bone Joint Surg Am 74:890–896, 1992.

Caspari R, Savoie F: Arthroscopic reconstruction of the shoulder: The Bankart repair. In McGinty J (ed): Operative Arthroscopy. New York, Raven, 1991.

Ellman H, Gartsman GM: Arthroscopic Shoulder Surgery and Related Procedures. Philadelphia, Lea & Febiger, 1993.

Gartsman GM, Roddey TS, Hammerman, SM: Arthroscopic treatment of multidirectional glenohumeral instability: 2- to 5-year follow-up. Arthroscopy 17:236–243, 2001.

Gartsman GM, Roddey TS, Hammerman, SM: Arthroscopic treatment of bi-directional glenohumeral instability: Two- to five-year follow-up. J Shoulder Elbow Surg 10:28–36, 2001.

Gartsman GM, Roddey TS, Hammerman, SM: Arthroscopic treatment of anterior-inferior glenohumeral instability: Two to five-year follow-up. J Bone Joint Surg Am 82:991–1003, 2000.

Gartsman GM, Taverna E, Hammerman, SM: Arthroscopic rotator interval repair in glenohumeral instability: Description of an operative technique. Arthroscopy 15:330–332, 1999.

Gartsman GM, Taverna E, Hammerman SM: Arthroscopic treatment of acute traumatic anterior glenohumeral dislocation and greater tuberosity fracture. Arthroscopy 15:648–650, 1999.

Gross RM: Open and Arthroscopic Glenohumeral Instability Repairs. New Orleans, American Academy of Orthopedic Surgeons, 1998.

Habermeyer P, Gleyze P, Rickert M: Evolution of lesions of the labrum-ligament complex in posttraumatic anterior shoulder instability: A prospective study. J Shoulder Elbow Surg 8:66–74, 1999.

Harryman DT, Sidles JA, Harris SL, Matsen FA: The role of the rotator interval capsule in passive motion and stability of the shoulder. J Bone Joint Surg Am 74:53–66, 1992.

Hayashi K, Thabit G, Bogdanske JJ, et al: The effect on nonablative thermal probe energy on the ultrastructure of joint capsular collagen. Arthroscopy 12:474–481, 1996.

Itoi E, Lee S-B, Berglund LJ, et al: The effect of a glenoid defect on anteroinferior stability of the shoulder after Bankart repair: A cadaveric study. J Bone Joint Surg Am 82:35–46, 2000.

Kohn, D: The clinical relevance of glenoid labrum lesions. Arthroscopy 3:223–230, 1987.

Lippitt SB, Vanderhooft JE, Harris SL, et al: Glenohumeral stability from concavity-compression: A quantitative analysis. J Shoulder Elbow Surg 2:27–35, 1993.

Lopez MJ, Hayashi K, Fanton GS, et al: The effect of radiofrequency energy on the ultrastructure of joint capsular collagen. Arthroscopy 14:495–501, 1996.

McIntyre LF, Caspari RB, Savoie FH: The arthroscopic treatment of posterior shoulder instability: Two-year results of multiple suture technique. Arthroscopy 13:426–432, 1997.

McIntyre LF, Caspari RB, Savoie FH: The arthroscopic treatment of multidirectional shoulder instability: Two-year results of a multiple suture technique. Arthroscopy 13:418–425, 1997.

McMahon PJ, Tibone JE, Cawley PW, et al: The anterior band of the inferior glenohumeral ligament: Biomechanical properties from tensile testing in the position of apprehension. J Shoulder Elbow Surg 7:467–471, 1998.

Morgan CD, Bodenstab AB: Arthroscopic Bankart suture repair: Technique and early results. Arthroscopy 3:111–122, 1987.

Morrey BF, Janes JM: Recurrent anterior dislocation of the shoulder. J Bone Joint Surg Am 58:252–256, 1976.

Neer CS, Foster CR: Inferior capsular shift for involuntary inferior and multidirectional instability of the shoulder. J Bone Joint Surg Am 62:897–908, 1980.

Neviaser TJ: The anterior labroligament periosteal sleeve avulsion lesion: A cause of anterior instability of the shoulder. Arthroscopy 9:17–21, 1993.

Nottage WM: Thermal probe–assisted shoulder surgery. Arthroscopy 13:635–638, 1997.

Pappas AM, Goss TP, Kleinman PK: Symptomatic shoulder instability due to lesions of the glenoid labrum. Am J Sports Med 11:279–288, 1983.

Richards RR, An KN, Bigliani LU, et al: A standardized method for the assessment of shoulder function. J Shoulder Elbow Surg 3:347–352, 1994.

Rodosky MW, Harner CD, Fu FH: The role of the long head of the biceps muscle and superior glenoid labrum in anterior stability of the shoulder. Am J Sports Med 22:121–30, 1994.

Rowe CR, Zarins B: The Bankart procedure: Long-term end-result study. J Bone Joint Surg Am 60:1–16, 1978.

Rowe CR, Zarins B: Recurrent transient subluxation of the shoulder. J Bone Joint Surg Am 63:863–872, 1981.

Savoie FH 3rd, Miller CD, Field LD: Arthroscopic reconstruction of traumatic anterior instability of the shoulder: The Caspari technique. Arthroscopy 13:201–209, 1997.

Speer KP, Deng X, Borrero S, et al: Biomechanical evaluation of a simulated Bankart lesion. J Bone Joint Surg Am 78:1819–1825, 1994.

Tibone JE, Lee TQ, Black AD, et al: Glenohumeral translation after arthroscopic thermal capsuloplasty with a radiofrequency probe. J Shoulder Elbow Surg 9:514–518, 2000.

Ticker JB, Bigliani LU, Soslowsky LJ, et al: Inferior glenohumeral ligament: Geometric and strain-rate dependent properties. J Shoulder Elbow Surg 5:269–279, 1996.

Warner JJ, Johnson D, Miller M, Caborn DN: Technique for selecting capsular tightness in repair of anterior-inferior shoulder instability. J Shoulder Elbow Surg 4:352–364, 1995.

Williams MM, Snyder SJ, Buford D Jr: The Buford complex—the "cord-like" middle glenohumeral ligament and absent anterosuperior labrum complex: A normal anatomic capsulolabral variant. Arthroscopy 10:241–7, 1994.

Wirth MA, Blatter G, Rockwood CA Jr: The capsular imbrication procedure for recurrent anterior instability of the shoulder. J Bone Joint Surg Am 78:246–59, 1996.

Wolf EM, Cheng JC, Dickson K: Humeral avulsion of glenohumeral ligaments as a cause of anterior shoulder instability. Arthroscopy 11:600–607, 1995.

Wolf EM, Eakins CL: Arthroscopic plication for posterior shoulder instability. Arthroscopy 14:153–163, 1998.

Wolf EM, Wilk RM, Richmond JC: Arthroscopic Bankart repair using suture anchors. Oper Tech Orthop:184–191, 1991.

Zuckerman JD, Matsen FA: Complications about the glenohumeral joint related to the use of screws and staples. J Bone Joint Surg Am 66:175–180, 1984.

5

Biceps Tendon Lesions

Biceps tendon lesions are an appropriate subject to bridge the transition from the glenohumeral joint to the subacromial space. Biceps lesions occurring at the glenoid attachment (superior labrum from anterior to posterior or SLAP lesions) are intimately involved in the treatment of glenohumeral instability, whereas biceps abnormalities in the region of the bicipital groove (subluxation and synovitis) are part of subacromial impingement. Biceps tenodesis may be part of my treatment for a massive rotator cuff tear or a subscapularis tear. Finally, I consider biceps tenotomy one of the options in the treatment of irreparable rotator cuff tears.

Proximal Biceps Lesions

Introduction

SLAP lesions represent an interesting and complex challenge to the shoulder surgeon. Patients with SLAP lesions present with a wide spectrum of clinical complaints, their physical examinations vary, clinical findings are nonspecific, and radiographic diagnosis is imprecise. At operation, the findings are variable, and the decision whether to repair the SLAP lesion requires a thorough understanding of the patient's clinical condition and shoulder pathophysiology.

Literature Review

Anatomy

The superior labrum has a wide variability of attachment. The anterior, inferior, and posterior labra are firmly attached to the glenoid, and separation of the labrum from the glenoid is pathologic. An exception to this is the normal sublabral hole that exists near the anterior superior glenoid (Fig. 5–1).

However, a normal superior labrum is not always attached, or it may have only a flimsy connection to the glenoid. If the glenoid underlying the superior labrum is covered with smooth cartilage and neither the superior labrum nor the glenoid demonstrates any evidence of trauma, I believe the superior labrum separation is a normal anatomic variant and not a pathologic lesion (Fig. 5–2).

Evidence of trauma includes fraying or tearing of the superior labrum or damage to the glenoid cartilage directly underneath the labrum separation. Superior labrum separation without evidence of trauma does not require repair. A SLAP lesion is an abnormal separation of the superior labrum from anterior to posterior and was first described by Snyder and colleagues, who described four variations. In a type 1 lesion, the superior labrum is attached to the glenoid rim, but there is fraying of the leading edge of the labrum. In a type 2 lesion, the superior labrum is detached from the glenoid. A type 3 lesion is similar to a type 2 lesion, but in addition there is a bucket-handle tear, whereas in a type 4 lesion, there is also a longitudinal split in the biceps tendon (Figs. 5–3 to 5–6).

As our experience has increased, we have observed many variations on these four basic lesions. This is particularly noted in regard to the glenohumeral ligaments. The middle and, rarely, the anterior inferior glenohumeral ligaments may have their only glenoid attachments through the superior labrum. SLAP lesions have also been identified in patients with full-thickness rotator cuff tears and in patients with glenohumeral instability. Some publications have addressed the lesion's frequency and our ability to diagnose this condition. Rodofsky and associates made an important contribution when they demonstrated the contribution of the superior labrum to anterior glenohumeral instability.

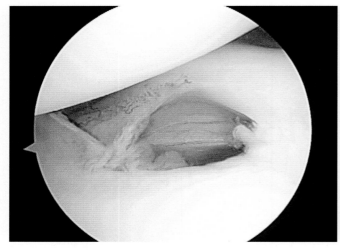

FIGURE 5–1. Normal anterosuperior labral hole.

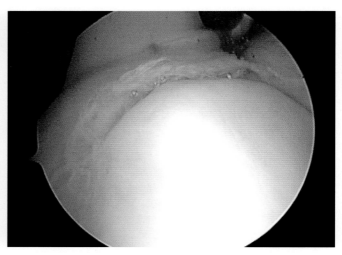

FIGURE 5–2. Normal superior labrum separation.

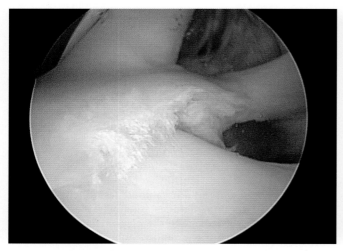

FIGURE 5–3. SLAP type 1.

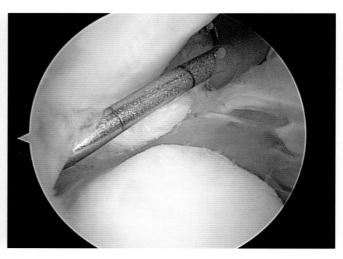

FIGURE 5–4. SLAP type 2.

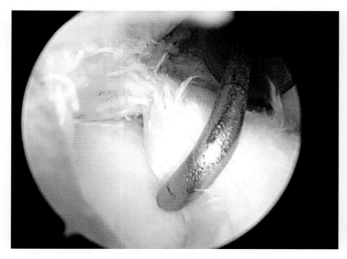

FIGURE 5–5. SLAP type 3.

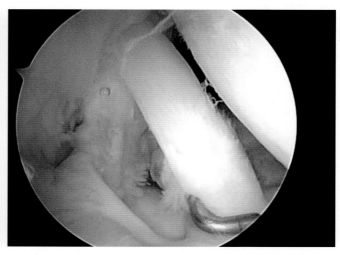

FIGURE 5–6. SLAP type 4.

Walch and associates, Jobe, and Morgan and Burkhart and their associates have discussed the role of the superior labrum in internal impingement.

It appears that SLAP lesions may cause shoulder pain from mechanical irritation of the interposed detached labrum between the humeral head and the glenoid. SLAP lesions alter glenohumeral joint dynamics and also contribute to shoulder pain and dysfunction in association with two other shoulder conditions: rotator cuff disease and glenohumeral instability.

Mechanical Irritation

Patients may present with symptoms of intermittent catching or locking of the shoulder during overhead sports or activities of daily living. The pain is sharp, severe, and localized vaguely as being "deep within the shoulder joint." Physical examination findings are variable. The examiner applying compression to the abducted shoulder and rotating the arm may reproduce the pain (Fig. 5–7). Placing the internally rotated arm in adduction and having the patient resist a downward force (O'Brien test) may be painful. The Speed test may be positive. A magnetic resonance imaging (MRI) study without contrast will rarely demonstrate a detached superior labrum, but with the addition of contrast material beforehand, the MRI seems to improve sensitivity (Fig. 5–8). The orthopedic surgeon who uses a high index of suspicion and excludes other more common causes of shoulder pain such as impingement, acromioclavicular joint arthrosis, and glenohumeral instability most commonly diagnoses SLAP lesions. Most SLAP lesions, however, are confirmed at arthroscopy.

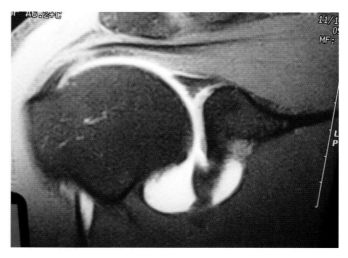

FIGURE 5–8. Magnetic resonance imaging with contrast.

Rotator Cuff Disease

SECONDARY IMPINGEMENT. SLAP lesions are infrequent in classic outlet impingement for stage 2 rotator cuff disease. I suspect SLAP lesions in younger patients who present with impingement symptoms and a type 1 or type 2 acromion. The MRI scan is normal, and usually the physical examination is consistent with impingement. Physical findings suggestive of a SLAP lesion are absent. In this setting, I carefully evaluate the superior labrum attachment at the time of arthroscopy. It appears that in certain patients the biceps tendon has a depressor effect on the humeral head and with loss of the biceps tendon attachment, the humeral head migrates superiorly enough to produce the symptoms of clinical impingement. Acromioplasty alone may not correct this condition, and SLAP repair is indicated. In this clinical setting, the surgeon should be aware that the SLAP lesion may cause or exacerbate subtle anterior inferior glenohumeral instability, and the "impingement" symptoms are secondary. Check carefully for subtle signs of anterior inferior instability such as labrum fraying, fissures, or minor separations.

SLAP LESION WITH AN ACUTE ROTATOR CUFF TEAR. With the advent and increasing use of arthroscopy, the glenohumeral joint is inspected routinely, and SLAP lesions are identified. SLAP lesions are not seen during an open rotator cuff repair, so their incidence has been underreported in publications dealing with open technique. They occur more frequently in younger patients after significant trauma. A typical example is a worker who falls backward and lands on his or her elbow with the shoulder in extension. The humeral head is driven superiorly, and, presumably, the biceps tendon attachment is avulsed from the glenoid. I repair SLAP lesions that are noted in the setting of an acute full-thickness rotator cuff tear.

CHRONIC FULL-THICKNESS ROTATOR CUFF TEAR. My experience is that SLAP lesions are found infrequently in patients with chronic full-thickness rotator cuff tears. My colleagues and I found an incidence of 2.5% (5 of 200), and we did not know whether the SLAP lesion predated the rotator cuff

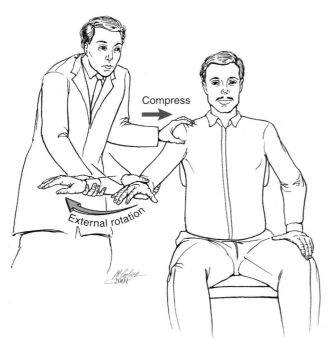

Compress

External rotation

FIGURE 5–7. Shoulder compressed and rotated.

tear, followed the tear, or was an independent entity. One of the reasons for repairing the rotator cuff tendons is to restore their ability to center the humeral head during overhead elevation. It seems reasonable to repair another possible source of humeral head depression, the biceps-labrum complex. Here again, theory collides with reality. My goal after rotator cuff repair is to restore full passive range of motion, but if the SLAP lesion is repaired, then I must restrict full external rotation so as not to disrupt the SLAP repair. Unless the SLAP lesion is significant, I prefer to repair the rotator cuff and not to repair the SLAP lesion.

Glenohumeral Instability

SLAP lesions contribute to glenohumeral instability directly and indirectly. Rodosky and associates demonstrated in the laboratory the decrease in force required to translate the humerus on the glenoid when a SLAP lesion is present. Pagnani and colleagues demonstrated in cadavers the increase in anterior posterior and superior inferior translation when a SLAP lesion is created. The presence of a SLAP lesion therefore contributes indirectly to glenohumeral instability, and it would seem reasonable to repair a SLAP lesion along with other lesions found during a glenohumeral reconstruction.

 — **Bankart and SLAP Variations**

The SLAP lesion also can directly affect glenohumeral stability. The anatomy of the glenohumeral ligament insertions is variable, and I have found instances in which the middle and even the anterior inferior glenohumeral ligaments are attached, not to the anterior inferior glenoid, but directly to the superior labrum. Superior labrum detachment removes the connection stabilizing the glenohumeral ligament from the glenoid. A SLAP lesion in such a patient is functionally a "Bankart" lesion, and I believe superior labrum repair is indicated.

Morgan and Burkhart and their associates presented a third type of relationship between SLAP lesions and glenohumeral instability. They postulated that repetitive overload stress in the throwing athlete creates a posterior superior SLAP lesion. The "bumper" and "suction-cup" effects of the labrum are destroyed, and posterior superior instability is the result. This type of instability can result in articular surface partial-thickness rotator cuff tears and can also allow anterior inferior glenohumeral instability. This is supported by the cadaver study by Pagnani and colleagues in which he found that an experimentally produced SLAP lesion resulted in increases in anterior posterior and superior inferior translation. My experience supports repair of the SLAP lesion in this setting.

 — **The Throwing Athlete**

Diagnosis

Patients with SLAP lesions may present with symptoms of mechanical abnormalities. They complain of locking or catching when they participate in athletics or vigorous activities of daily living. They also complain of painful catching or popping with passive shoulder compression and rotation. The relocation test may be positive. The physician may perform a variety of clinical tests, but in my experience they may not be painful when a SLAP lesion is present, and they can produce pain when no SLAP lesion exists (Fig. 5–9).

I believe these tests are helpful, but the examiner must put them in the context of the patient's clinical situation. Patients with SLAP lesions may present with findings typical of subacromial impingement or a full-thickness rotator cuff tear. The physical examination findings and patient complaints also may be consistent with glenohumeral instability. Patients may additionally have complaints of posterior superior subdeltoid pain when the arm is placed in abduction and external rotation in athletics or work.

I pay close attention to posterior shoulder soft tissue contracture and evaluate the shoulder internal rotation in neutral extension as well as in the scapular plane. Internal rotation may be quite limited. The source of the underlying soft tissue contracture is unclear because some patients may have significant loss of internal rotation yet also have excessive posterior glenohumeral translation. This suggests that in some patients the posterior capsule may be contracted, whereas others may have a normal or lax capsule with contracture of the posterior rotator cuff.

Morgan and Burkhart and associates believe that the posterior contracture is primary. With forceful internal rotation, the tight posterior capsule causes traction on the superior labrum and produces an avulsion injury (Fig. 5–10).

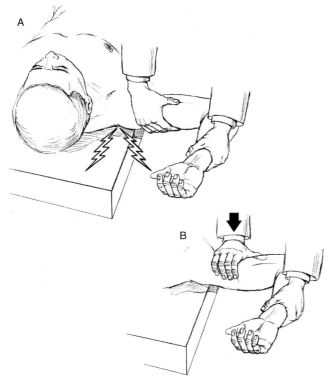

FIGURE 5–9. *A* and *B,* Relocation test.

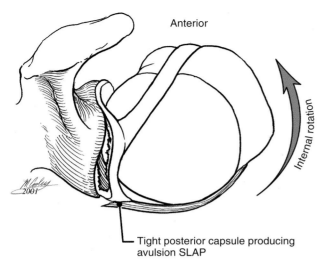

Anterior

Internal rotation

Tight posterior capsule producing avulsion SLAP

FIGURE 5–10. Tight posterior capsule producing avulsion.

Nonoperative treatment

Nonoperative treatment is directed at correctable, underlying causes of shoulder pain. Limitations of passive range of motion are corrected with appropriate stretching exercises. Impingement is treated with activity modification and selective rest of the shoulder. Glenohumeral instability is treated with exercises to strengthen the glenohumeral stabilizing muscles and to improve neuromuscular coordination, as described in Chapter 4.

Indications

SLAP lesions that produce mechanical symptoms of locking or catching are the least likely to respond to rehabilitation, and operation is indicated if symptoms are present for 3 to 6 months. Patients with SLAP lesions that coexist with glenohumeral instability or rotator cuff disease have indications for operations that are based on the underlying condition.

Contraindications

Contraindications are not based on the length of time before surgery, but rather on the decision whether to repair a SLAP lesion that is discovered at operation. Because patients with a SLAP repair require immobilization, I do not repair SLAP lesions that are found during operation for adhesive capsulitis or chronic rotator cuff tears.

Operative Technique

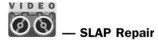 **— SLAP Repair**

Before a surgeon repairs a SLAP lesion, decisions must be made concerning two issues. Is the superior labrum separation from the glenoid a "lesion," or is it an anatomic vari-

ant? Second, what is the relationship between the labrum separation and the patient's clinical presentation?

Prior undergoing general anesthesia, patients receive an interscalene block to diminish postoperative pain. Patients are placed in the sitting position. The range of motion for external and internal rotation with the arm in 90 degrees of abduction and the range of external rotation with the arm in 0 degree of abduction are recorded. I examine the shoulder for anterior, inferior, and posterior translation and record the results. The shoulder is then prepared and draped routinely. The bony outlines of the acromion and coracoid process are palpated and are marked with a surgical marking pen.

The shoulder joint is entered with a cannula and blunt trocar through a posterior skin incision placed approximately 1.5 cm inferior and 2 cm medial to the posterolateral border of the acromion. The arthroscope is inserted into the glenohumeral joint. An anterior inferior portal is identified with a spinal needle so that the cannula enters the shoulder immediately superior to the subscapularis tendon and 1 cm lateral to the glenoid. The arthroscope is then inserted through the anterior portal, and the posterior structures are inspected. The arthroscope is then reinserted posteriorly (Figs. 5–11 to 5–17).

All structures within the glenohumeral joint are examined systematically. Lesions are variable and include tears of the rotator cuff (partial and complete), rotator interval lesions, biceps tendon fraying, and glenohumeral ligament tears. I specifically examine the labrum below the glenoid equator, anteriorly and posteriorly, for signs of fraying and detachment. Attention is then turned to the superior labrum.

An arthroscopic probe is useful to assess labrum attachment accurately because fibrous healing may have occurred after trauma. A normal labrum cannot be separated with the probe.

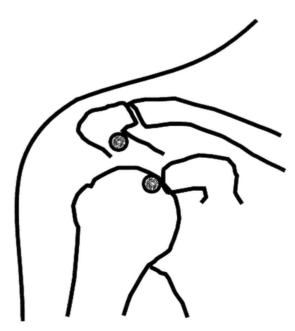

FIGURE 5–11. Anterior portal sites.

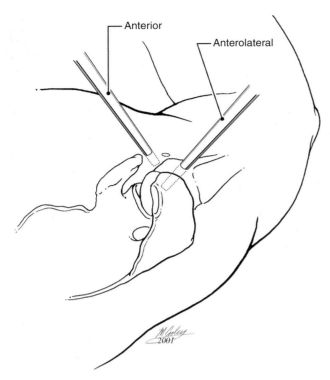

FIGURE 5–12. Superior portal placed more laterally if necessary.

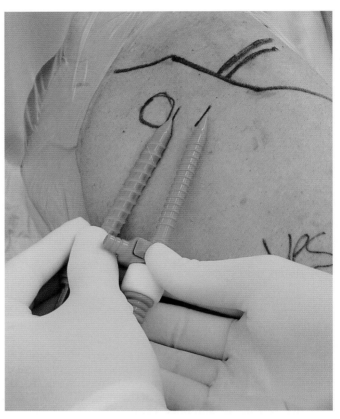

FIGURE 5–14. Cannula orientation.

SLAP 1 Lesions

I do not regard the minor fraying at the free edge of the labrum as pathologic and therefore do not perform any débridement.

SLAP 2 Lesions

If a SLAP 2 lesion is identified, an anterior superior portal is created. A spinal needle is inserted at the anterolateral acromial corner and enters the joint lateral to the biceps tendon. The second cannula is introduced. It is critical to

position the anterior superior cannula precisely. To obtain a proper angle for the bur and drill, this cannula must be placed as far laterally and superiorly as possible. I always use a spinal needle to identify both the entry point and angle for this cannula. The spinal needle should enter the joint close to the biceps exit from the glenohumeral joint and should approach the superior glenoid perpendicularly (Figs. 5–18 to 5–23).

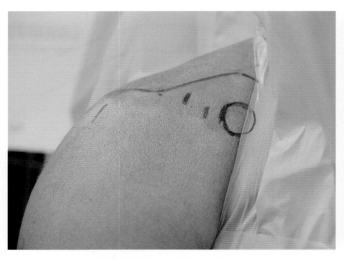

FIGURE 5–13. Skin markings.

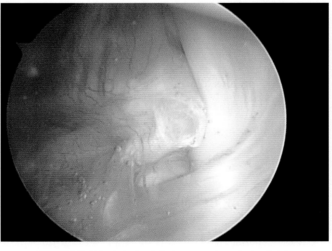

FIGURE 5–15. Anterior inferior cannula entering joint.

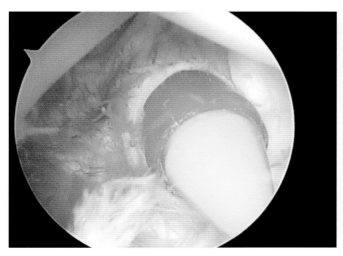

FIGURE 5–16. Anterior inferior cannula entering joint.

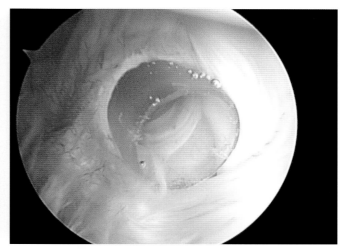

FIGURE 5–17. Anterior inferior cannula entering joint.

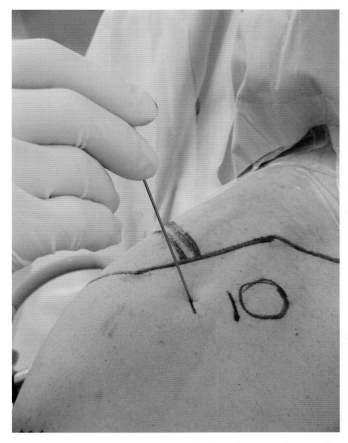

FIGURE 5–18. Angle for spinal needle insertion, anterior superior cannula.

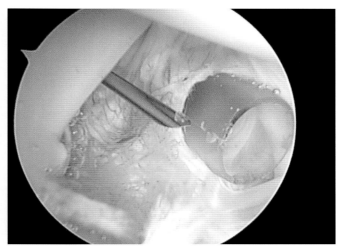

FIGURE 5–19. Spinal needle identifying site for anterior superior cannula.

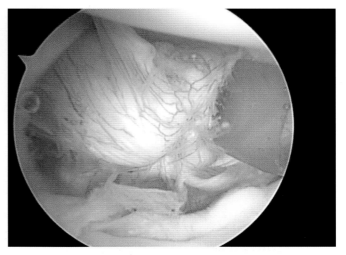

FIGURE 5–20. Anterior superior cannula entering through rotator interval.

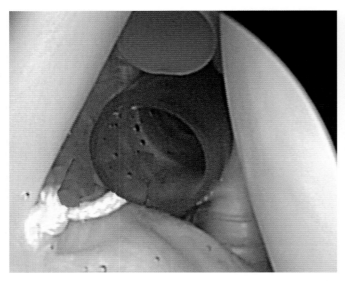

FIGURE 5–21. Cannula orientation.

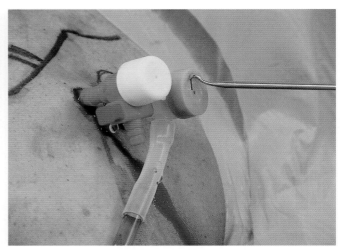

FIGURE 5–23. Cannula orientation.

I prefer suture anchor repair rather than the tack technique, because I am more comfortable with the fixation afforded by the anchors. Often, the superior labrum is robust, and the amount of tack inserted into the superior glenoid seems marginal. There are three drawbacks to the suture anchor method: (1) the surgeon inserts metal into the glenohumeral joint, (2) knot tying is necessary, and (3)

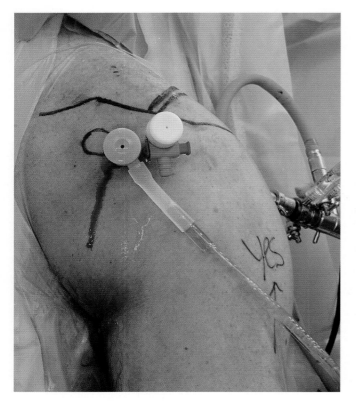

FIGURE 5–22. Cannula orientation.

the posterior of the two anchors appears difficult to insert. However, the superior glenoid bone in younger patients who require SLAP repair is strong, and with modern screw designs, the risk of anchor pullout is minimal. Knot tying is required, but it is a skill that can be mastered with practice. The surgeon can easily place an anchor posterior superiorly on the glenoid (through the anterolateral portal) if required. No additional portals are necessary.

I use a 4-mm power bur to abrade the glenoid beneath the detached superior labrum to expose cancellous bone. I usually insert it through the anterior superior portal because this gives me the best angle of approach. On occasion, the superior labrum is very meniscoid, with the labral margin extending down the glenoid and obscuring my view of the superior glenoid. In this situation, I insert the bur through the anterior inferior portal, and Dr. Hammerman (my assistant) inserts a probe through the anterior superior portal and retracts the labrum superiorly. This reveals the superior glenoid surface. Cancellous bone is exposed from the anterior to the posterior margins of the superior labrum detachment (Fig. 5–24).

Drill holes for the suture anchors are then made with a power drill. The drill is inserted through the anterior superior cannula, and the two drill holes are spaced proportionally along the length of the defect. I drill the anterior hole first and then the posterior hole. Because of the curvature of the glenoid, the posterior hole is more oblique than the anterior hole. As the posterior drill hole is moved posteriorly along the glenoid rim, it becomes more oblique. It is a matter of surgical judgment how much obliquity is permissible. The greater angle of approach causes the screw to be located more superficially in the bone. If the angle is unacceptable, there are two options: move the cannula more posteriorly so that it approaches the glenoid less acutely, or change the curvature of the superior glenoid rim.

If the superior labrum separation extends more posteriorly than normal, anchor placement is made easier with a technique modification. I believe that both the superior portal of Neviaser and a posterior superior portal pass through the substance of the rotator cuff tendons may lead to tendon rupture. When the SLAP lesion extends fur-

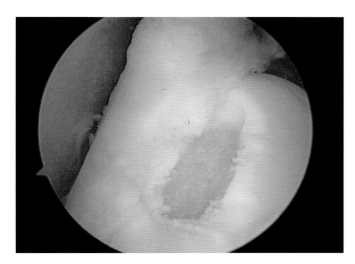

FIGURE 5–24. Bone preparation.

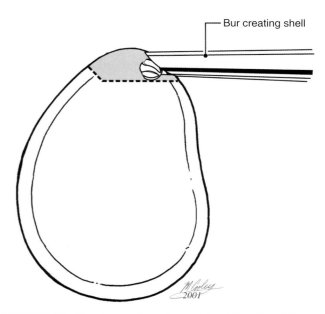

FIGURE 5–27. Abrade superior surface of glenoid to allow drill to penetrate.

ther posteriorly than normal, I try to move the anterior superior portal posteriorly. I use a spinal needle placed 1 cm posterior to the anterior acromial border. If the drill angle is still too acute, I insert a 4-mm round bur through the anterior superior portal and remove a small amount of glenoid bone to create a "shelf" whose face is now more perpendicular to the drill (Figs. 5–25 to 5–28).

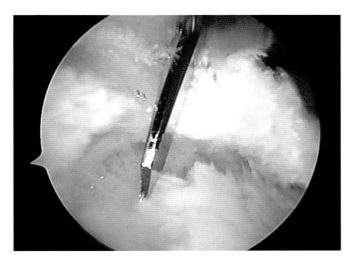

FIGURE 5–25. Drill, normal angle of approach.

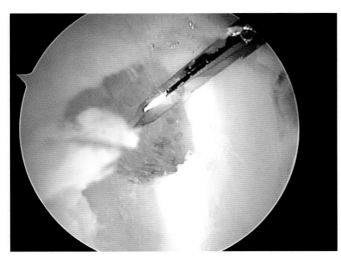

FIGURE 5–26. Drill, tangential angle.

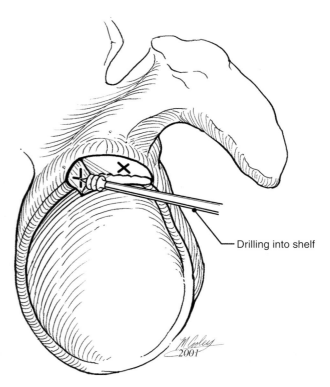

FIGURE 5–28. Anchor insertion.

The posterior anchor is inserted through the anterior superior cannula, and the two anchor sutures remain in this cannula. A Linvatec Spectrum (Largo, FL) instrument is then inserted through the anterior inferior portal. The Spectrum right-angled instrument is passed from the superior aspect of the detached labrum to the inferior aspect. Passing the suture from inferior to superior may result in detachment of the bucket handle as pressure is placed on the suturing device. Passing the suture in this direction also causes the nylon sutures to exit the suture passer and to move superiorly, thus making them harder to retrieve. Passing the sutures from superior to inferior places less stress on the labrum; the sutures exit the labrum and move inferiorly, thereby making their retrieval easier. However, it does require an additional surgical step because the surgeon must reverse the location of the suture loop.

The nylon suture is advanced fully into the glenohumeral joint, and the Spectrum instrument is withdrawn. A crochet hook is used to retrieve both suture ends. Insert the crochet hook through the anterior superior cannula. To avoid tangling the sutures, pass the crochet hook underneath (medial to) the sutures coming from the anterior inferior cannula. The loop portion of the nylon suture protrudes from the anterior inferior cannula, and the two free ends protrude from the anterior superior cannula. I prefer to repair the labrum with the suture knot on the superior surface of the labrum rather than bury the knot and interpose it between the detached superior labrum and its repair site. Therefore, it is necessary to reverse the direction of the loop. Loop a 0 monofilament suture, and use the nylon to pass the monofilament suture through the labrum.

The monofilament loop is now external to the anterior superior cannula, and the two free ends are external to the anterior inferior cannula. Place a hemostat on the two free ends of the sutures. A crochet hook retrieves one of the anchor's suture strands and brings it out the anterior inferior cannula. The remaining anchor suture (in the anterior superior cannula) is placed through the looped monofilament and is pulled through the labrum and out the anterior inferior cannula. Both sutures from the posterior anchor now exit the anterior inferior cannula (Figs. 5–29 to 5–38).

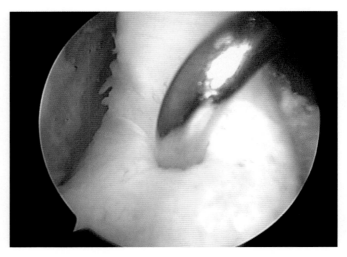

FIGURE 5–30. Spectrum suture passer.

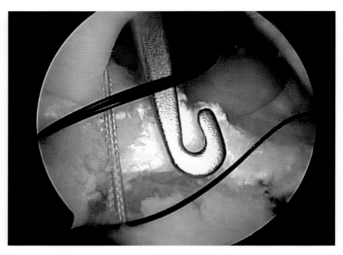

FIGURE 5–31. Retrieve nylon through anterior superior cannula.

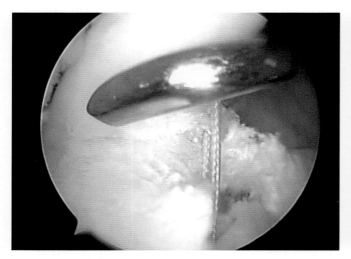

FIGURE 5–29. Spectrum suture passer.

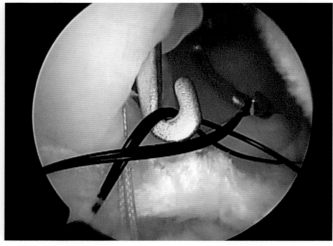

FIGURE 5–32. Bring nylon underneath.

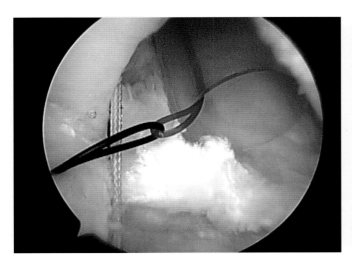

FIGURE 5–33. Reverse direction of loop.

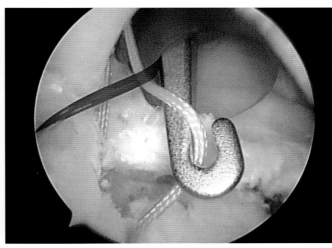

FIGURE 5–34. Move one suture strand from anterior superior cannula to anterior inferior cannula.

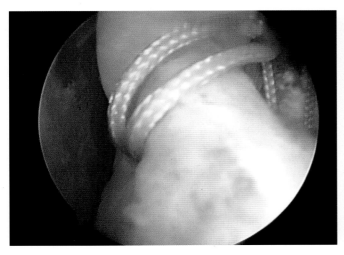

FIGURE 5–35. Pass anchor suture through labrum.

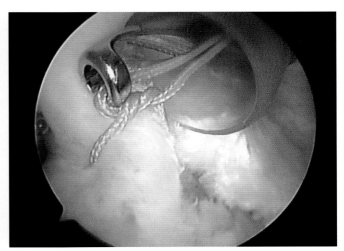

FIGURE 5–36. Tie knot.

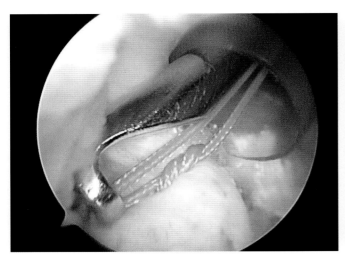

FIGURE 5–37. Post point.

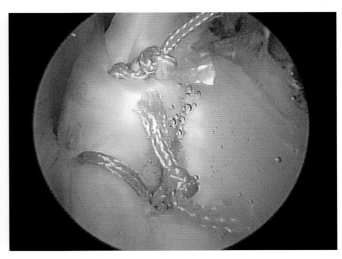

FIGURE 5–38. Completed repair.

Occasionally, the braided suture anchors do not pull smoothly through the labrum. Using additional force will cause the nylon passing sutures to tear. I prefer to use the technique developed by Dr. Hammerman. He threads the two free ends of the nylon suture through the knot-tying instrument and then advances the tip of the instrument near the labrum. Rather than pull the nylon sutures, he uses the knot-tying instrument to push the sutures through the labrum. Because the instrument is adjacent to the point where the sutures exit from the labrum, he is able to exert significant force without danger of suture breakage (Figs. 5–39 to 5–40).

The second anchor is inserted into the anterior drill hole through the anterior superior cannula. I insert the anterior anchor before I tie the posterior sutures because the anterior hole is obscured after the posterior sutures are tied. The posterior anchor sutures are tied with an arthroscopic knot-tying instrument through the anterior inferior cannula, and the sutures are cut with arthroscopic scissors. The anterior anchor suture is then placed through the anterior portion of the detached superior labrum, as described earlier, and the sutures are tied and cut.

SLAP 3 Lesions

If the bucket handle is less than one third of the labrum width, it is excised, and we repair the major portion of the superior labrum to the glenoid, as described earlier. If the bucket handle is one third or greater, then we repair the detached portion. The posterior anchor is inserted, and one limb of the suture-anchor suture is passed through the major portion of the labrum, as described earlier. Both suture strands, which are now in the anterior inferior cannula, are retrieved out the anterior superior cannula with a crochet hook. Failure to perform this step may result in the suture instrument's cutting the suture during the next portion of the operation. Place a hemostat on one of the suture limbs to identify which suture limb passes through the bucket fragment. The Spectrum instrument is then inserted through the anterior inferior cannula and pierces the

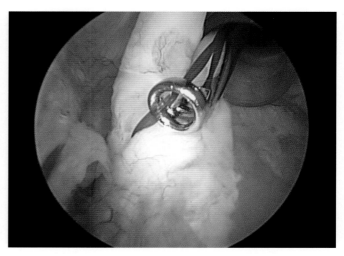

FIGURE 5–40. Advance into joint with knot pusher.

bucket handle from lateral to medial so as not to avulse the bucket fragment.

The free ends of the nylon suture are retrieved out the anterior superior cannula with a crochet hook. A 0 monofilament suture is used to reverse the loop. The first suture (already passed through the labrum) is transferred from the anterior superior cannula to the anterior inferior cannula, to minimize tangling. The second posterior anchor suture is then passed from the anterior superior cannula, through the labrum, and out the anterior inferior cannula. The sutures are tied and cut. This technique is repeated with the anterior anchor sutures to repair the anterior portion of the superior labrum and the anterior portion of the bucket-handle tear (Figs. 5–41 to 5–44).

SLAP 4 Lesions

If the longitudinal tear in the biceps tendon is less than one third of the tendon diameter, I excise the torn fragment. If

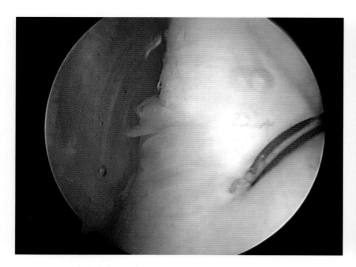

FIGURE 5–39. Anchor suture caught in labrum.

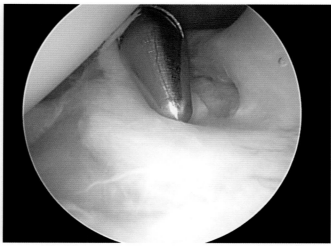

FIGURE 5–41. SLAP type 3.

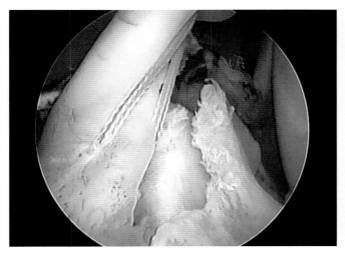

FIGURE 5–42. First anchor suture strand through major fragment.

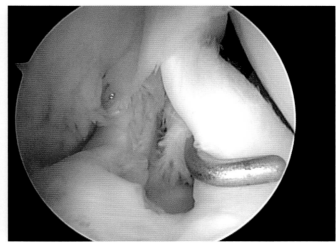

FIGURE 5–45. SLAP type 4.

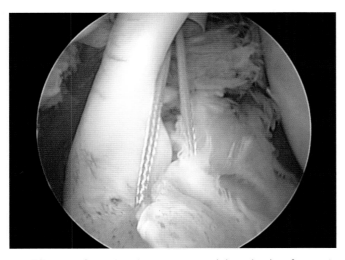

FIGURE 5–43. Second anchor suture strand through minor fragment.

the fragment is one third or greater, I repair the torn fragment to the major portion of the biceps tendon. The superior labrum is repaired first, as described earlier. The Spectrum instrument is used to place a No. 1 absorbable monofilament suture through the torn fragment and then through the major portion of the biceps tendon. The suture is then tied. One or two sutures are all that is necessary to accomplish the repair (Figs. 5–45 to 5–50).

Postoperative Treatment

The patient's arm is placed in a sling that is worn at all times except while bathing. At 2 weeks, active range of motion is allowed in all planes except external rotation in abduction. The sling is worn until week 4, at which time passive range of motion is started, with emphasis placed on posterior capsule stretching. Six weeks postoperatively, external rotation in abduction is allowed, and stretching continues. The patient is started on a progressive strengthening program

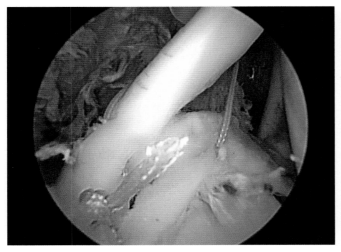

FIGURE 5–44. Completed repair.

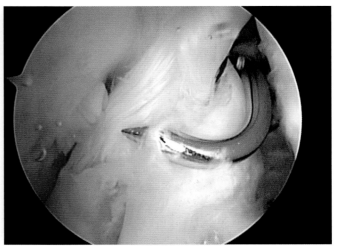

FIGURE 5–46. Biceps repair.

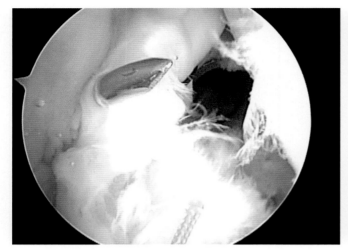

FIGURE 5–47. Biceps repair.

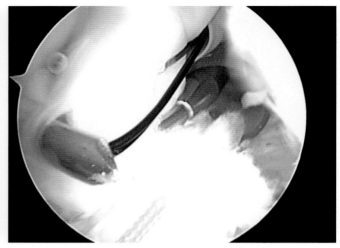

FIGURE 5–48. Biceps repair.

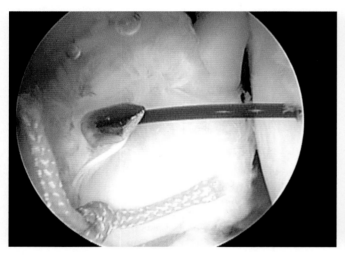

FIGURE 5–49. Biceps repair.

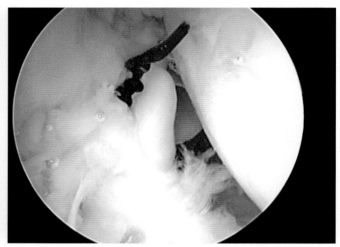

FIGURE 5–50. Biceps repair.

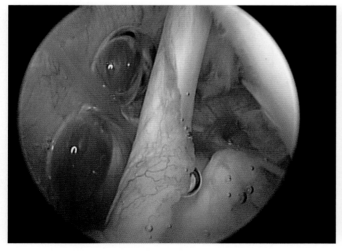

FIGURE 5–51. Biceps synovitis.

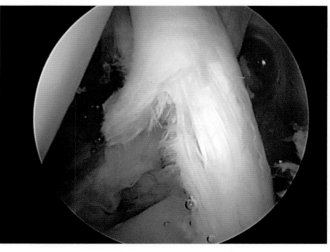

FIGURE 5–52. Biceps partial tear.

using surgical tubing for the deltoid, rotator cuff, scapular muscles, biceps, and triceps. Upper extremity sports are allowed 3 months after the surgical procedure, with the exception of throwing, which begins 4 months after operation. Throwing begins with low-velocity, short-distance throwing with the athlete concentrating on proper throwing mechanics. Distance and velocity are gradually increased until 7 months after operation, at which point I allow the patient to resume competitive throwing.

Biceps Lesions—Tendon Substance

Biceps tendinitis and partial tears are occasionally isolated causes of significant shoulder pain but are more commonly found in conjunction with subacromial impingement and rotator cuff tears. Although much has been described about arthroscopic subacromial decompression and rotator cuff repair, arthroscopic biceps treatment has been rarely mentioned. Biceps lesions requiring arthroscopic treatment include tendinitis, partial-thickness tears, and subluxation (Figs. 5–51 and 5–52).

Literature Review

The literature is sparse concerning arthroscopic treatment for biceps lesions because most patients respond to nonoperative care. Two methods of fixation for biceps tenodesis have been reported. We described our technique with suture anchors, and Boileau and associates described their experience with a bioabsorbable screw. Hawkins and Walch and colleagues questioned the value of any tenodesis operation. Their results suggest that equal or better results can be achieved with tenotomy. Regrettably, no prospective studies provide firm scientific support for one treatment method over the other. As of this writing, there is no published description of a method for arthroscopic biceps tendon stabilization for painful subluxation.

Diagnosis

The diagnosis of biceps tendinitis or partial tear is suggested on physical examination by patient complaints of pain in the area of the proximal biceps or of pain radiating down into the biceps muscle in the arm. These complaints are nonspecific and are commonly noted by patients with subacromial impingement syndrome. The primary (Neer) and secondary (Hawkins) impingement signs may also produce pain on physical examination. I have not found the Yergason test helpful and prefer the Speed test. Patients commonly describe painful popping or catching in the anterior shoulder area. A lidocaine injection into the area of the proximal biceps tendon sheath may be helpful in differentiating subacromial impingement from biceps tendinitis, but more commonly I find that it helps me to determine the *degree* to which the biceps lesion is producing pain. The definitive diagnosis is usually made on MRI or at the time of arthroscopic surgery. When reviewing the MRI findings, I pay particular attention to the subscapularis because biceps subluxation and tendinitis can be associated with partial-thickness tears of the articular surface of the subscapularis (Figs. 5–53 to 5–56).

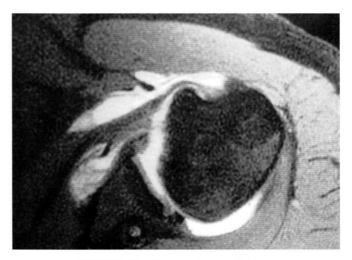

FIGURE 5–53. Subscapularis partial tear.

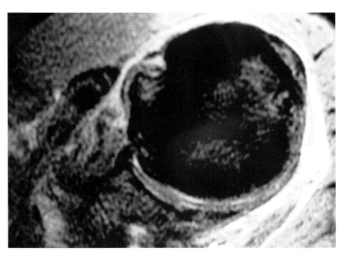

FIGURE 5–54. Subscapularis partial tear.

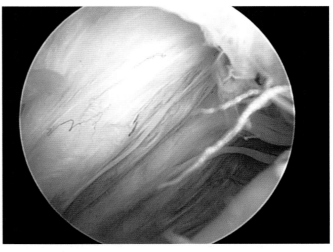

FIGURE 5–55. Subscapularis partial tear.

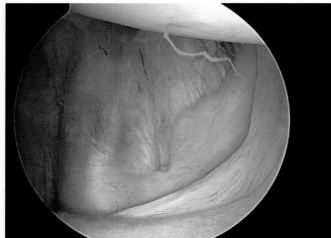

FIGURE 5–56. Subscapularis partial tear.

TABLE 5–1. INDICATIONS FOR TREATMENT	
Intact Rotator Cuff	
Biceps Lesion	*Treatment*
Inflamed	Tenosynovectomy
Partially torn < 50%	Repair
Partially torn > 50%	
Biceps quality good	Repair
Biceps quality poor	Ignore/tenotomy
Rotator Cuff Tear	
Biceps Lesion	*Treatment*
Biceps inflamed	Tenosynovectomy
Partially torn < 50%	Repair
Partially torn > 50%	
Biceps quality good/cuff repair good	Repair and stabilize
Biceps quality good/cuff repair poor	tenodesis
Biceps quality poor/cuff repair good	Tenotomy
Biceps quality poor/cuff repair poor	Tenotomy

Indications

Partial-thickness biceps tendon tears found within the glenohumeral joint are not an uncommon finding, and they may occur subsequent to a traumatic event or may be the result of chronic subacromial impingement. When the tear is less than 50% of the tendon width, the frayed edges are débrided. If the tear is greater than 50% of the tendon width, I repair the lesion with absorbable monofilament suture. It is very rare for the intra-articular portion of the biceps tendon to be frayed or partially torn so extensively that a repair is not possible. Such lesions occur closer to the bicipital groove. When the tendon is of good quality but subluxed medially, I prefer biceps stabilization, usually in combination with a subscapularis repair. Stabilization is a technique in which the biceps tendon is replaced within the bicipital groove and is maintained in this location by subscapularis or supraspinatus repair. If a biceps lesion is found in the area of the bicipital groove during subacromial decompression for a full-thickness rotator cuff tear, I believe there are four options available to the surgeon. The surgeon may choose to ignore the biceps lesion, or the surgeon may perform stabilization, tenodesis, or tenotomy. Because there is no scientific evidence to guide the orthopedic surgeon, treatment is dictated by personal preference. I have experience with all four options, but I have seen the best results with stabilization in younger patients in association with good-quality rotator cuff repairs and with tenotomy in older patients who have poor-quality rotator cuff tendons (Table 5-1).

Contraindications

I consider a complete tear of the biceps long head a contraindication to arthroscopic repair and, if necessary, prefer to perform an open tenodesis (Fig. 5–57). Because the remnant stump within the glenohumeral joint may cause mechanical symptoms, I perform an arthroscopic débridement of the biceps tendon portion back to the level of the superior labrum.

Operative Technique

 — Biceps Synovitis

Intra-articular Biceps Tendinitis

I use a standard posterior portal and enter the glenohumeral joint. I visualize the biceps tendon and areas of fraying, inflammation, or partial tear. An anterior portal is established and a probe is introduced so that the tendon can be pulled to bring the extra-articular tendon portion into view (Figs. 5–58 and 5–59). If the fraying or inflammation is localized to the intra-articular portion of the biceps tendon, a shaver is introduced through the anterior portal, and

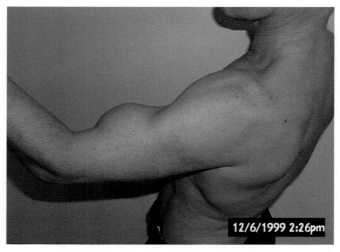

FIGURE 5–57. Patient with complete biceps tear.

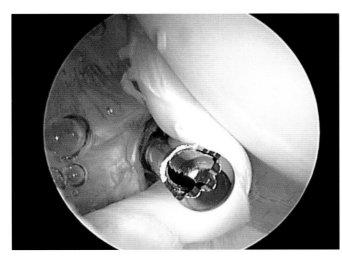

FIGURE 5–58. Shaver retracting biceps tendon.

débridement is performed. If a portion of the biceps tendon lesion lies within the bicipital groove, external to the glenohumeral joint, I prefer to use a subacromial approach to treat the lesion.

Intra-articular Biceps Tendon Partial Tear

This lesion is immediately observed on entry into the glenohumeral joint. I establish an anterior portal with an 8-mm cannula. If the biceps tear is the only lesion within the glenohumeral joint, I prefer to repair it with a one-cannula technique. I use a Spectrum right-angled instrument (or the Caspari suture punch) loaded with a monofilament suture and pierce through the entire tendon from the area of the tear flap toward the more normal tendon. I advance 15 to 20 cm of the suture into the joint and then withdraw the instrument. I grasp the free end of the suture with a crochet hook and withdraw it through the anterior cannula. I tie the

suture and repeat these steps for additional sutures as necessary, depending on the length of the tear area. There are other instruments that enable the surgeon to repair the biceps tendon, but they require two cannulas because one instrument is used to pass the suture and another instrument must then be inserted to retrieve the suture.

Subacromial Techniques

TENDINITIS AND PARTIAL-THICKNESS TEARS: INTACT ROTATOR CUFF. I use a standard posterior portal and enter the glenohumeral joint. The biceps tendon is visualized, and areas of fraying, inflammation, or partial tear are noted. I establish an anterior portal and introduce a probe to pull on the tendon to bring the extra-articular tendon within view.

I introduce a spinal needle percutaneously near the anterolateral acromial border and pierce the tendon just proximal to its exit from the joint. The needle is advanced until it is lodged in bone so that it does not dislodge when I remove the arthroscope from the glenohumeral joint and reinsert it into the subacromial space (Fig. 5–60).

I then remove the arthroscope from the joint and redirect it into the subacromial space. I locate the spinal needle and establish a lateral portal. I use scissors or a motorized shaver to divide the flimsy capsular tissue of the rotator interval and to expose the biceps tendon and the bicipital groove. I then insert an arthroscopic probe through the anterior portal and lift the biceps tendon from its groove and inspect it. If the tendon is intact and of good quality but inflamed, I perform a tenosynovectomy using a power shaver. If the biceps is partially torn less than 50% of its thickness, I repair it with monofilament sutures. If the biceps tendon is torn greater than 50%, and I wish to perform a tenodesis, I use the technique described in the next section.

BICEPS TENODESIS: PARTIAL THICKNESS BICEPS TEARS: ROTATOR CUFF TEAR. The biceps tenodesis is performed after the subacromial decompression but before the arthroscopic rotator cuff repair. Standard anterior and lateral portals are used. If the bicipital groove is flattened, as is common in

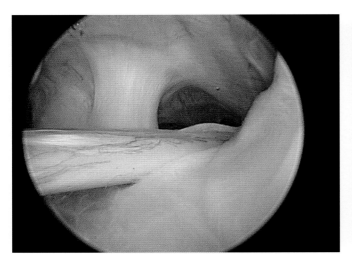

FIGURE 5–59. Extra-articular biceps pulled into view.

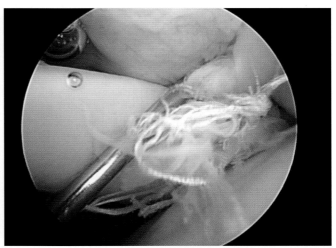

FIGURE 5–60. Spinal needle piercing biceps tendon.

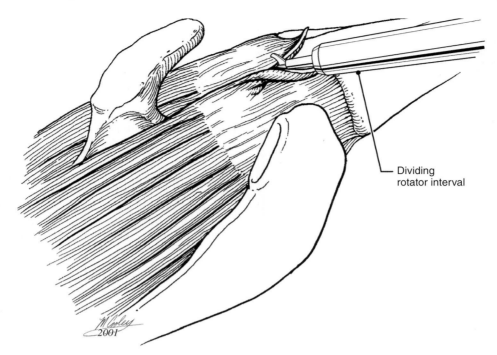

FIGURE 5–61. Division of rotator interval exposing biceps tendon.

chronic cuff tears, the tendon is retracted medially, and a 4-mm round bur is used to deepen the bicipital groove. I then insert two anchors into the center of the deepened groove. I place the first anchor distal to the supraspinatus insertion and the second anchor 10 mm distal to the first. These may be inserted through the anterior cannula, but often the angle is too oblique. If this is the case, I insert the anchors through a percutaneous stab wound. I use a spinal needle and pierce the anterior shoulder until the needle tip is within the bicipital groove and the angle of approach is satisfactory for anchor placement. I then incise the skin at this location and insert the suture anchor. A Caspari suture punch (loaded with a doubled 2–0 nylon suture) is inserted through the lateral cannula and pierces the biceps tendon. The 2–0 nylon suture is advanced and drawn out the anterior cannula. One limb of the first anchor suture is brought from the anterior cannula (or stab wound) to the lateral cannula and is passed through the biceps tendon using the nylon loop. This process is repeated with 5 mm from the first suture. A mattress suture has now been placed through the biceps tendon. This process is repeated with sutures from the second anchor, and the sutures are tied. I excise the intra-articular portion of the biceps tendon and repair the rotator cuff tear with arthroscopic technique (Figs. 5–61 to 5–69).

BICEPS STABILIZATION: INTACT ROTATOR CUFF. While viewing from the glenohumeral joint, I percutaneously insert a spinal needle through the rotator interval adjacent to the superior border of the subscapularis. I redirect the arthroscope into the subacromial space, locate the spinal needle, and establish a standard lateral portal. I use a shaver to débride any anterior bursal tissue and then create an anterior portal at the site where the spinal needle enters the

skin. If the subscapularis is completely torn and retracted, the biceps will be visible. If the subscapularis is torn only on its articular surface, I divide the tissue medial to the spinal needle with arthroscopic scissors. I move the arthroscope to the lateral portal to obtain a better view. I insert a round bur through the anterior cannula and abrade an area for the subscapularis repair medial to the biceps tendon. I then insert bone-suture anchors through the anterior portal into the area of abraded bone medial to the biceps tendon and use a crochet hook to bring retrieve the sutures out the posterior cannula. I introduce a Caspari suture punch

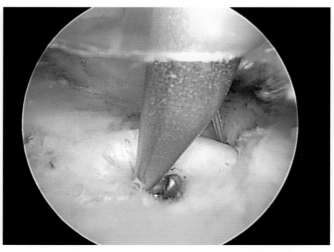

FIGURE 5–62. Identifying biceps tendon.

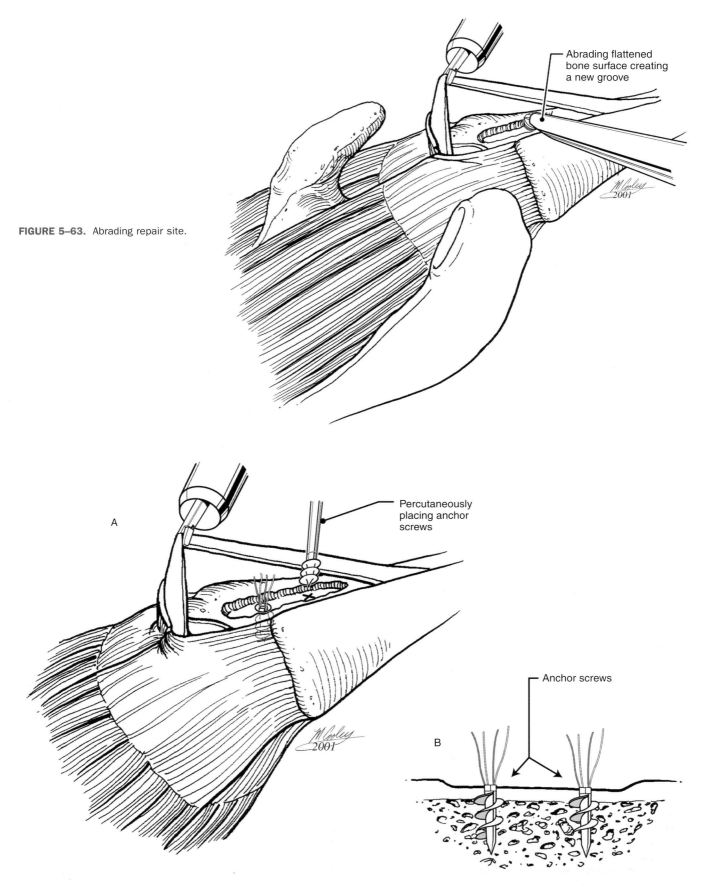

FIGURE 5–63. Abrading repair site.

Abrading flattened bone surface creating a new groove

A

Percutaneously placing anchor screws

Anchor screws

B

FIGURE 5–64. *A* and *B*, Anchor insertion.

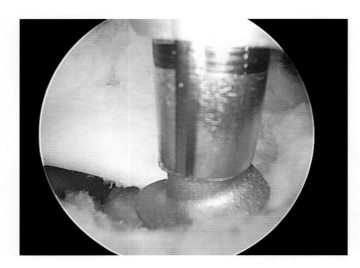

FIGURE 5–65. Anchor insertion.

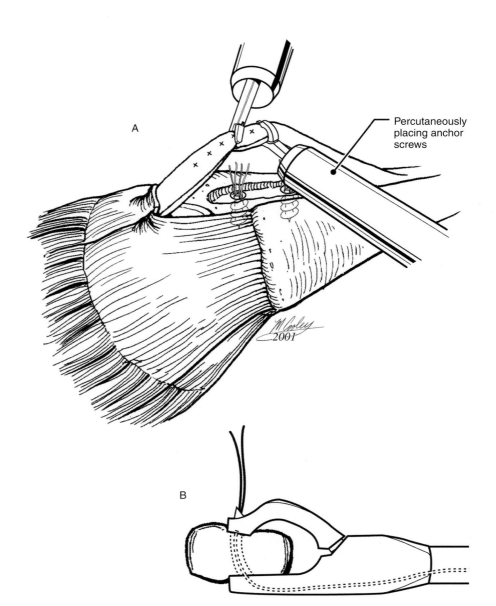

Percutaneously placing anchor screws

FIGURE 5–66. *A* and *B,* Suture placement.

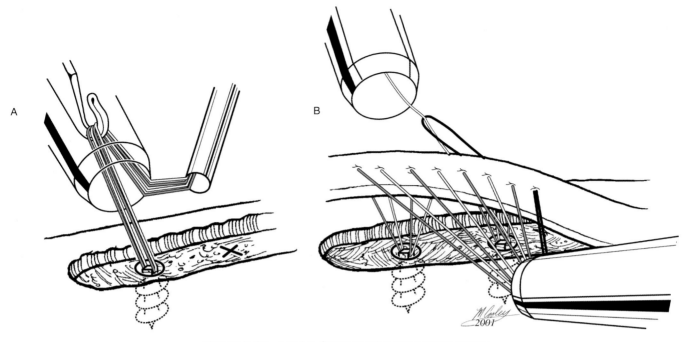

FIGURE 5–67. *A* and *B,* Suture spacing along biceps tendon.

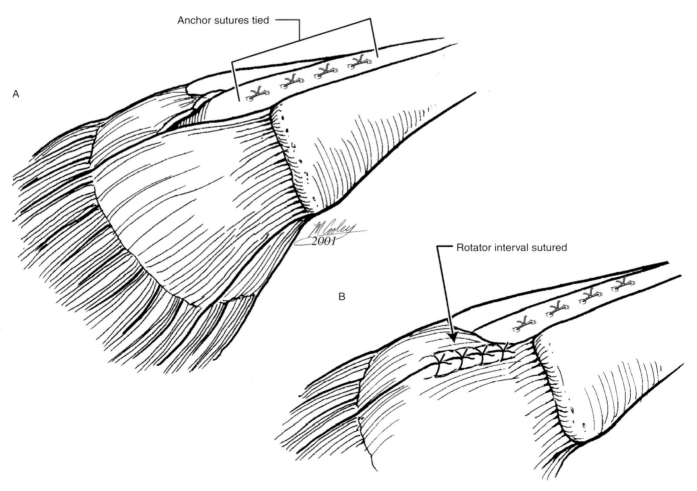

FIGURE 5–68. *A* and *B,* Sutures tied.

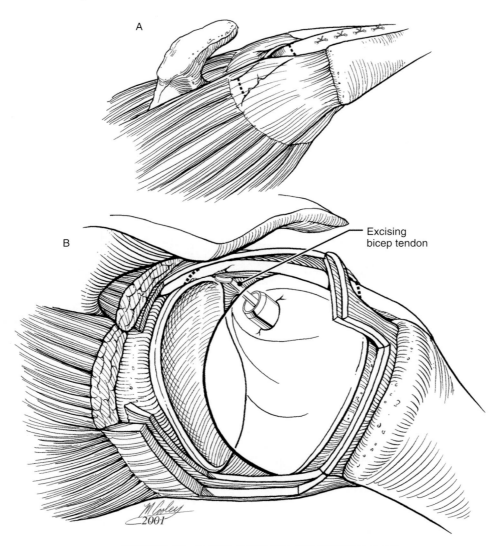

FIGURE 5–69. *A* and *B,* Excise intra-articular biceps stump.

through the anterior cannula and place the sutures in the subscapularis tendon following the technique previously described. My technique is to repair the subscapularis medial to the bicipital groove. Usually, the bicipital groove is flattened, and I use a round bur to deepen the groove and to repair the rotator interval with monofilament sutures (Fig. 5–70).

While viewing the repair, I put the patient's shoulder through a range of motion and record the safe limits of elevation and external rotation. I determine these motion limits by recording the point at which any tension develops at the repair site as I elevate and rotate the shoulder.

BICEPS STABILIZATION: ROTATOR CUFF TORN. In the presence of a rotator cuff tear, if the subscapularis is also torn, I perform a biceps tenodesis with the technique described earlier. If the subscapularis is intact, I perform tenodesis of the biceps before I repair the supraspinatus.

Tenotomy

 — Irreparable Rotator Cuff Tear

I have recently begun to appreciate the benefits of biceps tenotomy. Initially, I was skeptical of this philosophy because I was concerned about sacrificing an important structure. My tenotomy experience has been rewarding; I have observed major benefits in pain relief and no adverse effects. My indications for biceps tenotomy are a poor-quality biceps tendon with a partial tear greater than 50%. I consider tenotomy in this situation whether the rotator cuff is intact or torn. I tend to perform tenotomy more frequently if the patient is older or less active or if the nondominant arm is involved. Larger patients with less muscle definition note no cosmetic deformity.

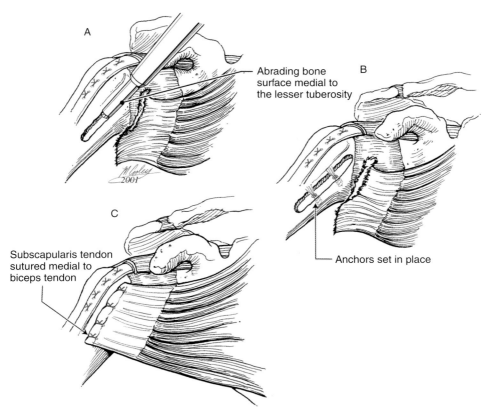

FIGURE 5–70. *A to C,* Subscapularis repair if necessary.

If the rotator cuff is intact, I establish two intra-articular anterior portals. I insert arthroscopic forceps through the anterior inferior cannula, grasp the biceps tendon, and pull the tendon into the glenohumeral joint as much as possible. I hold the tendon in this position, insert scissors through the anterior superior portal, and divide the tendon as far distally as possible. I then grasp the remaining stump of tendon distally and incise it near the superior labrum. The tendon stump is then retrieved out through the anterior inferior cannula. If the rotator cuff is torn, I perform tenotomy with the foregoing technique before I repair the rotator cuff.

Postoperative Treatment

Post-operative treatment for partial-thickness biceps tendon tears that are repaired and for tenodesis is similar to that for a full-thickness rotator cuff tear. However, passive range of motion (particularly external rotation) is allowed only within the safe limits recorded at the time of operation. I discourage active elbow flexion for 6 weeks. If I perform tenotomy, I make no changes in the normal postoperative rehabilitation for a rotator cuff repair.

Discussion

This technique of biceps tenodesis is applicable when the tendon is partially ruptured or subluxed. It is not applica-ble with complete rupture, because the distal tendon ordi-narily cannot be identified arthroscopically, and I prefer conventional open technique. The long-term results of tenotomy are unknown, and my enthusiasm is tempered by this knowledge. Nonetheless, tenotomy appears to offer excellent pain relief and improved function in selected patients.

Bibliography

Proximal Biceps Lesions (SLAP)

Gartsman GM, Taverna, E: The incidence of glenohumeral joint abnor-malities associated with full-thickness, reparable rotator cuff tears. Arthroscopy 13:450–455, 1997.

Kohn D: The clinical relevance of glenoid labrum lesions. Arthroscopy 3:223–230, 1987.

Maffet MW, Gartsman GM, Moseley B: Superior labrum–biceps tendon complex lesions of the shoulder. Am J Sports Med 23:93–98, 1995.

Morgan CD, Burkhart SS, Palmeri M, Gillespie M: Type II SLAP lesions: Three subtypes and their relationships to superior instability and rota-tor cuff tears. Arthroscopy 14:553–565, 1998.

Pagnani MJ, Deng XH, Warren RF, et al: Effect of lesions of the superior portion of the glenoid labrum on glenohumeral translation. J Bone Joint Surg Am 77:1003–1010, 1995.

Rodosky MW, Rudert MJ, Harner CH, et al: Significance of a superior labral lesion of the shoulder: A biomechanical study. Trans Orthop Res Soc 15:276, 1990.

Snyder SJ, Karzel RP, Del Pizzo W, et al: SLAP lesions of the shoulder. Arthroscopy 6:274–279, 1990.

Snyder SJ, Banas MP, Karzel RP: An analysis of 140 injuries to the superior glenoid labrum. J Shoulder Elbow Surg 4:243–248, 1995.

Vangsness CT Jr, Jorgenson SS, Watson T, Johnson DL: The origin of the long head of the biceps from the scapula and glenoid labrum: An anatomical study of 100 shoulders. J Bone Joint Surg Br 76B (6):951–954, 1994.

Walch G, Noel E, Donell ST: Impingement of the deep surface of the supraspinatus tendon on the posterosuperior glenoid rim: An arthroscopic study. J Shoulder Elbow Surg 1:238–245, 1992.

Biceps Lesions—Tendon Substance

Boileau P, Krishnan SG, Coste JS, Walch G: Arthroscopic biceps tenodesis: A new technique using bioabsorbable interference screw fixation. Tech Shoulder Elbow Surg 2:153–165, 2001

Dines DM, Warren RF, Inglis AE: Surgical treatment of lesions of the long head of the biceps. Clin Orthop 164:165–171, 1982.

Hitchcock HH, Bechtol CO: Painful shoulder: Observation on the role of the tendon of the long head of the biceps brachii in its causation. J Bone Joint Surg Am 30:263–273, 1948.

Gartsman GM, Hammerman SM: Arthroscopic biceps tenodesis: Operative technique. Arthroscopy 16:550–552, 2000.

Gartsman GM, Khan M, Hammerman SM: Arthroscopic repair of full-thickness rotator cuff tears. J Bone Joint Surg Am 80:832–840, 1998.

Neer CS: Anterior acromioplasty for the chronic impingement syndrome in the shoulder: A preliminary report. J Bone Joint Surg Am 54:41–50, 1972.

O'Donoghue DH: Subluxing biceps tendon in the athlete. Clin Orthop 184:26–34, 1982.

Post M: Primary tendinitis of the long head of the biceps. Clin Orthop 246:117–124, 1988.

Walch G, Boileau P, Noel E, et al: [Surgical treatment of painful shoulders caused by lesions of the rotator cuff and biceps, treatment as a function of lesions: Reflections on the Neer's concept]. Rev Rhum Mal Osteoartic 58:247–257, 1991.

Walch G, Nove-Josserand L, Boileau P, Levigne C: Subluxations and dislocations of the tendon of the long head of the biceps. J Shoulder Elbow Surg 7:100–108, 1998.

6

Stiffness

Four basic conditions produce shoulder stiffness and are amenable to arthroscopic treatment: idiopathic adhesive capsulitis, the diabetic stiff shoulder, post-traumatic stiffness, and postoperative stiffness. I discuss the treatment of the stiff, osteoarthritic shoulder in Chapter 7.

Idiopathic adhesive capsulitis is widely believed to be a painful but self-limiting condition that resolves after 1 to 2 years. Reports suggest that while many patients improve, they have significant limitations of movement and function. Additionally, many patients suffering from disabling pain are unwilling to wait for their condition to resolve and inquire about operative treatment. Shoulder stiffness in patients with diabetes seems to cause greater pain and is more refractory to nonoperative treatment than idiopathic stiffness. The impairment from post-traumatic stiffness is related directly to the severity of the trauma. Post-operative stiffness can be the result of excessive scarring in the area of surgical treatment (subacromial adhesions after rotator cuff repair, anterior glenohumeral capsular contracture after a Bankart procedure), but I have also seen profound glenohumeral joint contracture after surgical treatment that does not violate the capsule (Figs. 6–1 to 6–3).

Arthroscopic technique is advantageous in that it enables the surgeon to release intra-articular and subacromial and subdeltoid adhesions without dividing the subscapularis. Active range of motion can be started immediately postoperatively without concern for tendon dehiscence.

Literature Review

Olgilvie-Harris, Harryman, and Warner have published landmark articles describing their results. The results of arthroscopic treatment are generally successful, with the degree of improvement related to the patient's underlying condition.

Warner reported on 23 patients with idiopathic adhesive capsulitis treated with arthroscopic release. In that study,

the Constant score improved an average of 48 points. Flexion improved a mean of 49 degrees, external rotation 45 degrees, and internal rotation by eight spinous processes. Harryman documented improved patient satisfaction, function, and pain relief in a population of patients with diabetes, although the range-of-motion improvement was not as great as that seen in patients with idiopathic adhesive capsulitis.

Clinical Presentation

Patients with all types of adhesive capsulitis present with painful, limited shoulder motion. Pain at night interferes with sleep, and routine activities of daily living that require reaching overhead or behind the back are difficult and

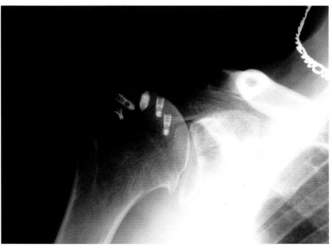

FIGURE 6–1. Postsurgical stiffness rotator cuff repair.

painful. Rapid movements cause especially severe pain. Most patients either recall a trivial antecedent injury or cannot recall an inciting event. Patients demonstrate both restricted passive and active motion such that the motion is usually less than 50% of that of the contralateral shoulder. Radiographs are normal, but mild osteopenia from disuse is typical.

Diagnosis

Numerous other shoulder conditions produce painful limited motion, but these are eliminated by patient history, physical examination, and radiographic evaluation. Patients with rotator cuff tears present with passive motion greater than active motion, weakness evident on manual muscle testing, and abnormal magnetic resonance imaging scans or arthrograms. Patients with osteoarthrosis have plain radiographs depicting loss of glenohumeral joint space (Fig. 6–4). Patients with post-traumatic stiffness may have malunited fractures, and those with postoperative stiffness may have internal fixation interfering with motion.

A thorough history that ascertains prior trauma or shoulder difficulties is important. Patients should be queried about diabetes and thyroid dysfunction. Evaluate and record passive range of motion in elevation, abduction, and external rotation (in adduction with the patient's arm at the side and in maximum allowable abduction). Measure internal rotation as the vertebral level to which the patient can reach with the extended thumb. Behind-the-back internal rotation is usually decreased, but occasionally it may be close to normal because internal rotation measured in this manner includes not only glenohumeral movement but also scapulothoracic motion. With prolonged shoulder stiffness, the scapulothoracic motion may be increased in order to compensate for the loss of glenohumeral rotation. For this reason, I use a more sensitive technique. I stabilize the scapula with one hand and abduct the arm as much as possible with the other. This maneuver eliminates scapulothoracic motion. I then record external and internal rotation in

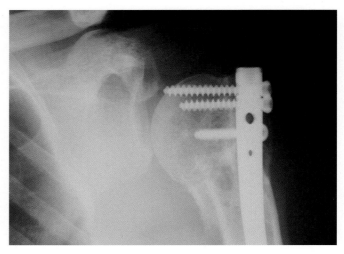

FIGURE 6–3. Post-traumatic and postsurgical stiffness after open reduction and internal fixation.

this maximally abducted position and compare it with the contralateral shoulder. I assess muscle strength in elevation and external rotation, and I obtain anterior posterior, axillary, and supraspinatus (scapular) outlet plain radiographs.

Indications

As a general principle, I consider operation if the patient has persistent pain and stiffness after 6 months of appropriate nonoperative care. I define severe stiffness as 0 degrees of external rotation and less then 30 degrees of abduction and moderate stiffness as a decrease of 30 degrees in either plane when compared with the contralateral shoulder. Although loss of internal rotation is clinically significant to the patient, I do not consider a loss of internal rotation in any plane as an indication for arthroscopic release. One exception is the throwing athlete. In these

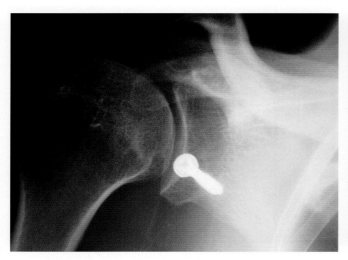

FIGURE 6–2. Postsurgical stiffness after a Bristow procedure.

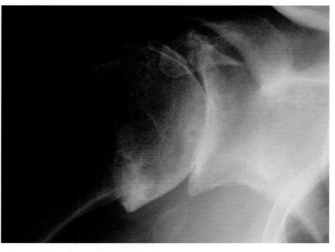

FIGURE 6–4. Osteoarthrosis.

patients, posterior contracture and decreased internal rotation may be the only lesion. I discuss the management of this special group in Chapter 5. If at 6 months stiffness persists, but pain has diminished, I continue nonoperative care for an additional 2 months in the event that the decrease in pain indicates that the stiffness is about to resolve or "thaw" spontaneously. If there is no improvement in the range of motion 2 months later, I consider operation. I have found external rotation to be the most important predictor of success or failure of nonoperative treatment. If at 4 to 6 months after the start of nonoperative treatment external rotation remains at neutral or worse, I do not recommend further nonoperative care, and I consider operation. I believe that persistent external rotation loss of such a degree indicates a stiff shoulder that will not respond to nonoperative care; therefore, earlier operative intervention is advisable.

Contraindications

Contraindications for arthroscopic treatment exist mainly in patients with postoperative and post-traumatic stiffness. Patients who have had surgical procedures for instability with subscapularis takedown or shortening may develop profound soft tissue contracture. The contracture in these patients is typically extra-articular between the subscapularis and the conjoined tendon. I have found open release a necessary addition to arthroscopic glenohumeral joint release. Patients with mildly malunited greater tuberosity or proximal humerus fractures can be treated arthroscopically, but patients with badly malunited fractures or internal fixation require open release, removal of hardware, and fracture osteotomy, as indicated. Patients in the inflammatory or contracting phase of idiopathic adhesive capsulitis should not undergo an operation because the surgical procedure may further accelerate the contracture. I measure range of motion sequentially and wait until the motion has stabilized.

Operative Technique

VIDEO
— **Contracture Release**

Examination under Anesthesia

After induction of anesthesia in the patient, examine both shoulders for range of motion in elevation, in abduction, and in external rotation in adduction. Place the shoulder in maximum abduction, and record internal and external rotation.

Manipulation

Before arthroscopic treatment, I attempt gentle closed manipulation. It is difficult to quantify the term "gentle," but I apply only a small amount of force to the shoulder in abduction and then in elevation. If the shoulder will respond to closed manipulation, it will move with minimal force. If I believe that motion is improving with abduction

and elevation, only then do I attempt to rotate the shoulder externally. Externally rotate the shoulder in maximum abduction and then in adduction. If motion continues to improve, begin internal rotation stretching. First internally rotate the shoulder in maximum abduction, and if the motion improves, then stretch the shoulder in cross-body adduction and finally in behind-the-back internal rotation. I believe the specific order of the motions is important because external rotation and internal rotation involve torsional stresses and can cause a spiral fracture to the humerus. If the shoulder does not respond to abduction and elevation, I do not attempt any rotational movements and proceed directly to arthroscopy. If the shoulder responds to manipulation but full movement is not achieved, I proceed to arthroscopy and release the remaining adhesions. If full range of motion is obtained after manipulation, I insert the arthroscope and confirm that the capsule is released completely. Some shoulders with full range of motion after manipulation have persistent capsular contracture. I believe that the manipulation only releases the extra-articular adhesions.

Joint Entry

Entry into the stiff shoulder is always difficult because, by definition, the joint volume is reduced. Forceful entry may damage the articular surfaces of either the glenoid or the humeral head.

The tight joint is difficult to identify with a spinal needle because the tight, thickened posterior capsule makes needle entry difficult and the generalized capsular stiffness limits the amount of fluid that can be injected. I have had better success with a standard metal cannula and a rounded trocar. Because the cannula and trocar are larger and stiffer than the spinal needle, I can palpate the posterior glenohumeral joint line with greater ease. The entry position is critical. Joint entry through the traditional "soft spot" (located at the level of the glenoid equator) increases the risk of cartilage surface damage. At this level, the glenohumeral joint space is narrowest, so that trocar entry is most difficult.

I prefer to enter the joint superiorly, among the superior glenoid, the rotator cuff, and the humeral head, where the joint space is wider (Fig. 6–5). Incise the skin and insert the cannula and trocar until you palpate bone. Then rotate the shoulder internally and externally as much as possible to determine whether the trocar tip rests on the humeral head (movement detected) or glenoid (no movement). I lower my hand (and elevate the trocar tip) until I can palpate the superior glenoid rim. Only then do I attempt to enter the joint (Fig. 6–6).

Once the arthroscope is in the glenohumeral joint, it is directed at the rotator interval. I insert a spinal needle percutaneously, lateral to the coracoid process, until I can see the needle enter the joint. I incise the skin and insert a plastic 5-mm cannula and trocar.

Rotator Interval

The first step in the operation is release of the rotator interval (Figs. 6–7 and 6–8). I use a motorized soft tissue resector to perform this step. The resector is inserted through the

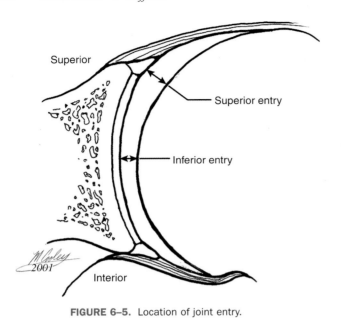

FIGURE 6–5. Location of joint entry.

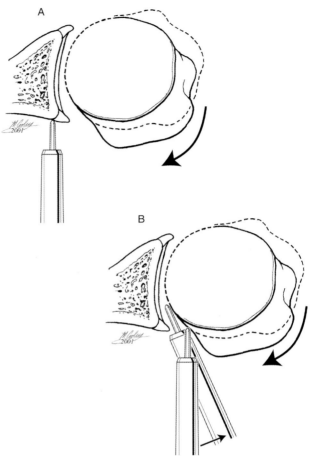

FIGURE 6–6. Palpate bone to determine entry point.

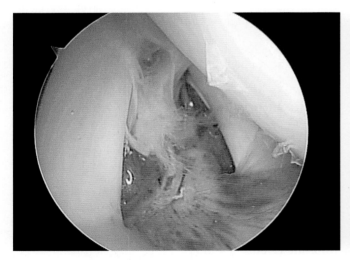

FIGURE 6–7. Contracted rotator interval.

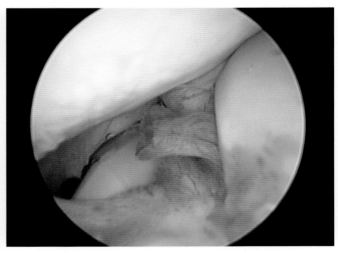

FIGURE 6–8. Synovitis rotator interval.

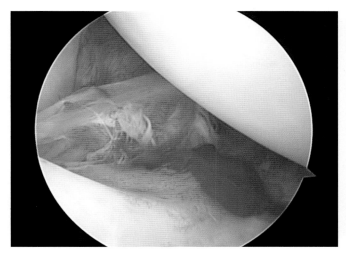

FIGURE 6–9. Contracted anterior capsule.

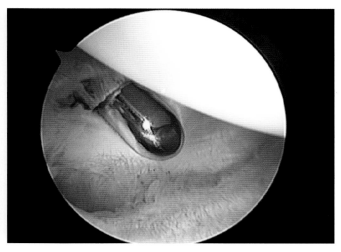

FIGURE 6–10. Identify superior portion middle glenohumeral ligament.

cannula into the joint, and then the cannula is backed out of the joint, to leave the resector tip in the rotator interval. Soft tissue is excised from an area bounded by the biceps tendon medially, by the superior border of the subscapularis tendon inferiorly, and by the humeral head laterally. Reintroduce the cannula into the joint, and remove the resector. Withdraw the arthroscope from the posterior cannula in the joint, to leave the cannula indwelling, and attempt a closed manipulation as described earlier. If full range of motion is obtained, reintroduce the arthroscope posteriorly, and verify that the capsule is divided and the humeral head is properly located. If full range of motion is not achieved, or if motion has improved but the capsule is not completely divided, proceed to the next step.

Anterior Capsule

Identify the point where the middle glenohumeral ligament crosses the subscapularis tendon (Fig. 6–9). It is important to separate the subscapularis tendon from the middle glenohumeral ligament, and I find electrocautery helpful to divide fibers of the middle glenohumeral ligament gradually until the tendinous portion of the superior subscapularis is visualized. Then insert a blunt dissector anterior to the middle glenohumeral ligament to separate the two structures. I use a Harryman soft tissue punch (Smith & Nephew Endoscopy, Andover, MA) to remove a 5- to 10-mm strip of anterior capsule. This includes the middle glenohumeral ligament and the superior portion of the anterior inferior glenohumeral ligament. Electrocautery may be used as an alternative for this portion of the procedure (Figs. 6–10 to 6–17). Usually, a small amount of increased lateral humeral head displacement results, and I then advance the arthroscope anteriorly and inferiorly so that I may see the posterior portion of the anterior inferior glenohumeral ligament and the inferior capsule more clearly. Advance the punch, place the bottom, blunt jaw exterior to the capsule, and divide it from anterior to posterior as far from the glenoid labrum as possible (Figs. 6–18 and 6–19). The level at which I stop the inferior anterior

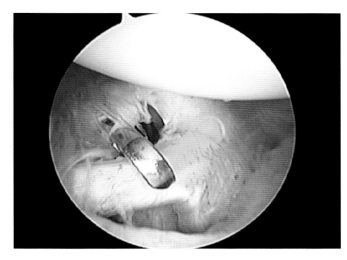

FIGURE 6–11. Divide superior portion middle glenohumeral ligament.

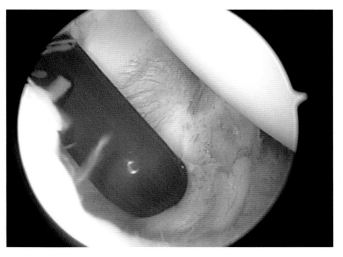

FIGURE 6–12. Cautery to middle glenohumeral ligament covering subscapularis.

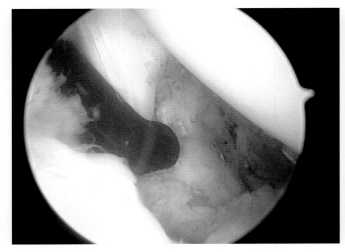

FIGURE 6–13. Cautery to middle glenohumeral ligament covering subscapularis.

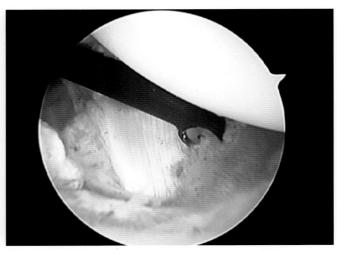

FIGURE 6–14. Cautery to middle glenohumeral ligament covering subscapularis.

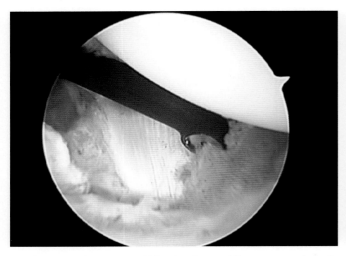

FIGURE 6–15. Cautery to middle glenohumeral ligament covering subscapularis.

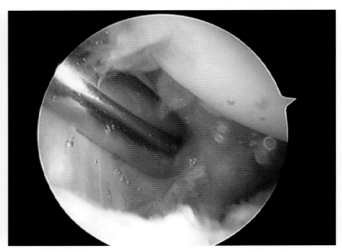

FIGURE 6–16. Blunt dissector anterior to subscapularis.

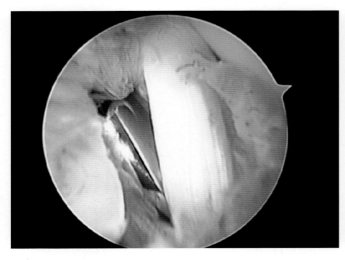

FIGURE 6–17. Blunt dissector posterior to subscapularis.

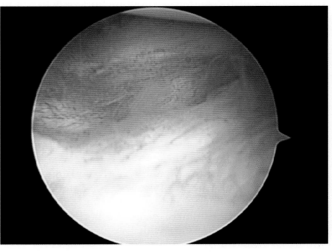

FIGURE 6–18. Contracted inferior capsule.

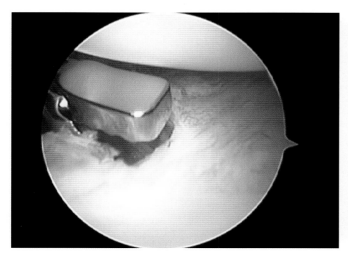

FIGURE 6–19. Capsular punch, anterior inferior capsule.

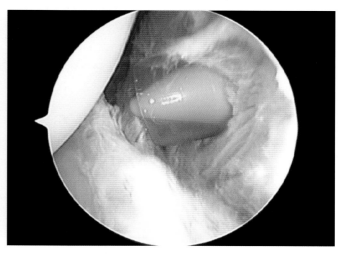

FIGURE 6–21. Insert large cannula posteriorly.

release depends on the amount of axillary pouch contracture. The tight pouch limits the degree to which I can safely advance the punch without applying excessive distraction to the glenohumeral joint. This is usually about the 5-o'clock position for a right shoulder. To gain access to and to release the axillary pouch safely, I then treat the posterior and inferior posterior areas of the capsule.

I remove the soft tissue punch and cannula from the anterior portal and insert a metal cannula and trocar in their place. I remove the arthroscope from the posterior portal and insert it anteriorly. Under direct vision, I insert the small plastic cannula and trocar posteriorly. The glenohumeral joint is usually too tightly contracted to allow me to insert a larger-diameter cannula. I insert a motorized shaver and resect 5 to 10 mm of posterior capsule, beginning superiorly and moving inferiorly (Fig. 6–20). Once I have resected the posterior capsule, I can easily insert a large-diameter cannula that will accommodate the capsular resection punch (Figs. 6–21 and 6–22).

I insert the punch and resect a 10-mm strip of the poste-rior inferior capsule. I resect the capsule 5 to 10 mm from the glenoid labrum to avoid any labral damage. The last step in the intra-articular portion of the procedure is complete release of the inferior capsule. Often, surgical division is not necessary because the last portion of the capsule may be released through a manipulation. I often use manipulation, to avoid placing instruments near the axillary nerve.

After I manipulate the shoulder, I reinsert the arthroscope to inspect the gap between the resected edges of the capsule and to confirm that the humeral head is normally located. If I cannot gain full range of motion with manipulation, I insert the arthroscope posteriorly and the cannula and punch anteriorly and resect the inferior capsule (Figs. 6–23 to 6–25).

Subscapularis

I do not believe there is any harm if the surgeon resects the superior tendinous border of the subscapularis to achieve

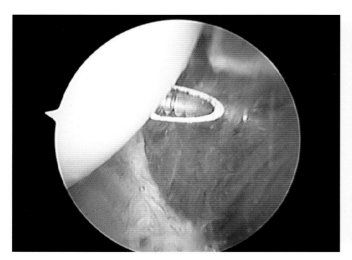

FIGURE 6–20. Shaver resecting posterior capsule.

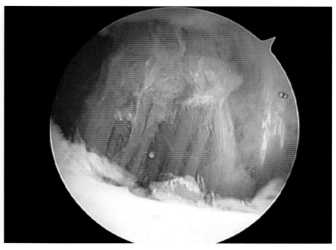

FIGURE 6–22. Complete posterior capsular resection with punch.

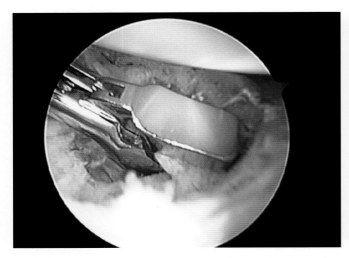

FIGURE 6–23. Return arthroscope to posterior portal and complete inferior capsular resection.

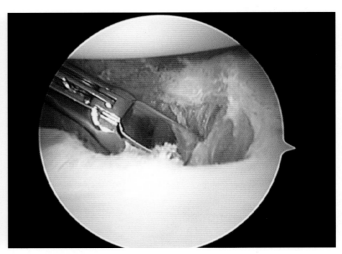

FIGURE 6–25. Inferior capsular resection.

full passive range of motion. I always use a blunt dissector to release any adhesions anterior and posterior to the subscapularis.

Subacromial Space

Introduce the arthroscope into the subacromial space. If the subacromial space is not clearly seen, insert a motorized soft tissue resector and remove bursa and adhesions (Fig. 6–26).

I do not advise an acromioplasty even if there is arthroscopic evidence of impingement, such as rotator cuff or coracoacromial ligament fraying. By definition, the patient with adhesive capsulitis cannot move the shoulder into the positions consistent with the clinical diagnosis of impingement. The raw acromial bone surface produced after acromioplasty creates the opportunity for postoperative adhesions and should be avoided.

Postoperative Care

I use the following pharmacologic techniques to reduce postoperative inflammation and adhesion formation. After I confirm the diagnosis of shoulder stiffness resulting from capsular contracture arthroscopically but before soft tissue resection, the anesthesiologist gives the patient 100 mg of hydrocortisone intravenously. I do not use intra-articular cortisone at the conclusion of the procedure because I believe that operative resection of the capsule will cause the steroid to extravasate and to lose its effectiveness. In patients with post-traumatic or postsurgical stiffness with subacromial adhesions requiring release, I inject 1 mg of hydrocortisone (Solu-Cortef) into the subacromial space at the conclusion of the operation. Postoperatively, I place the patient on a methylprednisolone (Medrol) dose pack. I do not use steroids in patients with diabetes.

Do not place the patient in a sling or immobilizer. Place

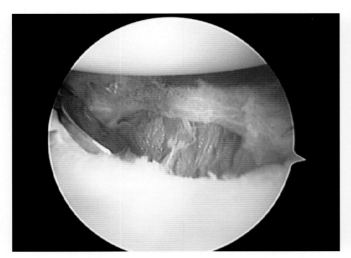

FIGURE 6–24. Inferior capsular resection.

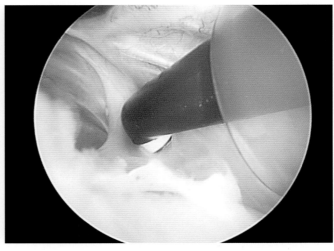

FIGURE 6–26. Remove subacromial adhesions if present.

a pillow under the axilla to keep the arm away from the chest, and encourage the patient and nursing staff to avoid placing the patient's arm in internal rotation. I admit patients to the hospital overnight. I use a continuous passive motion chair to maintain the full range of motion gained during the surgical procedure. Continuous passive motion begins the afternoon of the operation. I find it extremely helpful to visit the patient on the afternoon of the surgical procedure and to demonstrate that the patient now has full range of motion. This is easily done because the patient's shoulder is still anesthetized from the interscalene block. This visual demonstration of full movement impresses on the patient that the operation was successful. I emphasize that complete recovery depends on the patient's adherence to the postoperative rehabilitation program. On discharge from the hospital, the patient uses the chair four times daily for 1 hour each session. This regimen continues for 2 weeks. I then see the patient in the clinic, and if movement is satisfactory, the continuous passive motion chair is discontinued. Passive elevation while the patient is supine and external rotation with the aid of a dowel or pulley are continued. The patient is encouraged to use the arm actively for all activities and motions that are comfortable. I see the patient again at 6 weeks, 3 months, and 6 months postoperatively.

If the patient has not achieved full range of motion by 3 months, I offer a repeat contracture release. At this point, however, usually only gentle closed manipulation is necessary.

Bibliography

Griggs SM, Ahn A, Green A: Idiopathic adhesive capsulitis: A prospective functional outcome study of nonoperative treatment. J Bone Joint Surg 82:1398–1407, 2000.

Harryman DT, II: Arthroscopic management of shoulder stiffness. Oper Tech Sports Med 5:264–274, 1997.

Harryman DT, II: Shoulders: Frozen and stiff. Instr Course Lect 42:247–257, 1993.

Harryman DT, II, Matsen FA, III, Sidles JA: Arthroscopic management of refractory shoulder stiffness. Arthroscopy 13:133–147, 1997.

Ogilvie-Harris DJ, Myerthall S: The diabetic frozen shoulder: Arthroscopic release. Arthroscopy 13:1–8, 1997.

Scarlat MM, Harryman DT, II: Management of the diabetic stiff shoulder. Instr Course Lect 49:283–293, 2000.

Warner JJP: Frozen shoulder: Diagnosis and management. J Am Acad Orthop Surg 5:130–140, 1997.

Warner JJP, Answorth A, Marks PH, Wong P: Arthroscopic release for chronic refractory adhesive capsulitis of the shoulder. J Bone Joint Surg Am 78:1808–1816, 1996.

Warner JJP, Greis P E: The treatment of stiffness of the shoulder after repair of the rotator cuff. J Bone Joint Surg Am 79:1260–1269, 1997.

Warner JJP, Allen AA, Marks PH, Wong P: Arthroscopic release of postoperative capsular contracture of the shoulder. J Bone Joint Surg 79A:1151–1158, 1997.

7

Arthrosis— Glenohumeral Joint

Arthroscopic treatment of glenohumeral arthrosis is a controversial subject with little scientific evidence to guide the orthopedic surgeon. Currently, limited surgical options are available, but with increased knowledge and technology this will inevitably change. The surgeon will encounter lesions that include minor areas of chondromalacia in patients with glenohumeral instability and areas of full-thickness cartilage loss, as well as osteophytes in patients with avascular necrosis, rheumatoid arthritis, or osteoarthrosis.

Diagnosis

The diagnosis of osteoarthrosis, rheumatoid arthritis, or avascular necrosis is made clinically with a combination of patient history, physical examination, laboratory tests, and plain radiographs. I do not use arthroscopy to evaluate the glenohumeral joint and to "stage" the disease. In some situations, the cartilage lesions are unsuspected and are encountered during arthroscopic treatment for impingement, rotator cuff tear, or glenohumeral instability.

Nonoperative Treatment

Nonoperative treatment is largely palliative and consists of medication to diminish the inflammatory response and physical therapy to maintain or improve shoulder range of motion and strength.

Indications

Surgical indications vary with the underlying disease process. Arthroscopic synovectomy may be beneficial in the treatment of early rheumatoid arthritis. Synovectomy may retard the disease process and produce results similar to

those seen in treatment of the rheumatoid knee, elbow, and wrist (Fig. 7–1).

The earliest stage of avascular necrosis may be amenable to arthroscopic débridement and humeral head drilling. Before subchondral and articular surface collapse (stage 1 and early stage 2 disease), core decompression may produce outcomes similar to those in the hip. The potential for improved success may be greater than in the hip because the glenohumeral joint is non–weight bearing (Fig. 7–2). Débridement of cartilage flap tears may help the patient with chondromalacia whose symptoms are the result of mechanical locking and catching (Fig. 7–3).

Osteoarthrosis is probably the most common clinical cause of glenohumeral incongruity seen in the office. The source of pain in osteoarthrosis is multifactorial and consists of joint surface irregularity, mechanical disturbances from loose or displaced labrum fragments, loose bodies, synovitis, and joint contracture (Figs. 7–4 and 7–5).

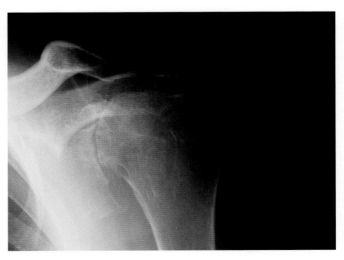

FIGURE 7–1. Rheumatoid arthritis.

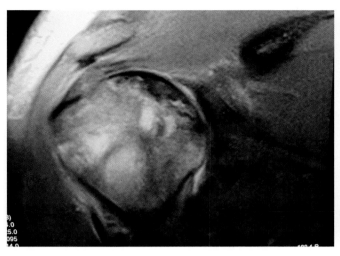

FIGURE 7–2. Avascular necrosis.

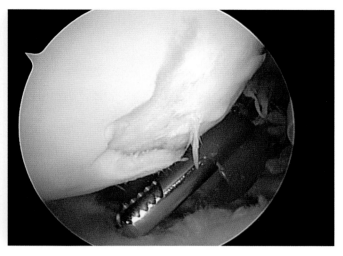

FIGURE 7–3. Débridement of cartilage fragments.

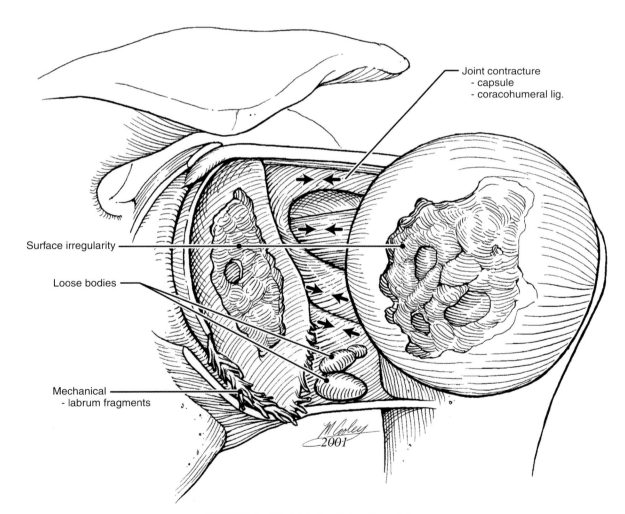

FIGURE 7–4. Sources of pain in osteoarthrosis.

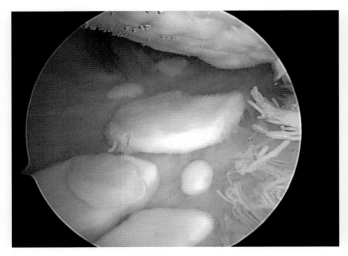

FIGURE 7–5. Loose bodies.

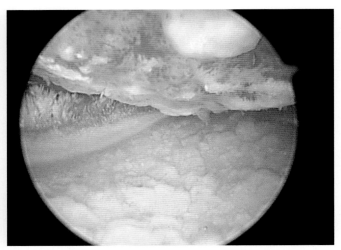

FIGURE 7–6. Osteoarthrosis at arthroscopy.

Arthroscopic lavage has been reported to achieve temporary limited benefit in pain relief because of either the placebo effect or alterations in the chemical composition of the glenohumeral joint fluid. The patient returns to the baseline state relatively quickly, and I do not perform or advise such a procedure. If the surgeon wishes to treat a patient with glenohumeral arthrosis arthroscopically, I believe the approach must be comprehensive and must include removal of loose bodies and labrum fragments, release of soft tissue contracture, and the restoration of joint surface congruity including the débridement of glenoid and humeral head osteophytes if necessary. Unless the surgeon is prepared for and is capable of dealing with all the factors involved, an arthroscopic approach seems unwarranted. The surgeon must also carefully explain the investigational nature of the procedure to the patient. Within these confines, I believe there are limited indications for arthroscopic treatment.

Contraindications

Contraindications to the arthroscopic treatment of arthrosis also vary with the underlying disease process. Synovectomy does not benefit the patient with articular incongruity. Core decompression cannot be expected to reverse bone collapse. Débridement of a small labrum tear will not help the patient with osteoarthrosis. I have also encountered many patients with pain and stiffness from osteoarthritis who had previously undergone a manipulation. This approach is not usually successful. Orthopedic surgeons must appreciate that although patients with idiopathic adhesive capsulitis and osteoarthritis have pain and decreased range of motion, these disorders have different causes and require different treatment. Patients with arthrosis have capsular contractures, as do patients with adhesive capsulitis, but they also have articular incongruity as an important cause of their shoulder stiffness.

Chondral Lesions

My approach is conservative for chondral lesions. I remove loose pieces and flap tears but do not drill or microfracture the bone surface. I gently abrade areas of cortical bone.

Osteoarthritis: Operative Technique

— Glenohumeral Joint Arthrosis

After the administration of anesthesia to the patient, I examine the shoulder for range of motion but do not attempt a closed manipulation (Figs. 7–6 and 7–7). I estab-

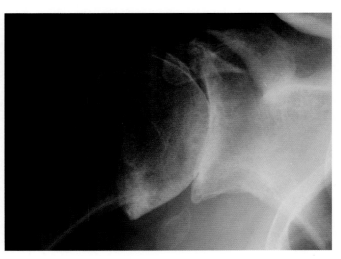

FIGURE 7–7. Osteoarthrosis.

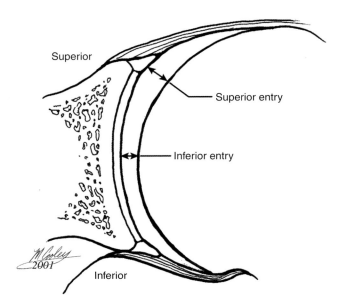

FIGURE 7–8. Greater space for trocar at superior aspect of glenohumeral joint.

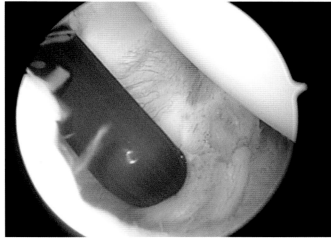

FIGURE 7–10. Cautery to define plane between subscapularis and middle glenohumeral ligament.

lish standard posterior and anterior portals and perform a complete glenohumeral joint inspection, observing particularly areas and degree of cartilage loss, labrum flap tears, rotator cuff fraying or tearing, and capsular contracture.

Entry into the glenohumeral joint is always difficult because of the loss of joint space from absent articular cartilage and soft tissue contracture. I insert the posterior cannula and trocar first and place the entry point more superiorly than normal, just inferior to the posterior acromion about 2 cm medial to the posterolateral acromial corner. The superior portal allows easier access to the glenohumeral joint at the level of the superior glenoid, so that the trocar does not have to enter the joint between the humeral head and the glenoid (Fig. 7–8). I prefer a plastic cannula and trocar to minimize articular damage, but often the capsule is so thick that the plastic trocar will not pene-

trate it. The anterior capsule is also difficult to penetrate, and sometimes it is necessary to use only the metal trocar (without the cannula) to create an entrance to the glenohumeral joint. I use a standard shaver to débride the rotator interval and to débride any labrum tears (Fig. 7–9).

I then perform a complete capsular release anteriorly, posteriorly, and inferiorly. I pay particular attention to the subscapularis because my experience with shoulder arthroplasty has convinced me how critical it is to restore subscapularis muscle excursion. The middle glenohumeral ligament is adherent to the posterior (articular) surface of the subscapularis, and I use cautery to identify the plane between the two structures (Fig. 7–10). Scissors are useful to divide firm bands of scar tissue, and I then use a blunt dissector to sweep any adhesions off the subscapularis muscle. The next step is to release adhesions from the anterior surface of the subscapularis, and for this maneuver I find the blunt dissector particularly useful (Fig. 7–11).

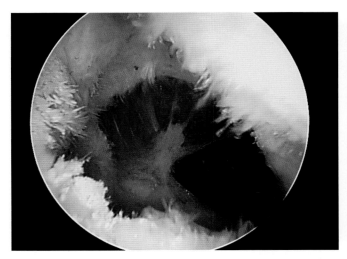

FIGURE 7–9. Rotator interval débridement.

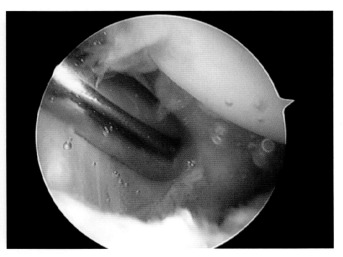

FIGURE 7–11. Soft tissue dissection anterior and posterior to subscapularis.

The third area of subscapularis release involves the connections between the subscapularis and coracoid. This portion of the operation is performed with the arthroscope in the glenohumeral joint after the rotator interval has been opened. The coracohumeral ligament is thickened and contracted and limits subscapularis excursion. This area is not normally seen during routine glenohumeral joint arthroscopy, but it can be visualized arthroscopically with the technique described later. After I excise the contracted tissue, open the rotator interval, and remove adhesions from the anterior and posterior surfaces of the subscapularis, the coracoid process comes into view. With scissors or a blunt dissector, I release any connections between the superior surface of the subscapularis and the coracoid.

The anterior and posterior capsular releases are similar to those I perform for adhesive capsulitis release, but the inferior release is different. With adhesive capsulitis, the inferior capsule can often be released by shoulder manipulation after the division of the anterior and posterior capsule. Patients with arthrosis have an extremely thickened inferior capsule, and such an approach is not successful. The inferior capsule must be divided with a capsular resector. This requires that the surgeon release the anterior inferior capsule from an anterior approach and the posterior inferior capsule from a posterior approach (Figs. 7–12 to 7–14). This step completes the soft tissue release, and I turn my attention to the bone surfaces of the glenoid and the humeral head.

The degree and type of glenoid wear are seen on preoperative imaging studies. Basically, two types of glenoid abnormalities are amenable to arthroscopic treatment. The first occurs when the glenoid conforms to the humeral head but the space is diminished. My goal is to increase space between the two structures. The second glenoid abnormality occurs when there is posterior glenoid erosion or step-off, usually resulting from chronic anterior contracture and posterior humeral head subluxation. Inspect the radiographs to determine both glenohumeral congruency and glenoid bone stock.

To create more space between the humeral head and a conforming glenoid, I place the arthroscope posteriorly and

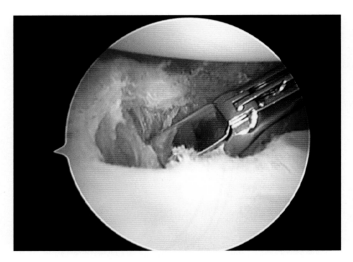

FIGURE 7–13. Inferior posterior capsular release.

the round bur through the anterior cannula. I begin removing bone 10 mm from the superior glenoid, and I remove a 2-mm strip from anterior to posterior. I then remove bone from that strip to the superior glenoid margin and take care not to damage the biceps-labrum anchor. I complete the glenoid bone removal by evening the glenoid from superior to inferior. It is usually necessary at some point to move the arthroscope anteriorly and the bur posteriorly to reach all areas of the glenoid and to create a level surface (Fig. 7–15).

To create a conforming glenoid surface when there is a posterior step-off, I follow the same general technique as described earlier, but I usually begin with the arthroscope in the posterior cannula and the power bur in the anterior cannula. I then remove the anterior surface from superior to inferior to eliminate the step-off and to create a smooth, uniform surface (Figs. 7–16 to 7–20).

After operation, patients begin continuous passive motion in a motorized chair. Patients undergo 1-hour sessions in the chair, four times daily for 2 weeks. During this

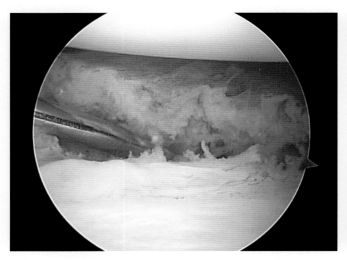

FIGURE 7–12. Anterior inferior capsular release.

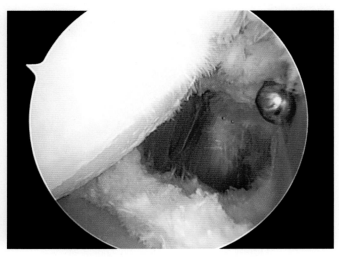

FIGURE 7–14. Posterior capsular release.

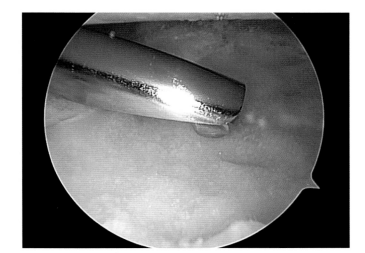

FIGURE 7–15. Bur in posterior portal. View from anterior portal.

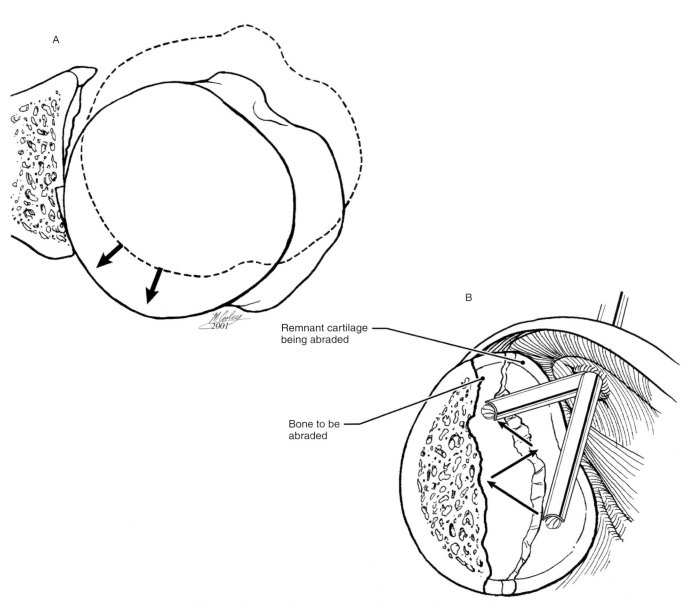

Remnant cartilage
being abraded

Bone to be
abraded

FIGURE 7–16. *A* and *B*, Posterior step-off and area of bone abrasion.

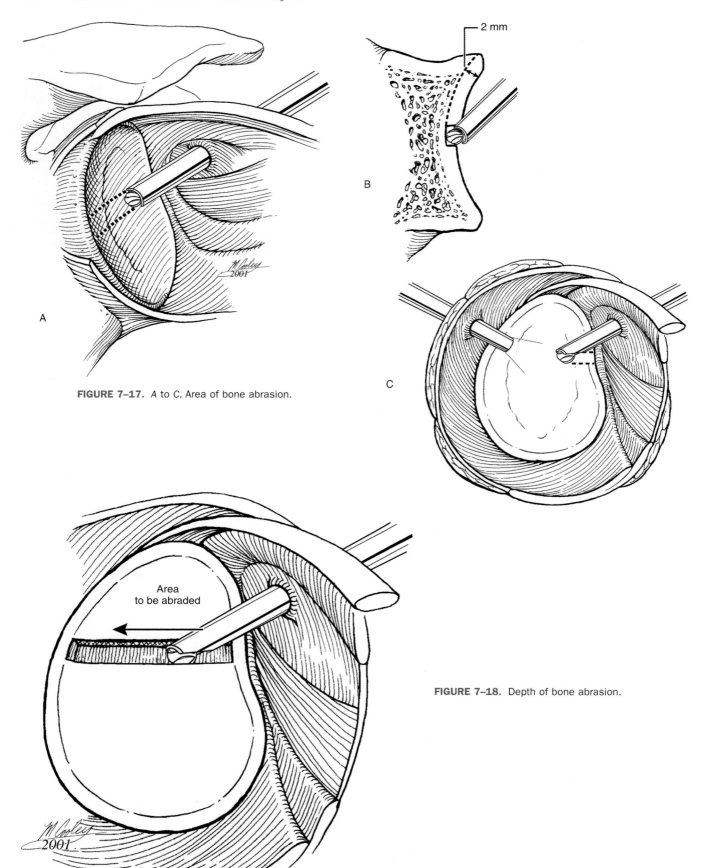

FIGURE 7–17. *A to C,* Area of bone abrasion.

Area
to be abraded

FIGURE 7–18. Depth of bone abrasion.

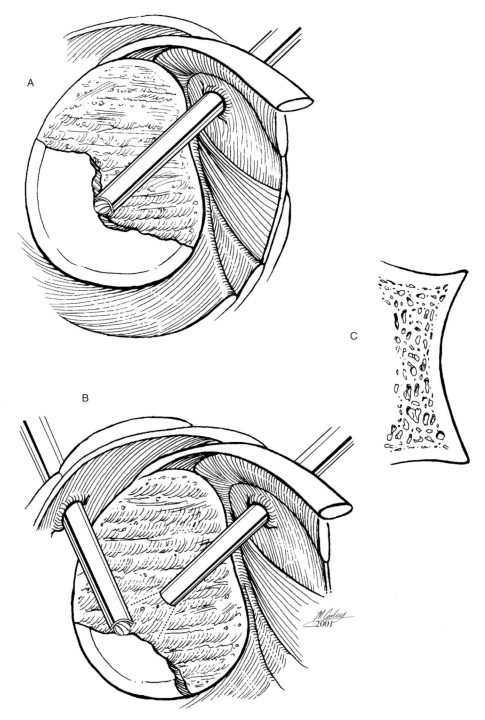

FIGURE 7–19. *A* to *C*, Abrasion arthroplasty.

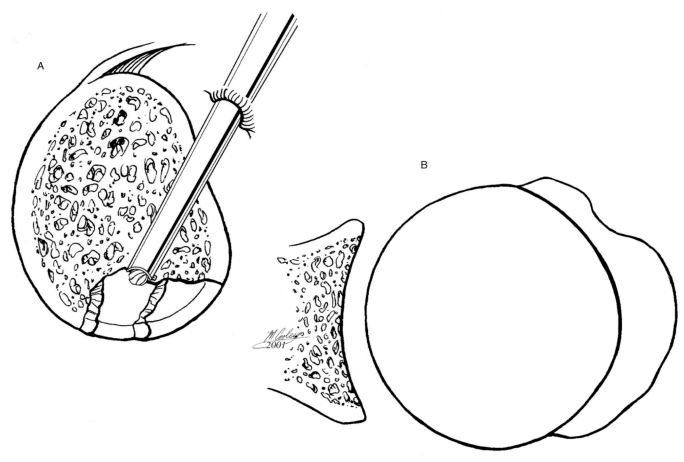

FIGURE 7–20. *A* and *B*, Completed abrasion arthroplasty.

time, active range of motion and activities are encouraged as much as pain allows. I continue to emphasize range of motion at each patient visit and start strengthening exercises when manual muscle testing is painless. To monitor disease progression, plain anterior posterior and axillary radiographs are obtained every 3 months for the first year, every 6 months for the next year, and then yearly.

The results are preliminary in this carefully selected and counseled group of patients, but so far they have been gratifying. Approximately 80% report satisfaction with the procedure and significant decrease in pain and increases in motion and function.

Rheumatoid Arthritis

As in other joints, synovectomy of the rheumatoid shoulder is most beneficial when it is carried out early in the disease before cartilage and bone have been destroyed and the rotator cuff has eroded. The patient's condition is staged according to the Steinbrocker Radiographic and Functional Classification, which is summarized here. Subsequent patient evaluation allows the surgeon to reassess the disease progression.

RADIOGRAPHIC CLASSIFICATION

Stage I: No destructive change; osteoporosis and soft tissue change only
Stage II: Mild or moderate erosive change or joint space reduction
Stage III: Joint markedly narrowed (less than 1 mm); extensive erosion and subluxation
Stage IV: Fibrosis or bony ankylosis

FUNCTIONAL CLASSIFICATION

Class I: Full function
Class II: Adequate function despite pain and limited motion
Class III: Very limited function
Class IV: Wholly incapacitated

The response is assigned to one of four categories:
Grade I: Complete remission
Grade II: Major improvement
Grade III: Minor improvement
Grade IV: No improvement or disease progression

Patients in the first two radiographic states and the first two functional classes have the best chance of benefiting from arthroscopic synovectomy and débridement.

Operative Technique

I enter the glenohumeral joint through a standard posterior portal and establish an anterior inferior and then an anterior superior cannula. Because of the bleeding that often occurs with rheumatoid synovectomy, the addition of the anterior superior cannula for outflow is helpful. A pump is essential. I use grasping forceps to remove large pieces of loose cartilage or soft tissue and a motorized resector to débride labrum flap tears. Because the synovium is vascular, I prefer to use the thermal coagulation probe to "paint" all areas of proliferative synovitis before resection (Fig. 7–21). I find that the whisker resector can allow me to perform a thorough synovectomy without violating the glenohumeral joint capsule (Fig 7–22).

I prefer to start the synovectomy inferiorly and to move to the anterior and then superior aspects of the joint. I move the arthroscope anteriorly and the resector posteriorly to complete soft tissue removal of the posterior inferior and posterior regions. I carefully inspect the subscapularis recess for additional synovitis or loose bodies. I then remove the arthroscope and, through the same posterior incision, insert it into the subacromial space. Bursal proliferation is often profound. I then remove the hypertrophic bursa and perform an arthroscopic subacromial decompression and acromioclavicular joint resection if indicated on clinical examination. Postoperative rehabilitation is identical to that described for treatment of the osteoarthritic glenohumeral joint.

Avascular Necrosis

The rare indication for arthroscopic treatment of avascular necrosis is limited to those patients with stage I or early stage II disease before any collapse has occurred. Based on the experience with core decompression in the hip, I have performed a similar procedure in these patients.

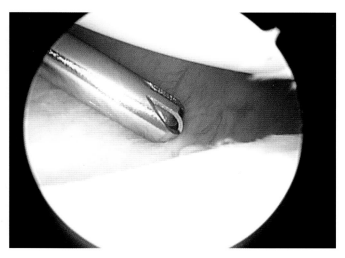

FIGURE 7–22. Whisker resector.

I place the guide pin from a hip compression set on the anterior shoulder and, with the use of fluoroscopic imaging, adjust the angle and direction of the pin until I obtain the correct position. I then mark the pin location on the lateral deltoid and incise the skin with a scalpel. To avoid injury to the axillary nerve, I use a hemostat to spread the deltoid fibers until I reach the lateral humeral cortex. A drill guide is placed into the wound until it rests on the humerus. I use biplane radiographic imaging to insert a guide pin in the center of the humeral head to within 3 mm of the articular surface. I place a cannulated drill over this and, under radiographic control, perform a single core decompression.

Postoperatively, patients are allowed unlimited active and passive range of motion, but no sport activity or heavy lifting is allowed for 3 months. I follow-up the patient with serial radiographs or magnetic resonance imaging studies as needed.

Bibliography

Billon JM, Hutsebaut K: Place de l'arthroscopie dans l'osteonecrose de l'epaule. Acta Orthop Belg 65(Suppl. 1):104, 1999.

Hayes JM: Arthroscopic treatment of steroid-induced osteonecrosis of the humeral head. Arthroscopy 5:218–221, 1989.

L'Insalata JC, Pagnani MJ, Warren RF, Dines DM: Humeral head osteonecrosis: Clinical course and radiographic predictors of outcome. J Shoulder Elbow Surg 5:355–361, 1996.

Mont M, Maar DC, Urquhart MW, et al: Avascular necrosis of the humeral head treated by core decompression. J Bone Joint Surg Br 75:785–788, 1993.

Nakagawa Y, Ueo T, Nakamura T: A novel surgical procedure for osteonecrosis of the humeral head: Reposition of the joint surface and bone engraftment. Arthroscopy 15:433–438, 1999.

Steinbocker O, Traeger CH, Batterman RC: Therapeutic criteria for rheumatoid arthritis. JAMA 140:659, 1949.

Weinstein DM, Bucchieri JS, Pollock RG, et al: Arthroscopic débridement of the shoulder for osteoarthritis. Arthroscopy 16:471–476, 2000.

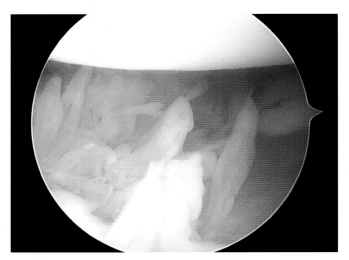

FIGURE 7–21. Rheumatoid synovium.

8

Periarticular Cysts

A recent development in shoulder surgery is treatment of periarticular shoulder cysts. With the increased use of magnetic resonance imaging (MRI), more cysts are diagnosed and more patients are referred for care. It is unknown whether this change represents a true increase in the incidence of cysts or merely reflects the sensitivity of MRI (Figs. 8–1 to 8–3).

Literature Review

It is the opinion of surgeons that the labrum tear is the cause of cyst formation. The proposed etiology is similar to that of a wrist ganglion because it is postulated that a labrum tear allows joint fluid to leak and to form an extra-articular accumulation. Communication between the glenohumeral joint and the cyst has been demonstrated, but as yet there is no evidence for this proposed origin. Iannotti and Ramsey described their approach for cyst treatment. They presented arthroscopic cyst decompression and labrum repair to treat patients with suprascapular neuropathy.

Diagnosis

Patients present with shoulder pain and/or weakness. These nonspecific symptoms do not point the examiner toward the diagnosis of a periarticular cyst. The surgeon should be suspicious when the findings are at odds with the typical presentation of patients with rotator cuff impingement or glenohumeral instability. Symptoms of a periarticular cyst may be the result of rotator cuff disease, labral disease, suprascapular nerve compression, or some combination of these conditions. Labrum detachment may cause rotator cuff symptoms as a result of contact against the posterior superior glenoid, and the patient may complain of posterior superior shoulder pain while throwing or during other activities that require the arm to be placed in abduction and external rotation (Fig. 8–4). Mechanical labral symptoms include sensations of locking, catching, or popping. Pain may prevent full muscular contraction and can result in weakness during lifting. Pressure from the cyst on the suprascapular nerve can cause pain or burning discomfort in the scapular region (Fig. 8–5).

Nerve compression can also result in weakness. The weakness may be difficult to detect because, over time, compensatory hypertrophy can develop in the teres minor muscle (Fig. 8–6). Although patients with advanced nerve compression may complain of weakness, in my experience, they usually present with more subtle findings. Suprascapular nerve compression initially causes mild weakness of the supraspinatus and infraspinatus. When patients perform overhead activities or movements, the weakened rotator cuff does not stabilize the humeral head adequately, and slight superior subluxation occurs. This results in com-

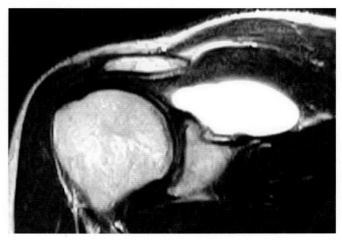

FIGURE 8–1. Superior location, coronal view.

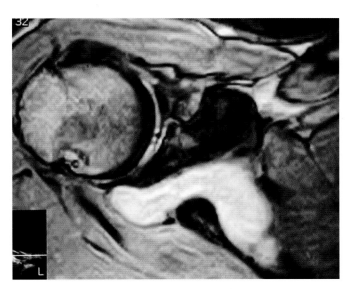

FIGURE 8–2. Transverse view.

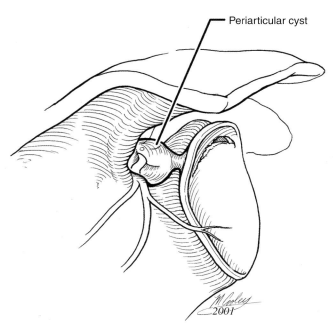

FIGURE 8–5. Suprascapular nerve compression.

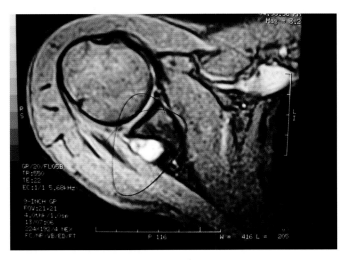

FIGURE 8–3. Posterior cyst.

plaints similar to those in patients with subacromial impingement.

None of these symptoms are diagnostic of a paralabral cyst, but they usually prompt the physician to order an MRI scan. Rotator cuff findings may be nonspecific or consistent with a partial-thickness rotator cuff tear. Superior or posterior superior labral detachment is noted. A cyst is seen in the posterior superior shoulder. The size is variable but typically measures 1 to 2 cm in diameter. The cyst may or not be seen communicating with the labrum tear. The cyst may be juxta-articular or located more superiorly in the region of the suprascapular notch. The surgeon should also be aware that the cyst may not be producing symptoms at all and may be an incidental finding. I believe it is important,

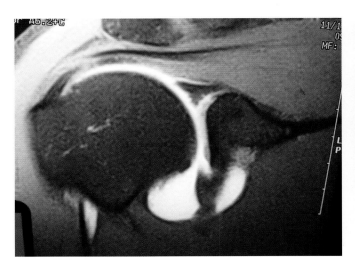

FIGURE 8–4. SLAP lesion.

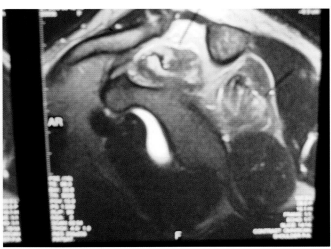

FIGURE 8–6. Atrophy, supraspinatus and infraspinatus. Teres minor hypertrophy.

when rotator cuff symptoms occur in a patient less than 50 years old, for the surgeon to order an MRI scan with contrast material. Without contrast material, the labrum lesion is usually not visible on an MRI scan.

Nonoperative Treatment

Treatment is directed at the underlying cause of the patient's symptoms. I treat patients with rotator cuff symptoms with selective rest, activity modification, nonsteroidal anti-inflammatory medication, and a home rehabilitation program focused on stretching the posterior shoulder structures and strengthening the shoulder-stabilizing muscles. Mechanical labral symptoms may be a result of subtle glenohumeral instability, so I have patients focus on exercises to improve the shoulder stabilizers. If the cyst is located near the posterior superior glenoid, I order electrodiagnostic testing to evaluate suprascapular nerve involvement. The test will detect the presence or absence of suprascapular nerve involvement as well as provide information about severity and location. Abnormalities of both the supraspinatus and infraspinatus point to a proximal lesion, usually at the suprascapular notch. Abnormalities limited to the infraspinatus are consistent with a more distal lesion, often at the spinoglenoid ligament.

Indications

I have been pleased with arthroscopic labrum repair for the treatment of perilabral cysts with or without suprascapular nerve involvement and recommend it as the treatment of choice. The underlying rationale of arthroscopic treatment is that the labrum tear allows the leakage of joint fluid extra-articularly and forms the cyst. With labrum repair, the joint seal is reestablished, and the cyst will resolve. There is anecdotal evidence for this view because some reports document MRI evidence of the disappearance of the cyst after labrum repair.

Indications depend on the cyst location and on associated conditions such as rotator cuff involvement and significant labral tearing. The anatomic alterations within the glenohumeral joint are often aggravated by subtle glenohumeral instability, and a 3- to 6-month period of home rehabilitation to strengthen the shoulder stabilizers is advised before operation is considered. If the cyst is causing nerve compression, based on physical examination and appropriate electrodiagnostic testing, the indications are different. In this situation, surgical intervention is considered more urgently rather than extensive rehabilitation. Spinoglenoid notch cysts are treated by arthroscopic labrum repair. Suprascapular notch cysts are treated by arthroscopic glenohumeral joint evaluation and labrum repair, if needed, followed by open decompression of the nerve and cyst excision.

My treatment is based on the degree of nerve involvement (as demonstrated by electrodiagnostic studies) and patient preference. If the nerve involvement is severe, I advise arthroscopic labrum repair and open cyst excision. Suprascapular nerve decompression is performed either at

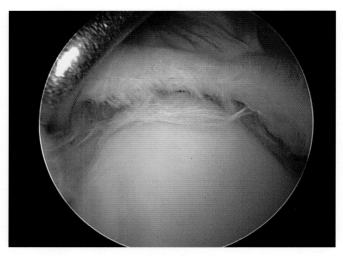

FIGURE 8–7. SLAP lesion.

the suprascapular notch or spinoglenoid ligament, as determined by preoperative electrodiagnostic examination. If the nerve involvement is minor, I advise arthroscopic labrum repair but give the patient the option of open cyst excision as described earlier or arthroscopic treatment alone. I counsel the patient that this arthroscopic treatment alone may be successful, but the possibility is that such treatment may not eliminate the cyst and later open treatment may be necessary. If MRI and electrodiagnostic testing performed 3 months after arthroscopic labrum repair show persistent disease, I perform an open cyst excision.

Operative Technique

The glenohumeral joint is entered posteriorly, and a routine anterior inferior portal is established. The labrum tear is usually located in the superior or posterior superior glenoid. I move the arthroscope to the anterior portal and carefully inspect the posterior superior aspect of the rotator cuff for signs of damage. If a grade 2 or 3 lesion is found, I mark the

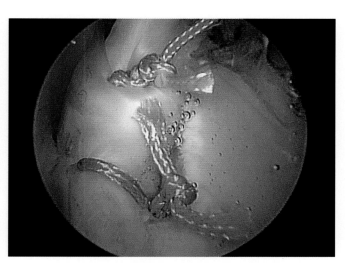

FIGURE 8–8. SLAP repair.

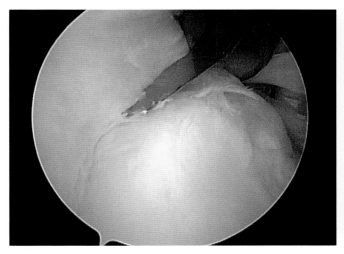

FIGURE 8–9. Chisel dissecting underneath superior labrum.

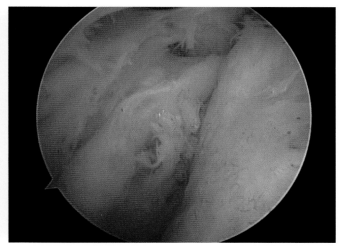

FIGURE 8–11. Suprascapular nerve.

area with a monofilament suture and (after labrum repair) inspect that area while viewing from the subacromial space. I perform a rotator cuff repair if there is also bursal-side partial tearing. If the rotator cuff is normal, than I proceed with labrum repair. The details of the repair are identical to those described for SLAP (superior labrum from anterior to posterior) lesions in Chapter 5 (Figs. 8–7 and 8–8).

If the labrum is separated only slightly, I use a chisel soft tissue instrument to dissect underneath the labrum (Fig. 8–9). In the experience of Iannotti and Ramsey, opening this area often leads directly to the cyst, and cystic fluid can be expressed into the joint. I still await this happy occurrence.

There are often soft tissue connections between the superior glenohumeral joint capsule and the posterior superior labrum. These may represent the pathway for synovial fluid from the joint to the cyst. Some surgeons cauterize this area to obliterate the connection, whereas others débride the area to open the connection and "decompress" the cyst (Fig. 8–10). Surgeon preferences dictate technique until there is ample scientific evidence to guide treatment.

Currently, I believe that labrum repair is the only necessary intra-articular treatment. I am concerned about thermal application or extensive soft tissue resection of the posterior superior capsule resulting from the proximity of the suprascapular nerve that lies approximately 1 cm medial to the glenoid rim. I carefully débride any soft tissue connections but keep the shaver near the glenoid (Fig. 8–11).

Variations of Technique

Other options for the treatment of the extra-articular cyst include open cyst excision and injection of cortisone into the cyst, usually under MRI guidance. The latter has been reported to cause cyst dissolution and may be performed preoperatively or postoperatively. Open cyst excision is more predictable but is associated with a higher morbidity rate.

Postoperative Treatment

Postoperative treatment is identical to that described for SLAP lesion repair described in Chapter 5.

Repeat MRI and electrodiagnostic testing are performed 3 months after operation.

Bibliography

Antoniou J, Tae SK, Williams GR, et al: Suprascapular neuropathy: Variability in the diagnosis, treatment, and outcome. Clin Orthop 386:131–138, 2001.

Chochole MH, Senker W, Meznik C, Breitenseher MJ: Glenoid-labral cyst entrapping the suprascapular nerve: Dissolution after arthroscopic debridement of an extended SLAP lesion. Arthroscopy 13(6):753–755, 1997.

Iannotti JP, Ramsey ML: Arthroscopic decompression of a ganglion cyst causing suprascapular nerve compression. Arthroscopy 12(6):739–745, 1996.

Levy P, Roger B, Tardieu M, et al: [Cystic compression of the suprascapular nerve: Value of imaging. Apropos of 6 cases and review of the literature]. J Radiol 78(2):123–130, 1997.

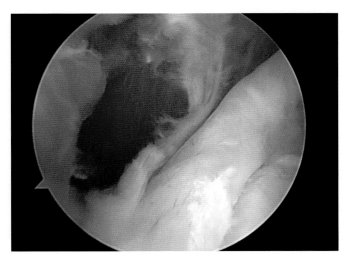

FIGURE 8–10. Opening cyst connection to glenohumeral joint.

9

Sepsis

Glenohumeral joint sepsis is an unusual indication for shoulder arthroscopy. In my experience, the arthroscope has greatly facilitated the management of this difficult condition. Treatment goals include obtaining fluid cultures and tissue biopsies to identify the infecting organisms and determining the extent of tissue involvement, followed by joint irrigation and débridement in a manner that minimizes morbidity and allows early functional recovery. Serial needle aspirations do not remove all joint debris, nor do they reach all loculations and infected clots. Arthrotomy enables thorough irrigation and débridement, but with increased soft tissue injury compared with arthroscopic treatment.

Literature Review

Most series on sepsis in various joints report the incidence of shoulder involvement as 3% to 12%. The most common organisms isolated are *Staphylococcus aureus* (61%) and *S. epidermidis* (17%), but polymicrobial infections are frequent (67%). In his series, Gelberman noted that all patients had significant underlying medical conditions such as alcoholism, liver disease, malignant disease, heroin addiction, or renal failure. Patients with acquired immunodeficiency syndrome and patients who have undergone shoulder replacement may also present with septic shoulders.

Diagnosis

All studies on shoulder pyarthrosis have noted a delay in establishing a diagnosis, because the clinical findings may be subtle. Patients are often afebrile and may complain of nonspecific shoulder discomfort. The white blood cell count may be normal, and the increase in the erythrocyte sedimentation rate is often not dramatic. I find the C-reac-

tive protein test to be far more sensitive. If doubt still remains about the possibility of glenohumeral sepsis, I advise arthroscopic evaluation; the risks of a negative arthroscopic examination are small when compared with the dire consequences of missed septic arthritis.

I obtain a consultation with an infectious disease specialist once I suspect the diagnosis of infection because this assistance is invaluable in the postoperative period. I have a general surgeon insert a catheter for long-term parenteral antibiotics after the patient is anesthetized in the operating room before I begin the arthroscopic operation.

Operative Technique

I establish a routine posterior portal and insert culture swabs into the joint before instilling fluid to obtain speci-

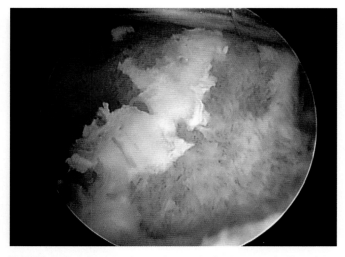

FIGURE 9–1. Infection after arthroscopic Bankart repair. Remaining glenoid articular cartilage.

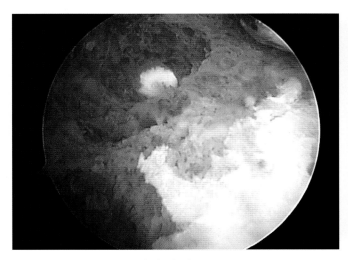

FIGURE 9–2. Anchor remnant.

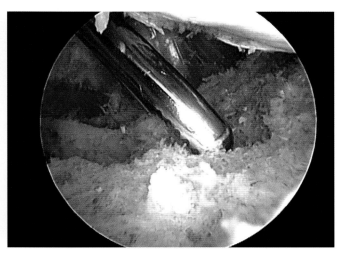

FIGURE 9–4. Bone defects in area of anchors.

mens for aerobic and anaerobic analysis. After the arthroscope is inserted posteriorly, I then create an anterior inferior portal and insert a large cannula. I use tissue-grasping forceps to obtain soft tissue specimens, which are then sent to the laboratory for frozen section, Gram stain, and culture and sensitivity testing. I find it helpful to alert the pathologist before the procedure so that a rapid reading of the Gram stain is performed. I use a motorized tissue resector to perform synovectomy and débridement of all involved areas throughout the glenohumeral joint. In my experience,

only a remnant of the rotator cuff is usually present (Figs. 9–1 to 9–4). I irrigate the joint copiously with 6 L of irrigation fluid. I then create an anterior superior portal and move the arthroscope to that location. I insert a hip suction tube through the posterior cannula and bring it out the anterior inferior cannula and repeat the process to insert a second suction drain. I move the arthroscope posteriorly and use a crochet hook to move one of the drains from the anterior inferior cannula to the anterior superior cannula. Through-and-through irrigation may be established with this technique. I inspect the subacromial space, perform débridement, and drain insertion as necessary. The drains are removed 48 hours postoperatively if the patient has responded. The operation is repeated as necessary until the infection is controlled.

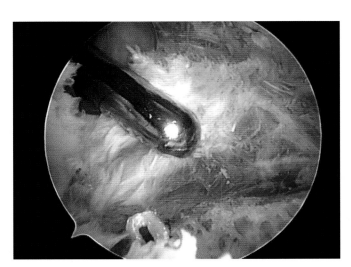

FIGURE 9–3. Débridement and synovectomy.

Bibliography

Gelberman RH, Menon JJ, Austerlitz MS, Weisman MH: Pyogenic arthritis of the shoulder in adults. J Bone Joint Surg 62A:550–556, 1980.

Gordon EJ, Hutchful GA: Pyarthrosis simulating ruptured rotator cuff syndrome. South Med J 75(6):759–762, 1982.

Master R, Weisman MH, Armbuster TG, et al: Septic arthritis of the glenohumeral joint: Unique clinical and radiographic features and a favorable outcome. Arthritis Rheum 20(8):1500–1506, 1977.

Parisien JS, Shaffer B: Arthroscopic management of pyarthrosis. Clin Orthop (275):243–247, 1992.

Ward WG, Eckardt JJ: Subacromial/subdeltoid bursa abscesses: An overlooked diagnosis. Clin Orthop (288):189–194, 1993.

Ward WG, Goldner RD: Shoulder pyarthrosis: A concomitant process. Orthopedics 17(7):591–595, 1994.

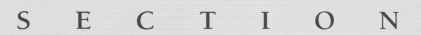

S E C T I O N

T H R E E

SUBACROMIAL SPACE SURGERY

Impingement Syndrome

Lesions of the subacromial space include rotator cuff tendinitis (impingement syndrome), partial-thickness rotator cuff tears, reparable full-thickness rotator cuff tears, massive rotator cuff tears, irreparable rotator cuff tears, rotator cuff arthropathy, and lesions of the acromioclavicular joint. Patients often present to the orthopedic surgeon's office with impingement syndrome, and this lesion is a common indication for arthroscopic surgery.

Clinical Presentation

Stage 2 impingement (chronic rotator cuff tendinitis) is a clinical syndrome. The patient complains of subdeltoid pain, often with radiation down the front of the arm into the biceps muscle. Night pain interferes with sleep, and pain occurs during activities as the arm passes through the painful arc of 70 to 100 degrees of abduction. Physical examination normally demonstrates full passive range of motion. Small limitations in elevation and behind-the-back internal rotation are limited by the patient's pain rather than by a true passive glenohumeral joint contracture. Active abduction and behind-the-back internal rotation are painful. Patients describe pain as they actively lower the arm after the examiner raises it passively. The primary and secondary impingement signs are positive, and pain is relieved with a subacromial lidocaine injection (impingement test).

Literature Review

Reports in the orthopedic surgery literature have described the arthroscopic management of stage 2 rotator cuff disease.

Several authors have reported 70% to 90% success rates with arthroscopic acromioplasty. All these authors stress that arthroscopic surgery is successful when impingement is the result of extrinsic compression on the tendon by the structures of the coracoacromial arch. It is not successful when impingement is intrinsic and results from the increased demand placed on the rotator cuff tendons in patients with glenohumeral subluxation. Other studies have compared open and arthroscopic techniques. Norlin found that the arthroscopic technique produced better results and a more rapid return of function. Van Holsbeeck and colleagues reported marginally better results with the open technique but advised arthroscopic decompression for patient convenience and satisfaction.

Diagnosis

The classic history of stage 2 impingement is one of shoulder pain with activities that place the shoulder in the painful arc of 70 to 100 degrees of elevation or abduction. Typical activities include reaching overhead (items on a high shelf), behind the back (fastening a brassiere or belt), or to the side (reaching for tickets in a parking lot, inserting ATM cards, using seat belts, or accessing alarm clocks).

Pain is localized to the subacromial region and radiates to the deltoid insertion and often anteriorly into the biceps. Night pain is noted regularly. The role of trauma is variable; some patients present with symptoms after major injury, but in many patients, pain occurs after repetitive activities without trauma or antecedent injury. Physical examination demonstrates a full or nearly normal range of passive motion. Localized tenderness in the area of the supraspinatus insertion can be demonstrated. Acromioclavicular joint tenderness should alert the examiner that this joint may be the primary source of disease because acromioclavicular joint arthritis may mimic stage 2 impingement or may coexist with primary impingement.

I carefully examine younger patients (less than 40 years old) for the presence of glenohumeral instability. In these patients, subacromial pain may be the result of traction rather than true stage 2 impingement. Three impingement signs consistent with stage 2 impingement have been described and are recorded as positive when subacromial pain is produced.

The primary sign occurs when the examiner places the patient's shoulder in maximum elevation. For the secondary sign, the shoulder is elevated 80 degrees and then is maximally internally rotated. The tertiary sign is subacromial pain with the shoulder in 90 degrees of abduction. The location of the pain during these maneuvers should be carefully noted. A patient with soft tissue pain from a rhomboid-trapezius spasm may have increased pain when each of these maneuvers is performed, but the pain will not be localized to the subacromial region.

After the physical examination, an impingement test may be performed. The test consists of local anesthetic injection into the subacromial space, followed by repeating maneuvers for the impingement signs. If the pain is eliminated or substantially reduced, the test is recorded as positive. The physician must remain aware that a positive test confirms only that the structures producing pain lie within the subacromial space and is not, in and of itself, diagnostic of impingement syndrome.

The diagnosis of impingement syndrome is clinical, and arthroscopy does not routinely play a role. Numerous conditions that mimic the clinical presentation of impingement are best diagnosed with arthroscopic techniques. Glenohumeral instability, articular surface partial rotator cuff tears, labrum tears, small areas of degenerative arthritis, posterior glenoid cuff impingement, and lesions of the rotator interval are examples. Glenohumeral instability may result in secondary traction tendinitis with a positive

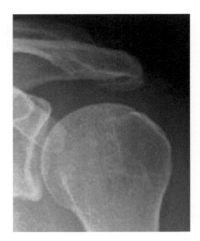

FIGURE 10–2. Anterolateral acromial spur.

impingement test. Successful surgical management does not involve shoulder decompression, but rather the treatment of the underlying glenohumeral instability. Other conditions that may mimic stage 2 impingement syndrome but that cannot be diagnosed with arthroscopic technique include acromioclavicular joint arthritis, cervical spine disease, and suprascapular neuropathy.

Acromial morphology is significant. Plain radiographic bone findings consistent with subacromial impingement include type 3 acromion, anterior acromial sclerosis, anteromedial spurs (ossification of the coracoacromial ligament), and inferior spurring of the distal clavicle. Magnetic resonance imaging (MRI) findings include tendinosis, bursitis, and lateral acromial downward sloping. In summary, the diagnosis of subacromial impingement that will respond to arthroscopic subacromial decompression should be based on extrinsic factors such as abnormal acromial shape, sloping, or spurs within the coracoacromial ligament or acromioclavicular joints (Figs. 10–1 to 10–4).

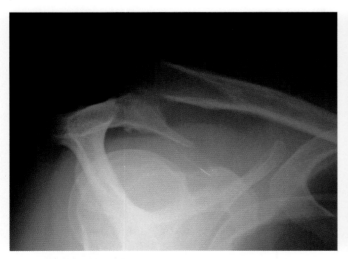

FIGURE 10–1. Type 3 acromion, scapular outlet view.

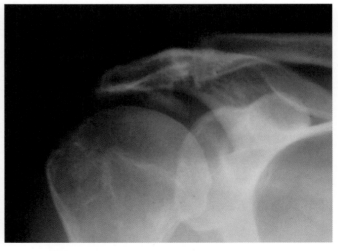

FIGURE 10–3. Coracoacromial ligament ossification.

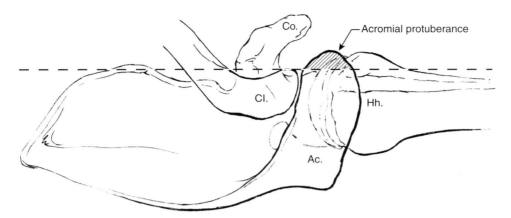

FIGURE 10–4. Anterior protuberance. Ac., acromion; Cl., clavicle; Co., coracoid; Hh., humeral head.

Indications

The indications for arthroscopic treatment and open surgery are identical: pain or weakness that interferes with work, sports, or activities of daily living and that is unresponsive to appropriate nonoperative treatment. The usual nonoperative regimen consists of oral anti-inflammatory medication, cortisone injections into the subacromial space (two or three, spaced 2 months apart), activity modification, selective rest, and a rehabilitation program. That program is designed to restore or maintain movement and to improve strength in the deltoid, in the scapular stabilizers, and in the rotator cuff. The recommended duration for this nonoperative approach varies in different publications, but it seems reasonable to consider surgery if the patient's pain continues for 12 months or is increasing in severity after 6 months. Additionally, an unusual indication for operative treatment is a superiorly displaced healed greater tuberosity fracture. Arthroscopic subacromial decompression treats the deformity by increasing clearance for the malunited bone.

The concept of acromioplasty itself is under debate; some surgeons believe that acromioplasty is unnecessary. Matsen believes that contact between the rotator cuff and acromial undersurface is normal and acromial spurs are the result of, but not caused by, primary tendon abnormality. He treats patients demonstrating stage 2 impingement by débriding abnormal bursa and adhesions and by initiating a vigorous rehabilitation program. Nirschl presented his views that impingement is an intrinsic tendinopathy and that acromioplasty is not needed. Currently, there is little scientific evidence to guide the orthopedic surgeon. The orthopedist who receives this information must evaluate it in conjunction with the numerous articles in the literature that report good results with acromioplasty and within the context of his or her own generally positive experience. We await well-designed, prospective, randomized studies to evaluate this question.

Acromioclavicular joint arthritis may also coexist with subacromial impingement. If the patient is symptomatic from acromioclavicular joint arthritis as determined on the preoperative clinical examination, acromioclavicular joint resection is performed. Acromioclavicular resection may be performed through the subacromial approach, although some surgeons prefer a direct approach into the acromioclavicular joint itself.

Contraindications

Pain occurring during abduction may result from causes other than the extrinsic mechanical factors of subacromial impingement. These causes include early rheumatoid arthritis, post-traumatic arthritis, and avascular necrosis. These are conditions with clear radiographic findings, however. A more unusual situation is the patient with chondromalacia resulting from early osteoarthrosis. Here the plain radiographic findings are normal, and the true origin of the patient's pain is discovered on arthroscopic examination.

Three common clinical entities may lead the surgeon to make an erroneous diagnosis: glenohumeral instability, adhesive capsulitis, and musculoskeletal pain syndromes. Fortunately, the surgeon can identify all with appropriate evaluation.

Probably the most common error is surgical treatment in patients with intrinsic tendinopathy that is secondary to glenohumeral instability. The repetitive overload of the rotator cuff tendons as they attempt to stabilize the glenohumeral joint causes inflammation and swelling of the tendons. Although the instability may be subtle, the pain from rotator cuff and bursa inflammation may be severe and may cause the patient to present for evaluation and treatment. The impingement signs and the impingement test are positive. These patients are usually less than 40 years old, and they have normal plain radiographs. In this setting, I proceed cautiously and advise a prolonged period of nonoperative care. Arthroscopic subacromial decompression without correction of the underlying glenohumeral joint lesions will fail.

The second most common error occurs when the patient has adhesive capsulitis. The diagnosis of adhesive capsulitis is straightforward when the disease is at its peak, but patients in the extremely early or late phases may have only a small loss of external rotation. This may be missed unless the examiner measures both shoulders. I carefully measure external rotation in maximum abduction and compare the side-to-side difference because this may be the first finding. The loss of external rotation does not allow the greater tuberosity to rotate away from the acromion during elevation and may mimic the clinical findings of impingement. Posterior capsular tightness leading to obligatory anterior superior humeral head translation may also cause this condition.

Musculoskeletal pain syndromes commonly cause pain in the scapular muscles, and these disorders can also be confused with subacromial impingement. The impingement signs may produce pain, but the pain is located in the scapular muscles or the trapezius and not in the classic locations.

Arthroscopic Findings

Most authors include glenohumeral joint inspection before arthroscopic subacromial decompression to examine for unsuspected lesions or to determine the status of the intraarticular structures. Imaging studies may have underestimated the extent of rotator cuff damage. Subtle Bankart or SLAP (superior labrum from anterior to posterior) lesions, labrum fraying, early adhesive capsulitis, and small areas of cartilage loss are some examples. Subacromial findings in stage 2 impingement are variable. The space may be clear, or a dense fibrous bursal reaction may exist. Impingement syndrome may exist even in the presence of a clear, well-defined subacromial space. In some patients, contact between the rotator cuff and the acromion produces pain but does not incite an inflammatory bursitis reaction. Tendon erosion, fraying, or partial-thickness tears may be found on the superior (bursal) surface of the cuff.

Erosions on the acromial undersurface near the anterior edge are frequently noted, as are small areas of inflammation. The surgeon may also observe coracoacromial ligament fraying. Although these findings are suggestive of subacromial impingement, they are not necessarily diagnostic.

Treatment

My arthroscopic treatment of stage 2 impingement involves examination with the patient under anesthesia to document range of motion and laxity, followed by inspection of the glenohumeral joint and treatment, if indicated, of any coexisting intra-articular lesions. Subacromial treatment includes excision of pathologic bursa to facilitate inspecting the surface of the tendons, to remove the space-occupying lesion, and to remove this inflamed, pain-producing structure. In most cases, treatment of the coracoacromial ligament involves resection from the lateral acromial border to the medial acromial border. Some surgeons prefer to divide, rather than to resect, the ligament. As noted earlier, some surgeons may elect not to perform acromioplasty or coracoacromial ligament resection but to limit their treatment to bursectomy. An inferior acromioplasty is performed, with the goal to convert the acromion to a flat (type 1) structure. This may be accomplished with a power bur placed in either the lateral or the posterior portal, depending on the surgeon's preference.

Anterior acromial recession is more controversial. This step involves removing the anterior acromial osteophyte or protuberance (i.e., all of the anterior acromion that projects anterior to the anterior border of the acromioclavicular joint). This part of the procedure is performed by some surgeons but not by others. I make my decision based on the amount of anterior projecting bone and the appearance of the anterior inferior acromion at the time of operation (see Fig. 10–4).

The acromioclavicular joint may contribute to impingement syndrome through formation of inferior acromioclavicular joint osteophytes. Inferior osteophytes may project downward into the rotator cuff tendons and may cause or exacerbate impingement. The presence of these osteophytes is documented on plain radiographic films or an MRI study. The osteophyte can be removed arthroscopically.

Operative Technique

 — Arthroscopic Subacromial Decompression

Anesthesia

I prefer a combination of general anesthesia and interscalene block.

Examination with the Patient under Anesthesia

I examine both shoulders for range of motion and translation. As noted previously, early (or late resolving) adhesive capsulitis or glenohumeral instability may mimic subacromial impingement. I have had the experience of a patient rapidly losing motion between the last office examination and the examination under anesthesia at the time of the surgical procedure.

Positioning

Although many surgeons are more comfortable with patients in the lateral decubitus position, I prefer to have them in the sitting position. The arm is allowed to rest naturally by the patient's side. I have not found traction necessary during this procedure or during any operations within the subacromial space.

Landmarks

I mark the surface anatomy of the clavicle, acromion, coracoid process, and scapular spine with a surgical marking pen. Mark the inferior surfaces of the bone because distances are measured from this point (Fig. 10–5).

Glenohumeral Joint Entry

I enter the glenohumeral joint posteriorly, as described in Chapter 3, and perform a complete inspection of the gleno-

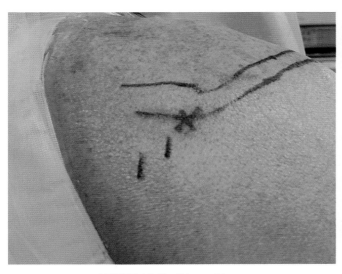

FIGURE 10–5. Skin markings.

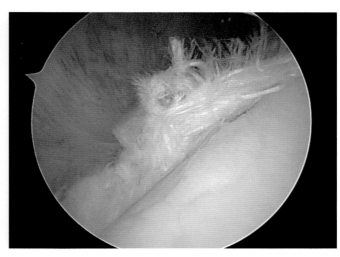

FIGURE 10–7. Labrum fraying.

humeral joint while viewing from the posterior portal. I then create an anterior portal, move the arthroscope anteriorly, and complete the diagnostic portion of the examination.

Glenohumeral Findings

Patients usually have few intra-articular signs of subacromial impingement. There may be fraying or erythema of the anterior supraspinatus. I carefully observe for findings that may mimic subacromial stage 2 impingement. These include a SLAP lesion (internal impingement), a Bankart lesion (anterior inferior glenohumeral instability), a contracted inferior capsular recess (adhesive capsulitis), or a rotator interval tear (anterior superior glenohumeral instability) (Figs. 10–6 to 10–12).

I use an arthroscopic probe and palpate the glenohumeral ligaments to assure myself that they are securely attached to both the glenoid rim and the humeral head. I have not

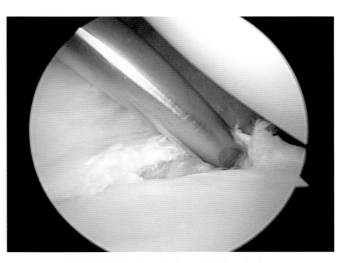

FIGURE 10–8. Nondisplaced Bankart lesion.

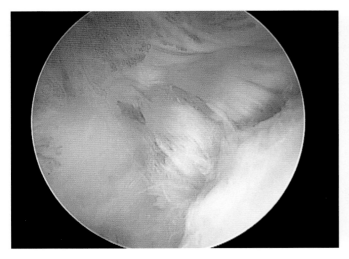

FIGURE 10–6. Partial-thickness rotator cuff tear.

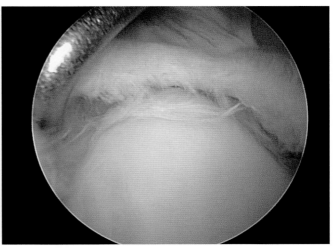

FIGURE 10–9. SLAP lesion.

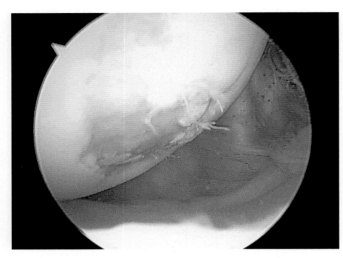

FIGURE 10–10. Humeral head cartilage lesion.

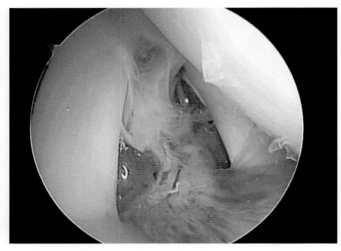

FIGURE 10–11. Contracted rotator interval.

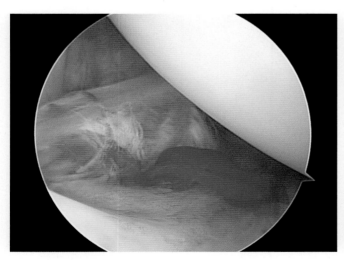

FIGURE 10–12. Contracted anterior capsule.

found it necessary to débride minor areas of labral fraying. I remove the instruments and cannulas and proceed to the subacromial space.

Subacromial Entry

I enter the subacromial space posteriorly and create a lateral working portal as described in Chapter 3. I verify my spatial orientation by rehearsing the movements that will be required during the operation. I touch the shaver tip to the acromion (lower my hand), the rotator cuff (raise my hand), anterior acromion (bring my hand toward myself), and posterior acromion (move my hand away from myself) (Figs. 10–13 to 10–21).

Subacromial Findings

Findings of subacromial impingement include erythema or fraying of the coracoacromial ligament or the bursal cuff surface. There is usually proliferative bursitis, although at other times the subacromial space may be clear. Adhesions may be present between the rotator cuff and the acromion or deep surface of the deltoid fascia. I sweep the cannula and trocar medially and laterally to release any significant adhesions (Fig. 10–22).

Bursectomy

If bursitis obscures the view, I remove it by turning the shaver tip away from the arthroscope (to avoid accidental damage to the lens) and positioning it midway between the acromion and the rotator cuff. I increase the suction slightly and begin shaving. As the bursa is removed, the subacromial space will become clear, and I will see the shaver tip. I gradually increase the suction on the shaver and continue to remove bursa. Do not shave medially because that area does not contribute to subacromial impingement, and shaving the well-vascularized bursa will result in bleeding that is difficult to control. Inadvertent débridement inferiorly and medially will also cause bleeding from the rotator cuff

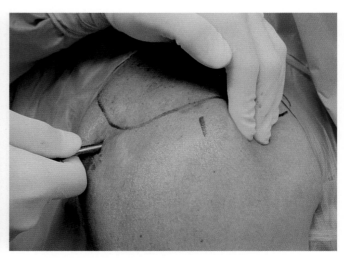

FIGURE 10–13. Palpate trocar.

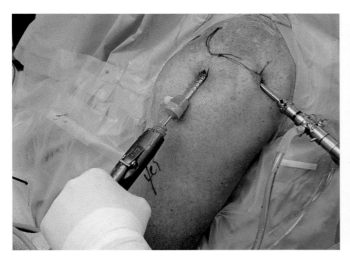

FIGURE 10–14. Palpate acromion.

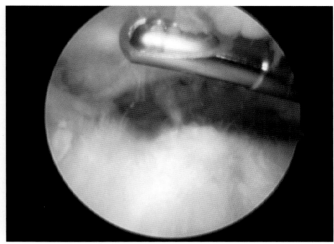

FIGURE 10–15. Palpate acromion.

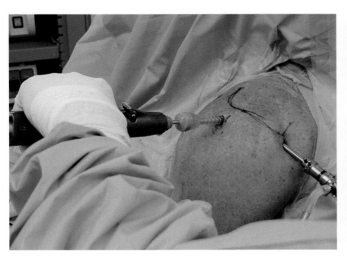

FIGURE 10–16. Palpate rotator cuff.

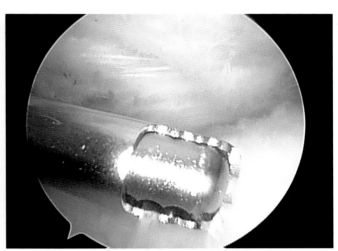

FIGURE 10–17. Palpate rotator cuff.

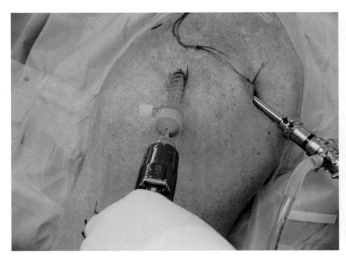

FIGURE 10–18. Palpate coracoacromial ligament.

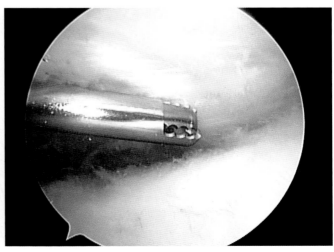

FIGURE 10–19. Palpate coracoacromial ligament.

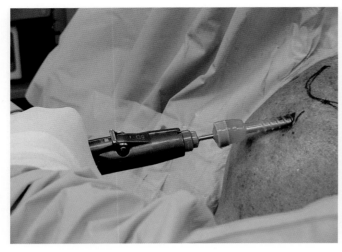

FIGURE 10–20. Move posteriorly.

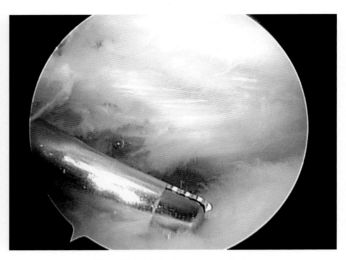

FIGURE 10–21. Move posteriorly.

musculature. Once the bursa is removed from the lateral, tendinous portion of the rotator cuff, I observe for adhesions anteriorly or laterally and remove these with scissors or a motorized resector until a complete view of the supraspinatus is possible (Figs. 10–23 to 10–29).

Coracoacromial Ligament

During subacromial decompression, the critical step is to identify the anterolateral acromion, which is usually covered by the coracoacromial ligament. Electrocautery is use-

ful for this portion of the procedure. I palpate the bone surface with the electrocautery tip (without power) and locate the anterior and then the lateral acromial borders. I place the electrocautery tip against the acromion approximately 1 cm posterior to the anterior bone margin and 1 cm medial to the lateral bone margin and ablate enough soft tissue until the bone is visible. I move anteriorly and laterally and remove more soft tissue and coracoacromial ligament until the anterolateral acromial border is clearly seen. I then sweep the coracoacromial ligament from the anterior inferior acromion until it falls inferiorly. This usually completes

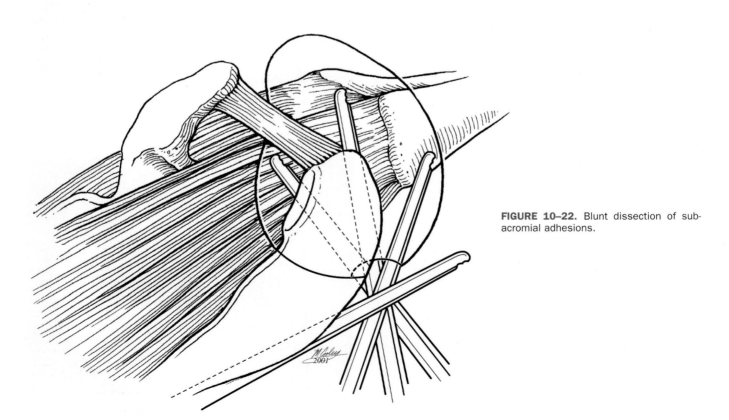

FIGURE 10–22. Blunt dissection of subacromial adhesions.

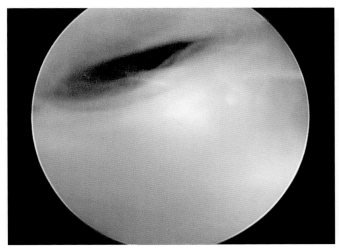

FIGURE 10–23. Posterior bursal curtain.

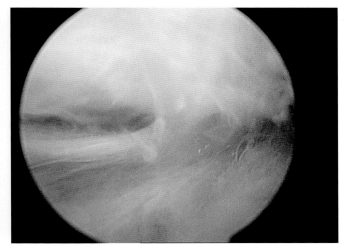

FIGURE 10–24. Bursa obscuring view of subacromial space.

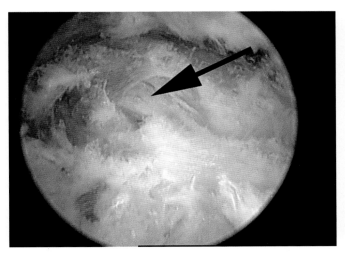

FIGURE 10–25. Musculotendinous junction (*arrow*).

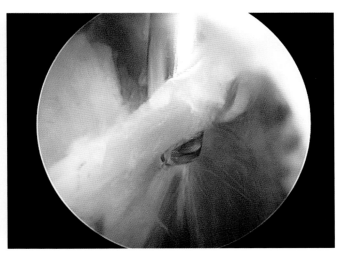

FIGURE 10–26. Subacromial adhesion.

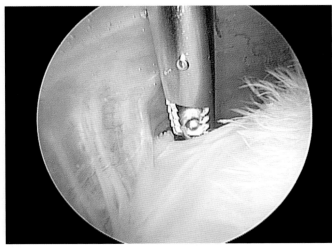

FIGURE 10–27. Resect adhesion.

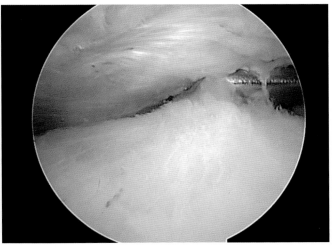

FIGURE 10–28. Bursal surface rotator cuff fraying.

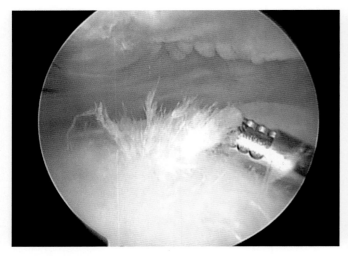

FIGURE 10–29. Bursal surface partial-thickness rotator cuff tear.

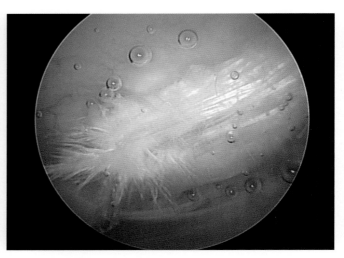

FIGURE 10–31. Coracoacromial ligament fraying.

my coracoacromial ligament release. Another technique is to use the power bur or shaver and gradually peel the soft tissue away from the acromion. If you wish to resect the ligament, you may now do so with more safety because the coracoacromial ligament is now a safe distance from the small branches of the thoracoacromial artery. If the surgeon believes that coracoacromial ligament release is preferable to resection, only the lateral portion of the coracoacromial ligament is resected, and the medial portion is left intact (Figs. 10–30 to 10–38).

Acromioplasty

I estimate the amount of necessary bone removal from preoperative radiographs. Anterior posterior radiographs may demonstrate anterolateral sclerosis and thickening. An apical tilt view may demonstrate ossification of the coracoacromial ligament with medial bony projection. The out-

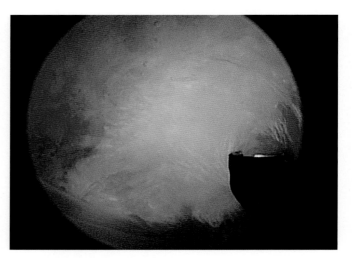

FIGURE 10–32. Coracoacromial ligament release.

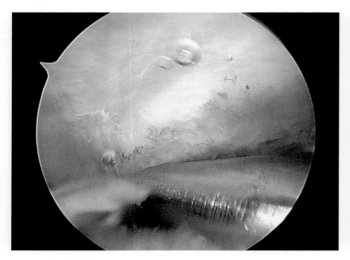

FIGURE 10–30. Coracoacromial ligament erythema.

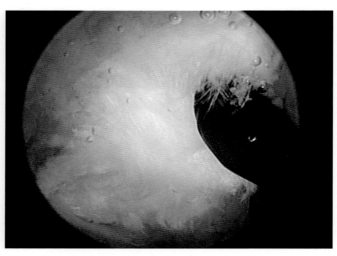

FIGURE 10–33. Coracoacromial ligament release.

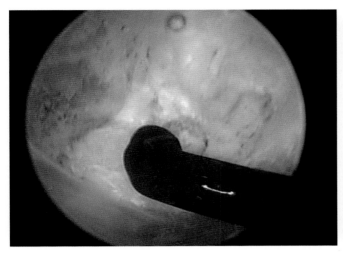

FIGURE 10–34. Coracoacromial ligament release.

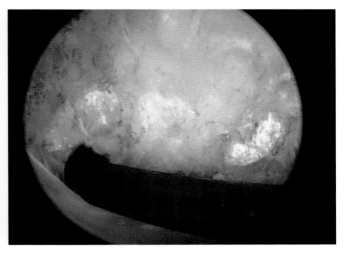

FIGURE 10–37. Identify medial acromion.

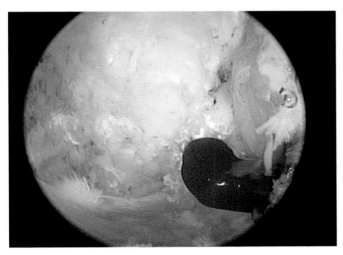

FIGURE 10–35. Identify anterolateral corner.

let view provides information about anterior acromial thickness.

Smaller patients require less bone removal than larger patients. The estimation of bone thickness and necessary bone removal to achieve a flat, type 1 acromion can help the surgeon avoid excessive bone removal or acromial fracture.

Before starting acromioplasty, the inferior bone surface should be free of soft tissue. I place the bur at the anterolateral bone margin and remove anterior inferior bone until the deltoid fascia is seen and the necessary amount of bone (as estimated from preoperative radiographs) is removed. I fashion the bone removal until the inferior acromial surface is flat and parallel to the floor. Only then do I continue medially. I remove bone from inferior to the superior.

Because the acromion is thicker medially than laterally, correspondingly more bone is removed medially. I remove bone until a flat surface is achieved, based on the view with the arthroscope in the posterior portal and angled upward. There are two additional ways to check the acromioplasty.

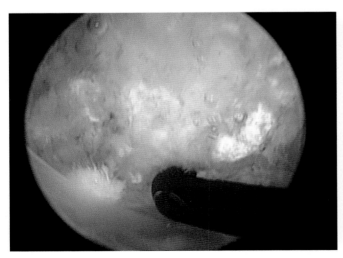

FIGURE 10–36. Identify anterior acromion.

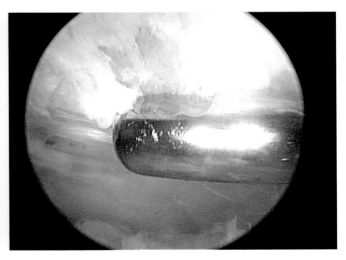

FIGURE 10–38. Soft tissue dissect with shaver.

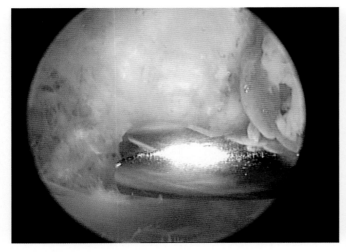

FIGURE 10–39. Bur oriented parallel to acromion undersurface.

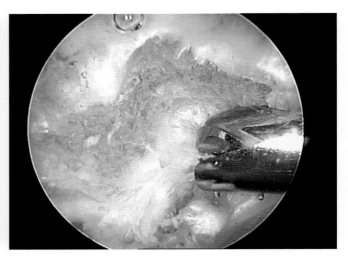

FIGURE 10–41. Resect bone more medially.

With the arthroscope in the posterior portal, the tip is placed up against the bone, and the arthroscope objective lens is rotated downward. This maneuver angles the beam parallel to the acromial undersurface, and bone projecting downward requires removal (Figs. 10–39 to 10–44).

Hemostasis

Bleeding control is vital to performing arthroscopic subacromial decompression. I avoid débridement of the medial subacromial space, where the bursa is well vascularized and the rotator cuff is muscular. The acromial branch of the thoracoacromial artery is located anterior to the coracoacromial ligament. A technique that decreases the likelihood of excessive bleeding includes use of a thermal cautery device for subperiosteal dissection of the coracoacromial ligament and for division of the ligament. When bleeding is encountered, I immediately seek to control it rather than proceed-

ing with the operation. I stop the outflow, advance the arthroscope with its inflow fluid stream as close to the site of bleeding as possible, and increase the pump pressure to tamponade the vessel. I bring the coagulation instrument into the space near the site of bleeding. I gradually decrease the pump pressure until the bleeding source is identified, and then I coagulate the area.

The foregoing thoughts are broad outlines of what is necessary. Because I believe this topic is so important, I would like to explain in detail how I perform an arthroscopic subacromial decompression.

Where to Start and When to Stop?

The question I am asked most frequently by orthopedic surgeons is this: Exactly where do I begin the acromioplasty, and how do I know when I have completed it successfully? The answer to this question is complex, but it begins with an understanding of acromial shape as it exists preoperatively and also as you wish it to appear after arthroscopic subacromial decompression. A basic problem is that we try to evaluate a three-dimensional structure such as the acromion with two-dimensional imaging. Therefore, multiple radiographic views are needed. An anterior posterior view gives the surgeon information about acromial thickness, anterior edge sclerosis, lateral slope, and medial ossification of the coracoacromial ligament. From this view, the surgeon gains an impression of how to perform the bone resection. Medial ossification of the coracoacromial ligament alerts the surgeon that more anterior and medial bone removal is needed. A lateral slope dictates more bone removal laterally than usual. The axillary view provides information about anterior acromial protuberance and an os acromiale, if present. The lateral or scapular outlet view demonstrates acromial thickness, slope, and shape. This view provides further information and guides the surgeon on how much anterior bone must be removed.

A thicker acromion dictates a greater amount of bone removal than a thin one, and from the radiograph or MRI scan, the surgeon can estimate how much bone removal is needed. Draw a line along the flat posterior portion of the

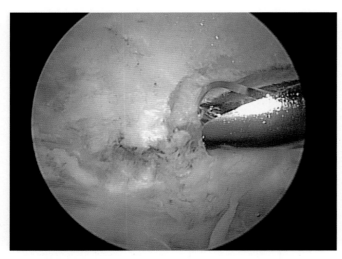

FIGURE 10–40. Begin resection anterolateral acromial corner.

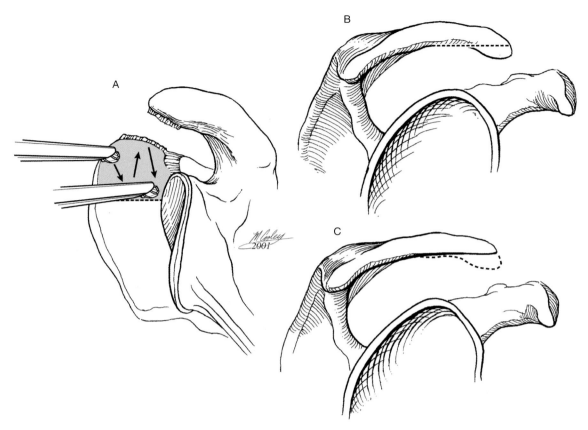

FIGURE 10–42. *A* to *C,* Pattern of bur movement.

acromion and extend it anteriorly past the anterior acromial edge. Bone inferior to that line must be removed to create a flat, type 1, acromion. A type 2 acromion can compromise the subacromial space and can result in impingement, particularly if the slope is more inferior then normal. After studying the three radiographic views listed earlier, the sur-

geon should understand the preoperative acromion in three dimensions.

Next, the surgeon must understand how the acromion must look after operation. The anterior posterior radiograph should show a thinner acromion with removal of anterior sclerosis and medial ossification. Lateral tilt, if

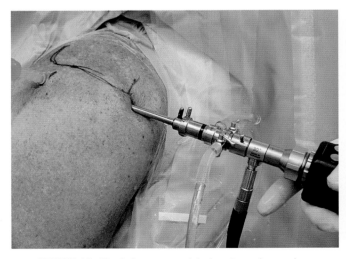

FIGURE 10–43. Arthroscope rotated up toward acromion.

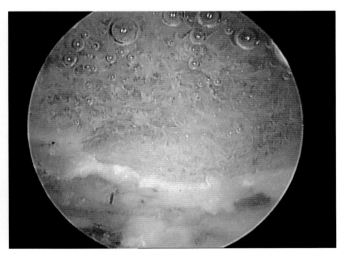

FIGURE 10–44. View of acromion.

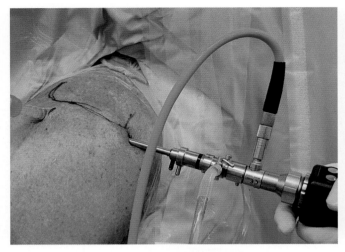

FIGURE 10–45. Arthroscope rotated toward rotator cuff. Beam parallel to acromion undersurface.

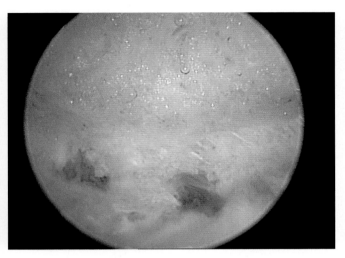

FIGURE 10–46. View of acromion.

present preoperatively, should be eliminated. The axillary view will show a more radiolucent acromion consistent with bone removal, and if the surgeon has removed an anterior projection, it will be absent. Probably the most helpful postoperative radiograph is the scapular outlet view. By comparing the preoperative and postoperative radiographs, the surgeon can judge the adequacy of bone removal.

Moving these concepts directly to the operating room requires that the surgeon first establish a clear view of the subacromial space. This requires bursectomy and hemostasis. Next, the soft tissue must be removed from the acromial undersurface so that the bone is visible. The next step is to identify the anterior and lateral acromial borders clearly, as described earlier. Only when these steps have been accomplished can the surgeon reliably and repeatedly perform an arthroscopic acromioplasty. I usually view the acromion with the arthroscope rotated superiorly, but at this point I tilt the arthroscope and advance it so that it touches the acromion and then rotate it so that the beam is parallel to the undersurface (Figs. 10–45 and 10–46). Bone projecting downward is bone that needs to be removed, and I estimate how many millimeters this represents. I place the acromionizer bur against the acromion, and this gives me a measure by which to judge the amount of bone removal needed. I then return the arthroscope to its original position and rotation and identify the anterolateral acromial corner both by inspection and palpation. Only when this area is clear and I can view the deltoid fascia anteriorly and laterally do I begin the coracoacromial ligament resection.

I use the electrocautery device to divide the coracoacromial ligament from the anterolateral acromion. I move medially, dissect the coracoacromial ligament from the anterior acromion, and let it fall toward the rotator cuff. During this portion of the procedure, if I encounter bleeding, I cauterize the vessel immediately. If I encounter a minor amount of bleeding, the temptation is to continue the operation. However, this small compromise in picture clarity gradually worsens, and if further bleeding occurs, it may be hard to find the offending blood vessels. Once I

have released the coracoacromial ligament attachment, I insert the soft tissue resector and remove the ligament until I reach the level of the medial acromion.

I then insert the acromionizer and begin at the anterolateral corner of the acromion. I increase the suction until I have a clear view, but I do not increase it too much because this will collapse the subacromial space. As I rotate the bur away from the arthroscope, I start the bur spinning before I touch the bone. If you rest the acromionizer on the bone and then start it, the bur tends to jump and can inadvertently strike the arthroscope lens. I hold the bur about 2 mm from the bone, engage the power, and then gently touch the bone. I apply gentle pressure and move the bur anteriorly, away from the arthroscope. Once I see and feel it break through the anterior cortex, I stop the bur and confirm that the deltoid fascia is visible. I then continue to work in this area and resect more bone superiorly until the anterolateral acromion is converted to a flat type 1 shape. I rotate the arthroscope objective lens 180 degrees as described earlier to confirm this. I then move medially and resect enough bone until this area is parallel to the anterolateral resection. I continue medially until I reach the medial margin of the acromion, where it forms the lateral border of the acromioclavicular joint.

As I resect bone medially, I advance the arthroscope and rotate it inferiorly and medially, always attempting to keep the area of bone resection centered in the picture. I usually resect the medial border of the acromion until the soft tissue of the acromioclavicular joint is visible. I have not had any significant problems with late acromioclavicular joint instability or pain with this approach.

I then move the arthroscope to the lateral portal to assure myself that I have created a type 1 acromion. The acromioplasty may be examined by inserting an instrument or probe and placing it flat against the acromial undersurface. Another technique, which Richard Hawkins and colleagues presented, is to enlarge the lateral portal enough to introduce the tip of a finger and to palpate the acromion digitally. This is a good technique to use when learning arthroscopic subacromial decompression.

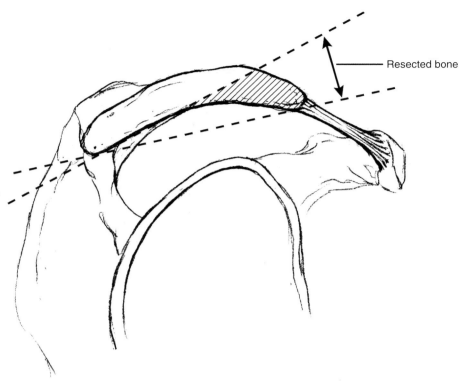

Resected bone

FIGURE 10–47. Orientation drawing for cutting block technique.

Variations of Technique

A variation of the standard acromioplasty is the posterior "cutting block" technique. You may find it helpful to draw on the preoperative scapular outlet view. Draw a line from the inferior margin of the posterior acromion to the inferior margin of the anterior acromion. Draw a second line from the inferior margin of the posterior acromion parallel to the inferior acromion. This should provide you with some guidelines to estimate the amount of bone removal. After the soft tissue is removed from the acromial undersurface,

move the arthroscope to the lateral portal and place the acromionizer bur in the posterior cannula. Advance the bur anteriorly and place it up against the acromial undersurface. Move the bur laterally and medially as you advance it anteriorly and remove bone. The alignment of the instrument shaft against the now flat acromion assures the surgeon that a type 1 acromion is now present (Figs. 10–47 to 10–51).

There is a danger of bone transection with the cutting block technique in patients with a thin or angulated acromion. Appropriate analysis of the preoperative scapular

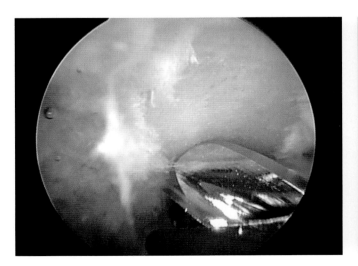

FIGURE 10–48. Bur posteriorly.

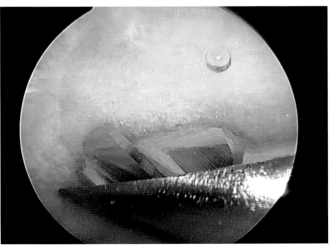

FIGURE 10–49. Advance bur.

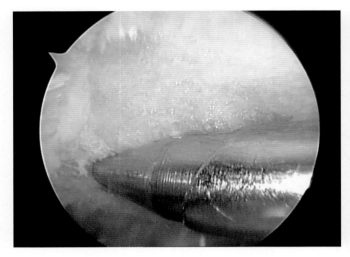

FIGURE 10–50. Test resection with trocar.

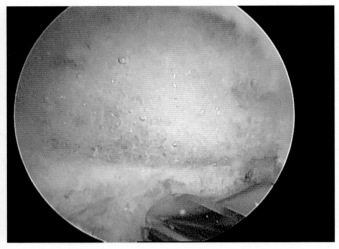

FIGURE 10–51. Completed acromioplasty viewed from lateral portal.

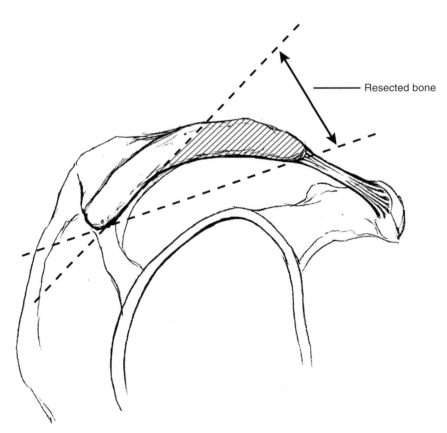

Resected bone

FIGURE 10–52. Curved acromion and danger of cutting block technique.

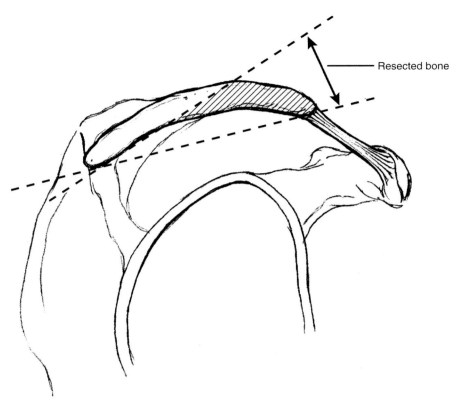

— Resected bone

FIGURE 10–53. Thin acromion and danger of cutting block technique.

outlet view should allow the surgeon to select the correct technique (Figs. 10–52 and 10–53).

Os Acromiale

An anatomic variation that the surgeon may encounter is the os acromiale (Fig. 10–54). The os represents a failure of the acromion to ossify completely and may be best diagnosed on the axillary radiograph. Three different treatments have been proposed. The surgeon may ignore the fragment, may excise it, or may perform internal fixation, and articles in the literature report good results with each method. I do not advocate excision unless the anterior fragment is extremely small. I perform internal fixation only if there is palpation tenderness over the fragment on the preoperative physical examination. I believe that, generally, the os is asymptomatic, and I therefore perform a routine acromioplasty.

Postoperative Management

Postoperative management after decompression for stage 2 impingement progresses rapidly after arthroscopic surgery because active motion can be started immediately without fear of deltoid detachment. The therapist instructs patients in passive range of motion in elevation and external rotation with a dowel rod. Active range of motion in all planes is encouraged. Strengthening may begin about 3 months postoperatively or sooner, once resisted manual testing of the operated shoulder muscles is painless.

Causes of Failure

Failures of Thought

The causes of failure after arthroscopic subacromial decompression are identical to those seen after open acromioplasty. Patients should understand that it may take 6 to 12 months to recover fully from the operation. I often see patients referred to me who have pain 1 to 2 months after

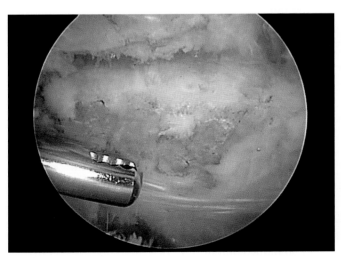

FIGURE 10–54. Os acromiale.

arthroscopic subacromial decompression. Both they and their surgeons are concerned about treatment failure. Counseling the patient about realistic expectations is valuable.

Improper Diagnosis

Shoulder pain as the arm passes through the painful arc is common to numerous diagnoses other than impingement syndrome. Early adhesive capsulitis with a loss of external rotation does not allow the greater tuberosity to rotate and to clear the acromion. Passive range of motion during examination under anesthesia demonstrates a loss of motion when compared with the contralateral side. The inferior recess and the rotator interval may appear contracted or inflamed on arthroscopic inspection.

Chondromalacia or early osteoarthrosis not detectable on plain radiographs can be diagnosed during the glenohumeral arthroscopic inspection. Acromioclavicular joint arthritis or osteolysis may irritate the rotator cuff and may result in a clinical presentation similar to that of impingement. Physical examination demonstrates local tenderness over the acromioclavicular joint and acromioclavicular joint pain with adduction and behind-the-back internal rotation.

Surgeons should be suspicious of the impingement diagnosis in patients less than 40 years old. Glenohumeral instability may cause traction tendinitis that may mimic impingement. At operation, the surgeon may observe an obvious Bankart lesion but should search for more subtle lesions.

In patients less than 40 years old, I carefully examine the glenohumeral joint for labrum fraying consistent with excessive glenohumeral translation. Rotator interval tears and SLAP lesions may also cause glenohumeral instability. Correction of the underlying instability is necessary.

Technical Failures

INADEQUATE DECOMPRESSION. At reoperation, the most common cause of failure is an inadequate acromioplasty or coracoacromial ligament release. The surgeon should pay close attention to the anterolateral acromial corner and must visualize this area clearly to ensure adequate bone removal.

EXCESSIVE DECOMPRESSION. This complication usually occurs in small female patients with a thin acromion. When the surgeon fails to study the preoperative scapular outlet view, the small bone size is not appreciated. A standard acromioplasty performed with the acromionizer bur in the lateral portal may excessively thin the acromion and may cause an intraoperative fracture or may result in a fracture during early postoperative rehabilitation.

An arthroscopic subacromial decompression performed with the cutting block technique with the acromionizer bur in the posterior portal may result in a complete anterior acromionectomy if the surgeon does not study the scapular outlet view carefully and appreciate the relative thinness or curvature of the acromion.

LATERAL ACROMIAL RESECTION. Lateral resection results from either a misunderstanding of the pathophysiology of subacromial impingement or a technical error. Lateral sub-

deltoid pain when the arm is abducted may prompt some surgeons to resect the lateral acromion. Poor visualization or disorientation may allow the surgeon to mistake the lateral for the anterior acromion.

Comparison of Open and Arthroscopic Approaches

Arthroscopy appears to have certain theoretical advantages over conventional open surgery. The skin incisions are smaller, and the cosmetic result is better. The procedure can be performed on an outpatient basis, which is more convenient for the patient and is less expensive for the third-party payer. Most patients can perform activities of daily living and can return to a sedentary job within days. Because the deltoid is not detached from the acromion, active range-of-motion exercises can be started as soon as tolerated. Perhaps more important is that the glenohumeral joint can be inspected. Although clinically important intra-articular lesions are not common, glenohumeral instability, labrum tears, partial-thickness articular surface rotator cuff tears, biceps tendon lesions, and arthritic changes in the glenoid and/or humeral head can be identified. These may well be overlooked with a conventional open approach; their accurate diagnosis and eventual treatment can clearly be of benefit in achieving the most optimal functional result for the patient. Arthroscopic subacromial decompression can be a difficult skill for many surgeons to master, and it is certainly harder to teach than open acromioplasty. Better hand-eye coordination is required. The ability to triangulate and to manipulate power instruments within millimeters of each other can be challenging.

The cost difference between outpatient arthroscopic surgery and inpatient open procedures may not be as great as perceived by patients, surgeons, and insurance carriers. Certainly, the cost of a hospital stay is avoided with arthroscopic surgery, but this is at least partially offset by the increased cost of the arthroscopic setup. The price of disposable instruments, tubing, and fluid is an important consideration. The operating room, recovery room, and surgeon's and anesthesiologist's fees constitute the largest portion of the expense. These charges are similar for both arthroscopic and open acromioplasty. It would seem logical that the arthroscopic approach allows patients to return more rapidly to a job that does not require heavy labor. This should have a substantial impact on cost analyses that take into account days lost from work; however, studies that systematically address this issue have not been performed. Furthermore, it appears that even in this area, the differences may only be slight. Many patients do not have manual labor jobs and can return to work when pain is adequately controlled. The ability to return to work seems to be less heavily influenced by the surgical findings. More important are social, emotional, and economic concerns, which are not influenced by the surgical technique.

Deltoid management differs between the open and arthroscopic approaches. The open approach requires a small amount of deltoid detachment and reattachment; therefore, the deltoid must be protected and allowed to heal, to avoid the debilitating complication of deltoid dehiscence. In contrast, the arthroscopic technique allows immediate active motion. Advocates of open techniques state that minimal deltoid removal from the acromion is required and that reliable techniques exist for the secure reattachment of the deltoid. Advocates of the arthroscopic approach argue that deltoid detachment is avoided with the arthroscopic approach; however, the arthroscopic technique also has the potential for deltoid injury. The deltoid fascial origin can be disrupted if an overly aggressive anterior or anterolateral acromioplasty is performed.

The impingement syndrome is a clinical diagnosis made on a combination of patient history, physical examination, and radiographic findings that can be treated successfully with arthroscopic subacromial decompression.

Impingement syndrome can be managed satisfactorily with arthroscopic techniques. Arthroscopy allows a complete inspection of the glenohumeral joint and enables the surgeon to diagnose and treat coexisting intra-articular lesions. The surgeon can perform a thorough bursectomy, a coracoacromial ligament resection, and an acromioplasty without the need for deltoid detachment.

Coracoid Impingement

VIDEO — **Coracoid Impingement**

Another cause of anterior shoulder pain with adduction is coracoid impingement. This unusual lesion is diagnosed by the patient's description of anterior shoulder pain with adduction of the internally rotated arm. There is tenderness over the coracoid process, and pain is increased when the examiner passively adducts the internally rotated shoulder. An injection of local anesthetic near the coracoid relieves the pain. Radiographs may be normal, but the axillary view may demonstrate pronounced lateral curvature or elongation of the coracoid process. Occasionally, MRI demonstrates compression of the subscapularis against the coracoid. If conservative care is not successful, then operation is indicated.

I inspect the glenohumeral joint and then redirect the arthroscope into the subacromial space. I create a lateral and an anterior portal and move the arthroscope to the lateral portal. I introduce the shaver through the anterior portal and perform a thorough bursectomy. I can then identify the subscapularis, the acromion, and the coracoacromial ligament. I advance the arthroscope and follow the coracoacromial ligament to the region of the coracoid process. I introduce a shaver through the anterior portal and palpate the coracoid process. I remove enough soft tissue so that I can see the coracoid bone, and then I insert a round bur to recess the coracoid distally and laterally until I have created sufficient space. I place the patient's arm in adduction and internal rotation and test the adequacy of the bone resection. Postoperative management is similar to that described earlier.

Bibliography

Altchek DW, Carson EW: Arthroscopic acromioplasty: Current status. Orthop Clin North Am 28:157–168, 1997.

Bonsell S: Detached deltoid during arthroscopic subacromial decompression. Arthroscopy 16:745–748, 2000.

Budoff JE, Nirschl RP, Guidi EJ: Debridement of partial-thickness tears of the rotator cuff without acromioplasty: Long-term follow-up and review of the literature. J Bone Joint Surg Am 80:733–748, 1998.

Caspari RB, Thal R: A technique for arthroscopic subacromial decompression. Arthroscopy 8:23–30, 1992.

Checroun AJ, Dennis MG, Zuckerman JD: Open versus arthroscopic decompression for subacromial impingement: A comprehensive review of the literature from the last 25 years. Bull Hosp Jt Dis 57:145–151, 1998.

Ellman H, Harris E, Kay SP: Early degenerative joint disease simulating impingement syndrome: Arthroscopic findings. Arthroscopy 8:482–487, 1992.

Ellman H, Kay SP: Arthroscopic subacromial decompression for chronic impingement: Two- to five-year results. J Bone Joint Surg Br 73:395–398, 1991.

Gartsman GM: Arthroscopic acromioplasty for lesions of the rotator cuff. J Bone Joint Surg Am 72:169–180, 1990.

Gartsman GM, Bennett JB, Blair ME, et al: Arthroscopic subacromial decompression: An anatomic study. Am J Sports Med 16:45–53, 1988.

Hawkins RJ, Plancher KD, Saddemi SR, et al: Arthroscopic subacromial decompression. J Shoulder Elbow Surg 10:225–230, 2001.

Holsbeeck Van J, DeRycke G, Declercq M, Martens, et al: Subacromial impingement: Open versus arthroscopic decompression. Arthroscopy 8(2):173–178, 1992.

Kim SH, Ha KI: Arthroscopic treatment of symptomatic shoulders with minimally displaced greater tuberosity fracture. Arthroscopy 16:695–700, 2000.

Matthews LS, Blue JM: Arthroscopic subacromial decompression: Avoidance of complications and enhancement of results. Instr Course Lect 47:29–33, 1998.

Morrison DS, Frogameni AD, Woodworth P: Non-operative treatment of subacromial impingement syndrome. J Bone Joint Surg Am 79:732–737, 1997.

Norlin R: Arthroscopic subacromial decompression versus open acromioplasty. Arthroscopy 5(4):321–323, 1989.

Rockwood CA, Matsen FA III: The Shoulder. Philadelphia, W.B. Saunders, 1998, pp 755–764.

Sampson TG, Nisbet JK, Glick JM: Precision acromioplasty in arthroscopic subacromial decompression of the shoulder. Arthroscopy 7:301–307, 1991.

T'Jonck L, Lysens R, De Smet L, et al: Open versus arthroscopic subacromial decompression: Analysis of one-year results. Physiother Res Int 2:46–61, 1997.

11

Partial-Thickness Rotator Cuff Tears

Partial-thickness rotator cuff tears represent a most interesting and difficult type of shoulder lesions. Partial-thickness rotator cuff tears may characterize a transition from subacromial impingement to full-thickness rotator cuff tears, but they also can be found in patients with glenohumeral instability. Because the same anatomic lesions can be caused by two different mechanisms, the surgeon must determine the cause and treat the partial-thickness rotator cuff tear accordingly.

Literature Review

In a group of throwing athletes (average age, 22 years) treated with arthroscopic débridement alone without decompression, Andrews and colleagues reported 85% good or excellent results. Snyder found 47 partial tears in a group of 600 patients undergoing shoulder arthroscopy and advocated débridement without decompression if the tear was confined to the articular surface. Arthroscopic subacromial decompression was added if the tear was present on both the articular and the bursal surfaces. In our series on treatment of partial-thickness rotator cuff tears, Milne and I reported that tears of less than 50% tendon thickness with outlet impingement responded well to arthroscopic subacromial decompression, whereas tears greater than 50% required repair. Partial-thickness rotator cuff tears found in patients with glenohumeral instability required instability correction and then rotator cuff repair or arthroscopic subacromial decompression, depending on the extent of the individual lesions.

Diagnosis

Patients with partial-thickness rotator cuff tears may present with signs and symptoms typical of rotator cuff disease. Pain localized deep to the lateral deltoid muscle (sub-deltoid pain) is present when the shoulder is elevated through the painful arc during activities of daily living. Night pain is also a regular feature. Examination demonstrates normal active and passive range of motion with positive impingement signs. Subacromial anesthetic injection relieves the pain. A critical feature of the examination is the amount of pain and weakness observed when resisted manual muscle testing is performed. Significant pain and weakness with resisted external rotation or elevation are relative indications for early operative intervention. Plain radiographs resemble those in patients with impingement syndrome or full-thickness tears. Most commonly, the diagnosis is made with magnetic resonance imaging (MRI). I have found that the use of intra-articular gadolinium increases the sensitivity of the MRI in patients with partial-thickness rotator cuff tears (Figs. 11–1 and 11–2). Often, a partial-thickness tear is only found at the time of arthroscopic examination of the glenohumeral joint.

Nonoperative Treatment

In the absence of significant subacromial space compromise from a type 3 acromion, nonoperative treatment is indicated and is identical to that prescribed for patients with impingement syndrome. Patients are instructed to avoid painful positions and activities. Nonsteroidal anti-inflammatory medication may help pain at night. If there are losses of passive motion, appropriate stretching exercises are indicated.

Indications

If pain persists after 9 to 12 months or is increasing after 6 months of nonoperative treatment, operative intervention is considered.

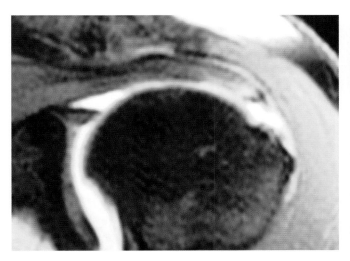

FIGURE 11–1. Partial-thickness rotator cuff tear, coronal view.

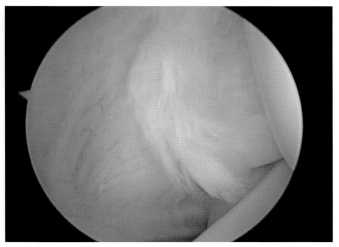

FIGURE 11–3. Supraspinatus tear grade 1.

Operative Technique

Operative Findings

The clinical findings in patients with partial-thickness rotator cuff tears are related both to the severity of the tear and to other lesions within the joint. Most tears are located on the articular surface; approximately 75% of these are in the supraspinatus tendon, 20% are in the infraspinatus tendon, and 5% are in the teres minor tendon. The depth or severity of tendon tears is grade 1 (less than one fourth of the tendon thickness) in 45% of cases, grade 2 (less than one half of tendon thickness) in 40%, and grade 3 (more than one half of tendon thickness) in 15% (Figs. 11–3 to 11–7).

The finding of chondral defects on the articular surfaces of the humeral head or the glenoid or the presence or labrum tears or separations is suggestive of glenohumeral instability and should prompt the surgeon to consider

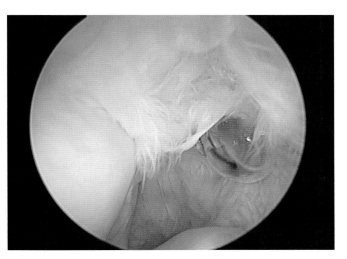

FIGURE 11–4. Supraspinatus tear grade 2.

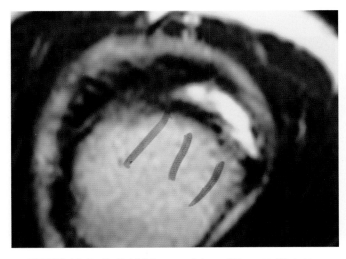

FIGURE 11–2. Partial-thickness rotator cuff tear, sagittal view.

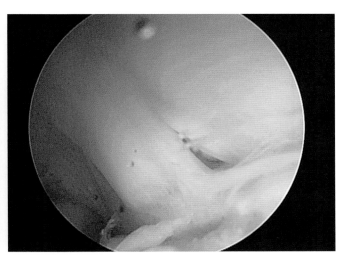

FIGURE 11–5. Supraspinatus tear grade 3.

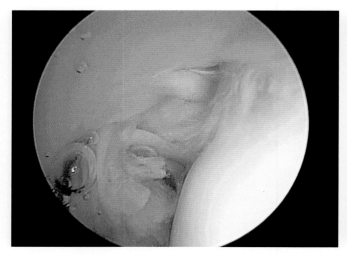

FIGURE 11–6. Supraspinatus tear grade 3.

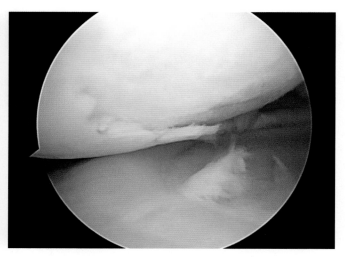

FIGURE 11–8. Chondral defect, humeral head.

whether the partial-thickness rotator cuff tear is coexistent with other clinical diagnoses (Figs. 11–8 and 11–9).

Intraoperative Decision Making

Three options are available for the arthroscopic treatment of partial-thickness rotator cuff tears: (1) débridement of the partial-thickness tear alone, (2) débridement of the tear with subacromial decompression, and (3) open or arthroscopic repair of the partial-thickness tear combined with subacromial decompression.

Four factors must be considered in the arthroscopic management of partial-thickness rotator cuff tears: (1) size and depth of the tear, (2) patient's desired activity level, (3) bone structure, and (4) the cause of the tear. No one factor solely determines treatment; the clinician's ability to analyze the effects of all the factors involved leads to appropriate management. I have found the following guidelines and thought processes helpful in my treatment of these troublesome lesions. The most critical decision is whether the tear can be treated by arthroscopic decompression alone or whether this must be accompanied by tendon repair. There

is no general agreement on how the area (length and width) of the tear should influence the surgeon. Most authors recommend surgical repair if 50% or more of the depth of the tendon substance is involved. I have always found this statement to be only partially helpful because I have not found any author's description of how the surgeon *precisely* determines the depth of tendon involvement. My practice is to débride the area until I observe normal tendon fibers. I then use the known dimensions of the shaver to *estimate* the depth of the lesion. I assume that the normal tendon thickness is 5 to 8 mm and use that to estimate the tear depth.

Sedentary patients with partial tears are more likely to do well with decompression alone; active patients are more likely to benefit from tendon repair. Patients with structural bone abnormalities (e.g., hooked acromion, inferior acromioclavicular joint osteophytes, anterior acromial spurs) are more likely to benefit from decompression. Patients with glenohumeral instability require correction of the lesions responsible for excessive translation. These factors are considered in light of patient preference. Some patients prefer tendon repair if it can more reliably effect a

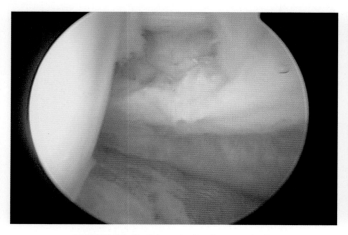

FIGURE 11–7. Infraspinatus tear grade 3.

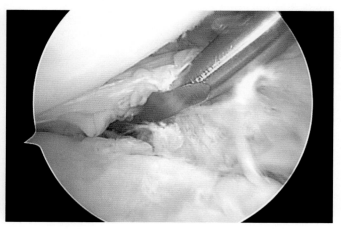

FIGURE 11–9. Small Bankart lesion.

cure; others may chose débridement or decompression because that approach offers fewer lifestyle inconveniences. At each end of the decision-making spectrum, treatment is less controversial. Active patients with normal bone shape and tears involving more than 50% of the tendon thickness are best treated with surgical repair. Sedentary patients with acromial spurring and tears involving less than 50% of the tendon thickness can be treated successfully with arthroscopic decompression alone. It is in the middle area that treatment is less well defined. Surgeon experience and patient preference, rather than scientific data, appear to dictate treatment.

Most partial-thickness tears appear on the articular surface of the rotator cuff tendon and are not visible during inspection of the bursal surface, such as occurs during an open procedure. It would seem, therefore, that the incidence of partial-thickness tears has been underestimated in the literature dealing with open shoulder surgery. Several techniques have been proposed to aid in diagnosing articular surface partial-thickness tears during open procedures. The techniques involving intra-articular fluid injection depend on the surgeon's ability to appreciate fluid egress from the cuff (saline injection) or staining of the cuff tissues with blue dye (methylene blue injection). These events signal a partial-thickness tear and should prompt the surgeon to split the cuff longitudinally to find the defect. Some surgeons incise the rotator cuff longitudinally if no defect is found but a tear is suspected on the basis of clinical or radiologic evaluation. Using such a longitudinal split, exposure is limited, and the articular surface of the cuff is not well visualized. Inspection of the cuff's articular surface is better performed through arthroscopic technique, because the entire cuff can be easily inspected, and the location, size, and depth of the tear can be appreciated. The tear can be marked with a suture so that the surgeon can locate the lesion during subsequent subacromial inspection.

Articular Surface Partial-Thickness Tears

 — Partial Rotator Cuff Tear

When an articular surface partial thickness rotator cuff tear is noted during the diagnostic examination, the surgeon should establish an anterior portal and should introduce a motorized shaver. Remember that you visualize the synovial lining, not the tendon, during the initial inspection. Perform a limited débridement to establish the length, width, and depth of the tear clearly. Some surgeons believe that the partial-thickness rotator cuff tear is always an intrinsic tendinopathy, and débridement stimulates a healing response. I am not comfortable with an "always" approach to partial-thickness rotator cuff tears, and I débride the partial tear to determine its size. If, based on the criteria discussed earlier, I decide that repair is necessary, I may use the shaver to complete the tear until the shaver enters the subacromial space. Usually, I perform a limited débridement and, while viewing from the glenohumeral joint, percutaneously insert a spinal needle into the area of partial tear. Generally, the area of needle insertion is near

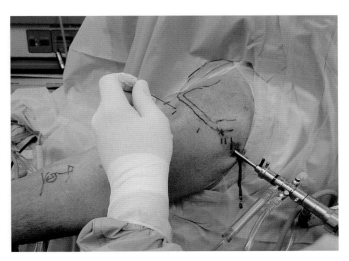

FIGURE 11–10. Percutaneous spinal needle insertion.

the anterolateral corner of the acromion because most articular surface partial-thickness rotator cuff tears are located in the anterior portion of the supraspinatus. If the tear is located more posteriorly, the needle insertion point will move further posteriorly.

I note the precise position of the needle within the tear and note how far the tear extends anteriorly, posteriorly, medially, and laterally from the needle. I then insert an absorbable monofilament suture through the needle and remove the needle (Figs. 11–10 to 11–14).

I then remove the arthroscope from the glenohumeral joint and insert it into the subacromial space. If I can see the monofilament suture, I create the lateral portal so that the cannula enters the subacromial space near the suture. If I cannot see clearly because of proliferative bursitis, I insert a spinal needle percutaneously to enter the subacromial space in the approximate area of the tear. I have a general idea of the tear's location and size based on examination of the rotator cuff tendon from the glenohumeral joint. I insert the

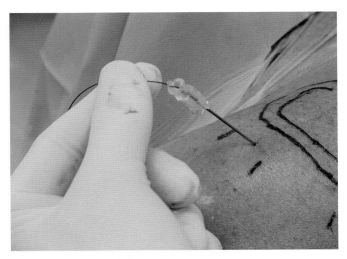

FIGURE 11–11. Pass monofilament suture through needle.

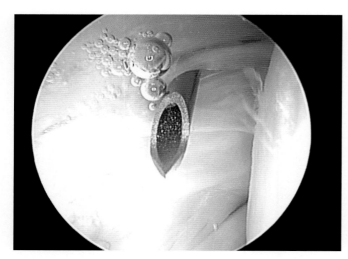

FIGURE 11–12. Needle through partial-thickness rotator cuff tear.

cannula and shaver and carefully remove bursal tissue beginning medial to the tear location until I can see the marking suture. Palpate the area of partial tear and you will appreciate the difference in tendon quality in the area of partial tear when compared with normal tendon.

I place the shaver near the point where the marking suture exits the tendon and remove the suture while holding the shaver firmly against the tendon. I begin débriding the tendon near its insertion into the greater tuberosity until I enter the joint. I use the shaver to palpate underneath the tendon and to determine the area of detachment (Figs. 11–15 to 11–17).

I remove the smallest amount of tendon possible because excessive débridement shortens the tendon. If the surgeon attempts to repair it to its anatomic insertion site, the result will be a repair under too much tension. This can lead to postoperative stiffness. I try to limit the débridement to 5 mm or less.

If, because of tendon damage, more débridement is nec-

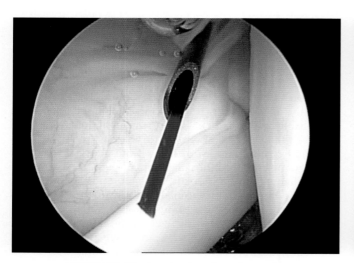

FIGURE 11–13. Insert suture through needle.

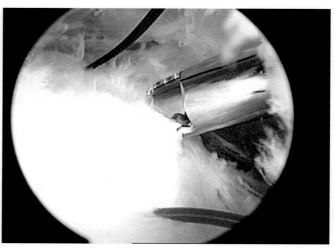

FIGURE 11–15. Anterior and posterior suture for larger partial-thickness rotator cuff tear, subacromial space.

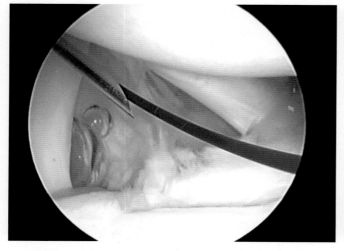

FIGURE 11–14. Advance sufficient suture into glenohumeral joint.

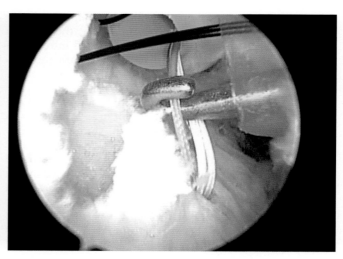

FIGURE 11–16. Rotator cuff repair.

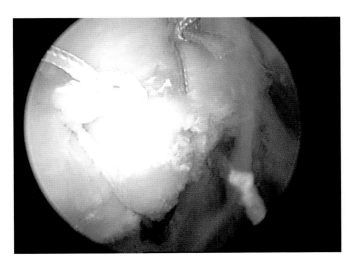

FIGURE 11–17. Rotator cuff repair, lateral view.

essary, I believe the surgeon should not repair the tendon edge laterally at its anatomic insertion site, but more medially. This approach will preserve the normal resting length of the torn cuff tendon and will decrease the incidence of tendon rupture and postoperative stiffness that result from a tendon repair under too much tension. A more medial repair requires that the bone-suture anchors are positioned correspondingly medial to their normal position. Once the articular surface partial-thickness rotator cuff tear is converted to a full-thickness tear, the surgeon can perform a standard rotator cuff repair.

Variations of Technique

Posterior Lesions

Partial-thickness rotator cuff tears are most often located on the articular surface of the anterior supraspinatus tendon. However, there is a subset of lesions located posteriorly, either in the posterior supraspinatus tendon or in the infraspinatus tendon. Because this area of the rotator cuff does not contact the anterior acromion during elevation, it does not seem likely that these lesions can be explained by the classic theory of outlet impingement. MRI studies have demonstrated *physiologic* contact between the posterior rotator cuff and the posterior superior glenoid during maximum abduction and external rotation. Therefore, contact that the surgeon observes between the rotator cuff and the glenoid on MRI or during arthroscopy is not necessarily pathologic. What is not clear at this time is why, in some patients, this contact does not produce pain, whereas other patients have significant symptoms. If the patient's complaints and physical examination findings demonstrate pain with abduction and external rotation localized to the posterior glenoid margin, the surgeon must search for an explanation. Walch and Jobe discussed the nature of posterior articular surface rotator cuff tears and introduced the term *internal impingement.*

A single theory to explain the etiology of internal impingement is unclear at this time. One theory is that anterior inferior glenohumeral instability occurs as a primary event. The resulting excessive translation causes a traction lesion on the posterior rotator cuff tendon as the rotator cuff is called on to stabilize the humeral head.

Another theory is that excessive anterior translation increases the frequency and degree of the normal physiologic contact, so that over time *compressive* pathologic tendon and labrum lesions occur when the arm is placed in abduction and external rotation. Another line of reasoning is that internal impingement is caused by superior posterior instability. The posterior contracture that occurs in throwing athletes causes traction on the posterior superior labrum. Because of a traumatic event or repetitive microtrauma, the biceps tendon–glenoid labrum anchor is detached. The loss of superior posterior stabilization allows superior posterior migration of the humeral head and rotator cuff. The resulting traction produces a rotator cuff tear.

Some surgeons believe that instability is not necessary for the development of internal impingement, and simple repetitive compression of the posterior rotator cuff between the humeral head and the glenoid is sufficient to cause damage. Another view is that a decrease of the normal 25 to 35 degrees of humeral retroversion leads to increased contact between the humeral head and the superior posterior glenoid.

I think we find ourselves in a situation similar to that confronting orthopedic surgeons in their search for an "essential" lesion to explain anterior inferior glenohumeral instability. We have learned that anterior inferior glenohumeral instability is actually a final result of numerous different causes. My own view is that all these conditions can produce internal impingement, but in an individual patient one of them is predominant. It is the task of the surgeon to identify which cause is responsible for pain. The analysis and diagnosis are difficult. Once the cause of the internal impingement is determined, the treatment is relatively straightforward (Figs. 11–18 to 11–21).

The preoperative evaluation should document the directions and degrees of translation, and the surgeon must compare them with the uninvolved shoulder. I test the amount of internal rotation with the patient's arm in 90 degrees of abduction in both the coronal and scapular planes. Radiographs and an MRI scan are usually necessary to determine the degree of rotator cuff involvement and the amount of humeral retroversion. At arthroscopic evalua-

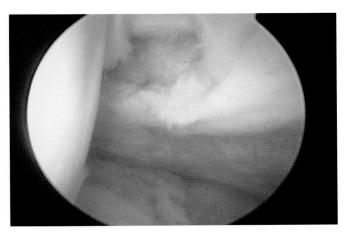

FIGURE 11–18. Posterior partial-thickness rotator cuff tear.

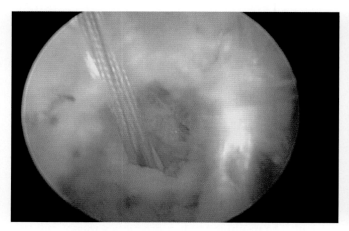

FIGURE 11–19. View from subacromial space.

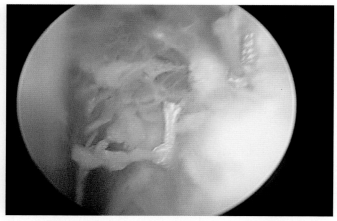

FIGURE 11–21. Rotator cuff repair, lateral view.

tion, I determine the direction and degree of humeral head translation and search for any signs that this translation is pathologic. I carefully evaluate all areas of the labrum for detachment, fraying, or tearing and assess the competency of the glenohumeral ligaments and the rotator interval. I then examine the posterior rotator cuff and evaluate the contact that exists between the cuff and the superior posterior glenoid when I place the patient's arm into abduction and external rotation. Gentle débridement may demonstrate a minor lesion of the synovial lining or tendon, but it may also reveal a near full-thickness tendon tear. I continue the posterior examination to evaluate the status of the posterior inferior glenohumeral ligament.

If the primary shoulder problem is one of instability, I perform an arthroscopic correction, and if the rotator cuff tear is minor, it is reasonable to treat lesser degrees of partial-thickness rotator cuff tear with débridement alone. If the partial-thickness rotator cuff tear is grade 2 or 3, I mark it with a needle and suture and view the lesion from the subacromial space. I complete the tear and repair it with standard technique.

Bursal Surface Partial-Thickness Tears

Articular surface partial-thickness rotator cuff tears have a varied etiology, and treatment is individualized. Bursal surface partial-thickness rotator cuff tears are almost always the result of chronic subacromial impingement. The surgeon should convert these lesions to full-thickness tears and should repair them with standard technique.

Postoperative Treatment

Patients with partial-thickness rotator cuff tears treated with débridement alone undergo rehabilitation similar to patients with arthroscopic subacromial decompression for subacromial impingement. A modification is made for strengthening. I do not strengthen the involved muscle for at least 3 months or until manual muscle testing does not produce pain. At that point, the muscle can be rehabilitated routinely. If a partial-thickness rotator cuff tear is converted to a full-thickness rotator cuff tear, rehabilitation proceeds as described in Chapter 12.

Bibliography

Andrews JR, Broussard TS, Carson WG: Arthroscopy of the shoulder in the management of partial tears of the rotator cuff: A preliminary report. Arthroscopy 1:117–122, 1985.

Barber FA, Morgan CD, Burkhart SS, Jobe CM: Current controversies. Point counterpoint. Labrum/biceps/cuff dysfunction in the throwing athlete. Arthroscopy 15:852–857.

Esch JC: Arthroscopic subacromial decompression: Results according to the degree of rotator cuff tear. Arthroscopy 4:241–249, 1988.

Fukuda H: Partial-thickness rotator cuff tears: A modern view on Codman's classic. J Shoulder Elbow Surg 9:163–168, 2000.

Gartsman GM: Partial thickness rotator cuff tears—evaluation and treatment. Current Orthopaedics 14(3):161–166, 2000.

Gartsman GM, Milne J: Partial articular surface tears of the rotator cuff. J Shoulder Elbow Surg 4:409–416, 1995.

Snyder S: Partial thickness rotator cuff tears: Results of arthroscopic treatment. Arthroscopy 7:1–7, 1991.

Weber SC: Arthroscopic debridement and acromioplasty versus mini-open repair in the treatment of significant partial-thickness rotator cuff tears. Arthroscopy 15:126–131, 1999.

Wright SA, Cofield RH: Management of partial-thickness rotator cuff tears. J Shoulder Elbow Surg 5:458–466, 1996.

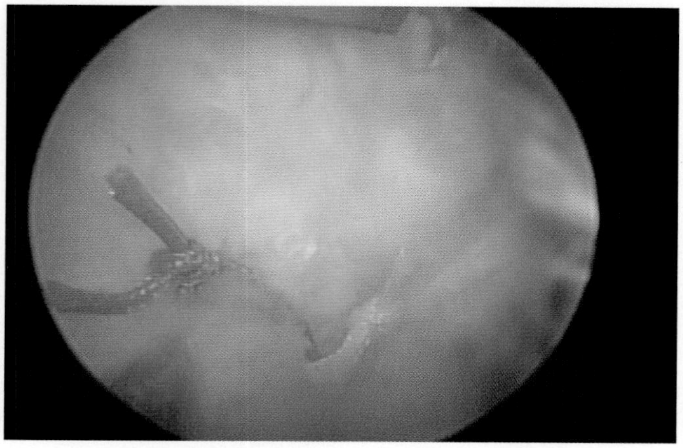

FIGURE 11–20. Rotator cuff repair, posterior view.

12

Full-Thickness Rotator Cuff Tears

An arthroscopic rotator cuff repair consists of the following elements: glenohumeral joint inspection, subacromial space inspection, partial bursectomy, assessment of rotator cuff tendon reparability, identification of tear geometry, coracoacromial ligament resection, acromioplasty, greater tuberosity repair site preparation, anchor placement, suture placement, and knot tying. Each of the individual elements can be accomplished arthroscopically; however, uniting them into a single operation requires strict adherence to a systematic operative technique.

Literature Review

Since the early 1990s, the repair of full-thickness rotator cuff tears has undergone a transition from open techniques, to combined open and arthroscopic methods (mini-open repair), and, most recently, to repairs using arthroscopic techniques exclusively. During this time, orthopedic surgeons have documented successful results with arthroscopic treatment of rotator cuff lesions such as stage 2 impingement and partial-thickness rotator cuff tears. Orthopedic surgeons now use arthroscopic techniques for many of the elements that comprise operative repair of a full-thickness rotator cuff tear. Arthroscopic acromioplasty, coracoacromial ligament release, bursal resection, and adhesion removal are now routinely performed.

When arthroscopic subacromial decompression is performed for a full-thickness tear without repair of the cuff defect, several authors have noted generally poor outcomes in most patients. Most current clinical data support the concept that subacromial decompression should be combined with tendon repair in patients with chronic full-thickness tears.

A technique that combines the arthroscopic evaluation of the glenohumeral joint and arthroscopic acromioplasty with open repair of the full-thickness rotator cuff tear is the mini-open method. Good results were described in initial studies by Blevins and colleagues, with 57 of 64 patients satisfied (89%), and by Paulos, with 16 of 18 patients with good to excellent results (88%). These authors were careful to point out that the limited incision used in the repair restricted this technique to the management of smaller, less retracted tears located in the anterior portion of the rotator cuff (supraspinatus and anterior half of the infraspinatus).

Orthopedic surgeons performing the mini-open repair have gained valuable experience toward the arthroscopic repair of full-thickness tears. The ability to assess the appearance of rotator cuff tears and to measure their size, tendon quality, and reparability arthroscopically has increased. Arthroscopic instruments, suture anchors, and suturing and knot tying techniques have also advanced. In other arthroscopic reconstruction procedures such as those for glenohumeral instability, orthopedic surgeons have developed expertise in relevant techniques such as arthroscopic bone preparation for soft tissue attachment, suture anchor placement, and knot tying. Collectively, these developments have allowed us to eliminate the open portion of the mini-open technique and to perform the repair using an all-arthroscopic technique.

Snyder and Gazielly documented their results using arthroscopic methods similar to those described in this chapter. Snyder presented 41 of 47 of patients (87%) with excellent and good results, and Gazielly reported on 15 patients with improvements of the Constant score from 58.1 to 87.6. My colleagues and I have reported similar results, and I summarize them later.

Diagnosis

The clinical presentation of patients with full-thickness rotator cuff tears is similar to that of patients with stage 2 impingement, although complaints of weakness, particularly with overhead activity, may be greater. Plain radiographs are essential to evaluate the shoulder for glenohumeral arthritis, superior migration of the humeral head, acromioclavicular joint arthritis, inferior acromioclavicular joint spurs, and acromial shape. Magnetic resonance imaging (MRI) provides information about the size and retraction of the rotator cuff tear. More important, MRI provides information about the degree of atrophy in the rotator cuff muscles (Figs. 12–1 to 12–4).

The findings from the clinical examination are most commonly correlated with those from radiologic studies (arthrography or MRI to make the diagnosis). Arthroscopy can be used as well to diagnose the presence and size of a complete rotator cuff tear, although no authors have suggested that this approach be used routinely. The arthroscope is most useful in diagnosing complete tears in patients who have false-negative imaging studies. False-negative results occur most frequently with arthrography, particularly if the synovial lining remains intact, or with MRI if the tear is smaller than 1 cm. I have found the injection of contrast material (gadolinium) before MRI to be helpful in increasing the accuracy of this imaging technique, particularly in patients with partial-thickness rotator cuff tears.

Nonoperative Treatment

The basic elements of nonoperative treatment are similar to those for patients with stage 2 impingement. They consist of selective rest and activity modification (avoiding painful activities and positions), nonsteroidal anti-inflammatory medication to reduce pain, and a home rehabilitation program designed to correct deficits of motion (with passive stretching) and strengthening of the uninvolved shoulder muscles.

The presence of a full-thickness rotator cuff tear is not necessarily an absolute indication for operation. I believe that some patients can be successfully managed with nonoperative care. Those patients have good-quality rotator

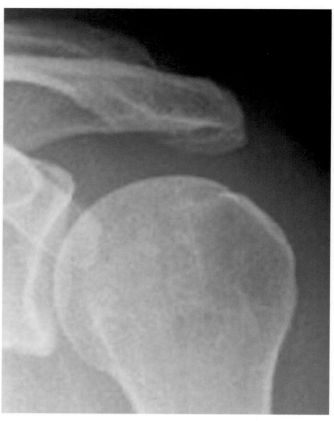

FIGURE 12–2. Anterolateral acromial spur.

cuff tendons, they report a specific injury that caused the onset of their symptoms, and they have little tendon retraction noted on MRI. I treat these patients nonoperatively and observe their progress monthly for 3 to 6 months. At this point, if their pain is controlled and they have good function, I will defer operation.

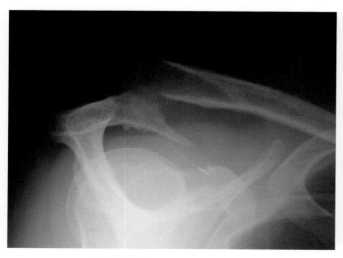

FIGURE 12–1. Type 3 acromion.

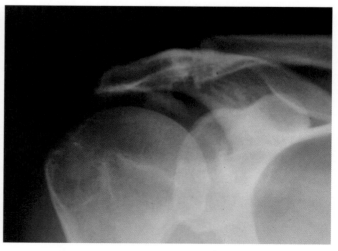

FIGURE 12–3. Ossification coracoacromial ligament.

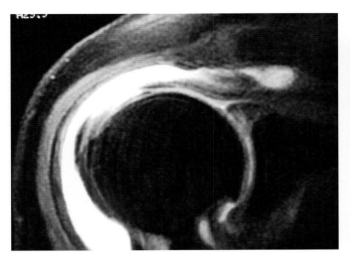
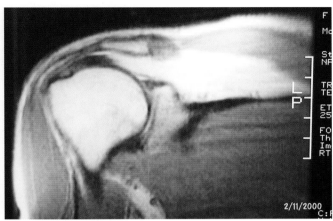

FIGURE 12–4. *A*, Full-thickness rotator cuff tear. *B*, Supraspinatus atrophy.

Indications

The indications for arthroscopic rotator cuff repair are identical to those for an open repair, and the surgeon should not in any way alter or "broaden" them in the mistaken view that arthroscopic repair is a lesser procedure. Although the skin incisions are smaller and the deltoid is left attached, arthroscopic repair incorporates all elements of open repair. I have repaired all sizes and shapes of rotator cuff tears with arthroscopic technique and have not performed any open repairs in the last 1200 operations. I have also found it helpful to present the patient with printed information outlining the postoperative rehabilitation and activity limitations that will occur.

Contraindications

Patients who are unable to tolerate either the surgical procedure or the postoperative rehabilitation of an open procedure are not candidates for an arthroscopic rotator cuff repair. Poor tendon quality, musculotendinous retraction, and muscular atrophy are not improved with arthroscopy.

Operative Technique

 — **Small Rotator Cuff Tear**

 — **Medium Rotator Cuff Tear**

 — **Large Rotator Cuff Tear**

 — **Reverse-L Rotator Cuff Tear**

 — **Tendon-to-Tendon Longitudinal Repair**

 — **Anterior Posterior Longitudinal Tears**

Anesthesia

I use interscalene block anesthesia supplemented with general anesthesia. Regional anesthesia allows for a decreased use of anesthetic agents. This approach minimizes postoperative side effects and allows for excellent pain relief in the postoperative period, so that the patient may begin physical therapy immediately after operation. General anesthesia eliminates unwarranted movement resulting from patient discomfort on the operating table.

Positioning

I prefer that the patient be in the sitting position because the orientation of the shoulder is similar to that seen during open procedures, and easy access is afforded to the anterior, lateral, and posterior aspects of the shoulder. I pay particular attention to the inclination of the acromion. The surgeon should position the patient so the acromion is as horizontal as possible (Fig. 12–5). The amount of posterior acromial slope varies from patient to patient, and failure to position the patient so the acromion is parallel to the floor causes the surgeon to direct the arthroscope more vertically and to have to work "uphill." Patient positioning is greatly facilitated by the use of the Schloein patient positioner (Orthopedic Systems, Inc., Union City, CA), and the patient's arm is controlled with a McConnell arm holder

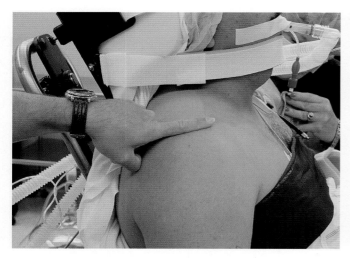

FIGURE 12–5. Acromion parallel to floor.

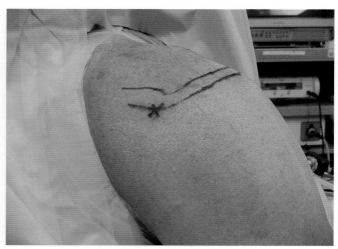

FIGURE 12–7. Posterolateral acromion.

(McConnell Orthopedics, Greenville, TX). The Schloein positioner speeds patient positioning and allows excellent access to the posterior shoulder without translating the patient off the side of the operating table. The McConnell arm holder allows the surgeon to position the patient's arm without occupying the assistant and is invaluable in maintaining proper arm rotation so that the repair site is directly underneath the operating cannula (Fig. 12–6).

Portals

Three portals are used. The posterior portal is 1.5 cm medial and 1.5 cm inferior to the posterolateral acromial border. The lateral portal is made 1 cm posterior to the anterior acromial border approximately 2 to 4 cm lateral to the acromion, and the anterior portal is made 2 cm anterior to the anterolateral acromion. The posterior portal is made superior to the traditional point of entry in the "soft spot" so that the arthroscope enters the subacromial space paral-lel to and just underneath the acromial undersurface. This maximizes the distance between the arthroscope and the rotator cuff tear and improves the surgeon's ability to determine tendon tear size and geometry (Figs. 12–7 and 12–8).

The lateral portal should allow the cannula (8-mm) to enter midway between the humeral head and the acromion. This location facilitates acromioplasty and also enables the surgeon to tilt the cannula inferiorly toward the humeral head so that the surgeon may easily place suture anchors in the greater tuberosity for rotator cuff repair (Figs. 12–9 and 12–10).

The anterior cannula (6-mm) is used for outflow and for retrieving sutures, but it may also be used for insertion of an anterior anchor. This cannula is inserted after the acromioplasty. Identify the precise location with a spinal needle so the center of the cannula is parallel to the tendon repair location. If the cannula is too medially placed, it is difficult to retrieve sutures from the anchors, because the patient's head will interfere. Conversely, nylon suture

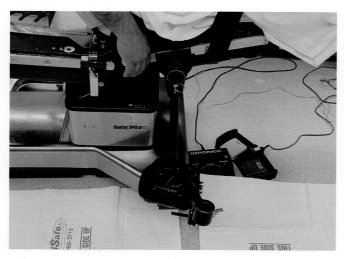

FIGURE 12–6. McConnell arm holder base.

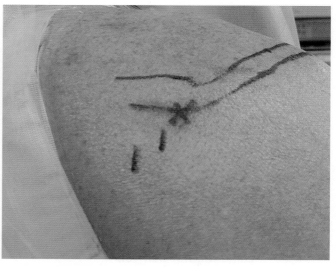

FIGURE 12–8. Soft-spot entry, my preferred entry site.

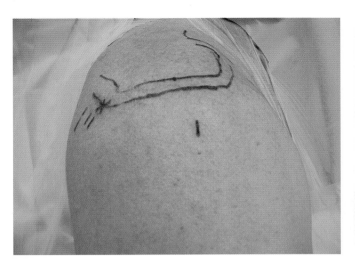

FIGURE 12–9. Lateral portal.

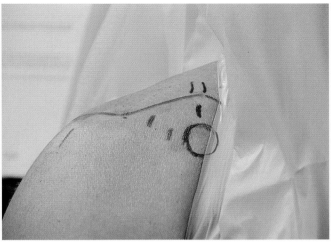

FIGURE 12–11. Anterior portals.

retrieval from the bursal rotator cuff surface is difficult if the anterior cannula is located too laterally (Figs. 12–11 to 12–16).

Glenohumeral Joint

I first determine the range of motion and stability of the shoulder with an examination while the patient is under anesthesia and then perform an arthroscopic glenohumeral joint inspection. Intra-articular lesions in patients with complete tears found during open rotator cuff repair are poorly and incompletely visualized, thus precluding ade-

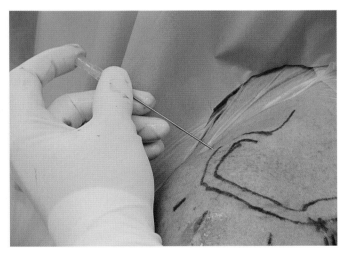

FIGURE 12–12. Establish anterior portal location with spinal needle.

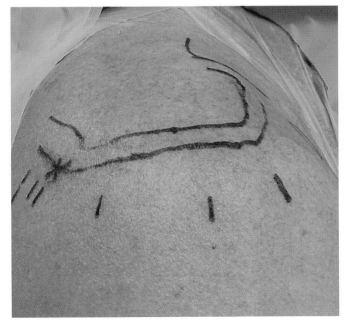

FIGURE 12–10. Accessory lateral portals.

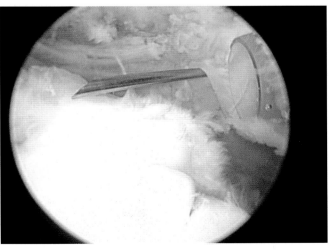

FIGURE 12–13. Needle too lateral.

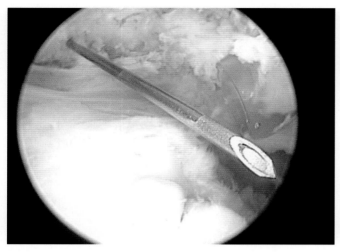

FIGURE 12–14. Needle too medial.

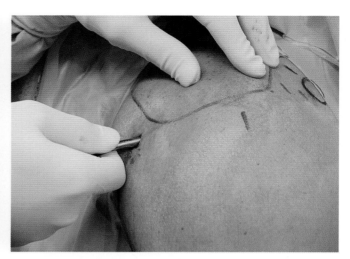

FIGURE 12–17. Palpate inferior acromion.

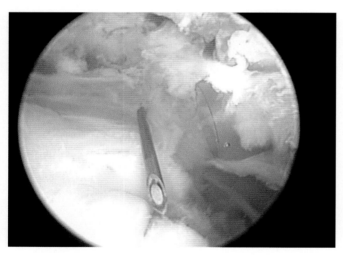

FIGURE 12–15. Needle parallel to rotator cuff edge.

quate comparison with arthroscopic findings. Most arthroscopic studies report abnormalities such as focal synovitis, partial biceps-tendon tears, arthritic changes in the humeral head or glenoid, labrum tears, and loose bodies. It is uncertain whether these intra-articular lesions arise because of the cuff tear or they merely accompany the cuff tear and occur during normal aging. Arthroscopic findings including arthritic changes, synovitis, and biceps tendon tears are often seen in patients, usually older, with irreparable tears. Not surprisingly, these findings occur with a higher frequency than in patients with partial or complete rotator cuff tears that are reparable. Overall, glenohumeral joint abnormalities occur in 12.5% of patients and include osteoarthrosis, biceps tendon tears (partial or complete), labrum tears, labrum separations (SLAP or superior labrum from anterior to posterior lesions), synovitis, and capsular contracture. On completion of the glenohumeral joint inspection the arthroscope is removed from the joint.

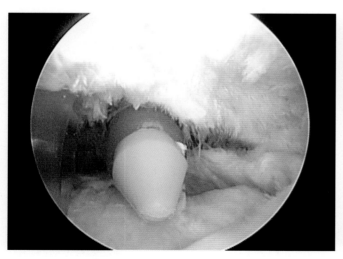

FIGURE 12–16. Anterior cannula.

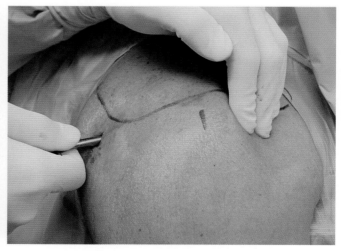

FIGURE 12–18. Palpate anterior acromion.

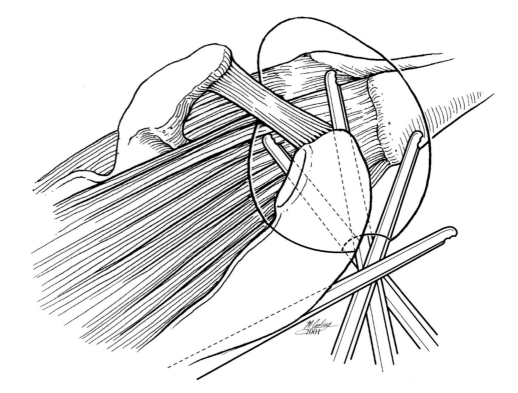

FIGURE 12–19. Sweep.

Subacromial Space

The cannula and trocar are then redirected through the same posterior skin incision into the subacromial space. I palpate the acromial undersurface with the cannula and sweep the cannula medially and laterally to make certain that no portion of the rotator cuff is adherent to the acromion (Figs. 12–17 to 12–19). The arthroscope is then inserted, and usually the space is easily seen. The camera is oriented so that the acromion appears horizontal and parallel to the floor, and I try to maintain this orientation throughout the procedure. I also try to maintain maximum distance between the arthroscope and the tendon lesion, because this helps the surgeon best appreciate the extent of the tendon tear (Fig. 12–20). The lateral portal is located with a spinal needle. Insert the needle percutaneously and

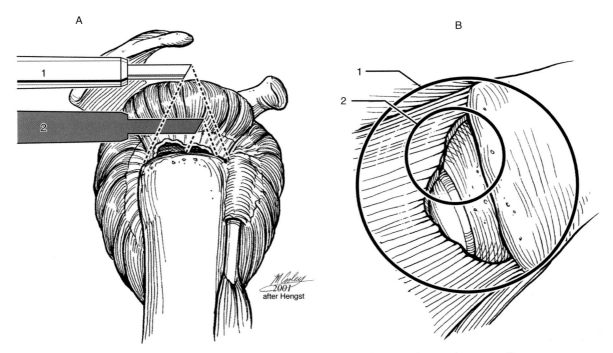

FIGURE 12–20. *A* and *B*, Maintain distance between arthroscope lens and rotator cuff.

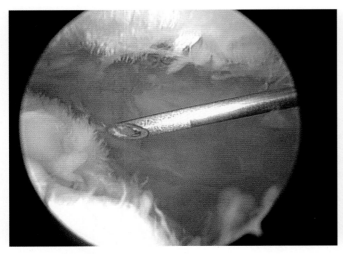

FIGURE 12–21. Insert needle parallel to acromion.

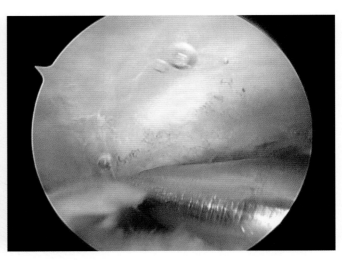

FIGURE 12–23. Coracoacromial ligament erythema.

direct it so that it is 1 cm posterior to the anterior acromial border and positioned midway between the acromion and the greater tuberosity (Fig. 12–21). A cannula is then inserted.

The first goal is clear visualization of the subacromial space. Bursa that obscures visualization is removed with a power shaver (Fig. 12–22). The surgeon should cautiously remove only the bursa that interferes with visualization and should not alter the appearance of the rotator cuff or acromion. Bursal tissue is involved in the healing response, and complete bursectomy appears unwarranted. Once the bursa is removed, the acromion and coracoacromial ligament are examined for signs of impingement such as erythema, fraying, and fibrillation (Figs. 12–23 and 12–24).

Tear Classification

The arthroscope is then rotated so that it points directly down at the rotator cuff tear. With small- to medium-sized

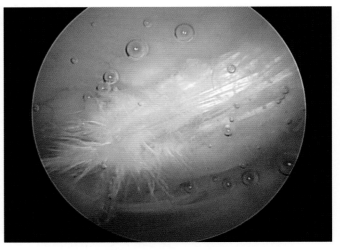

FIGURE 12–24. Coracoacromial ligament fraying.

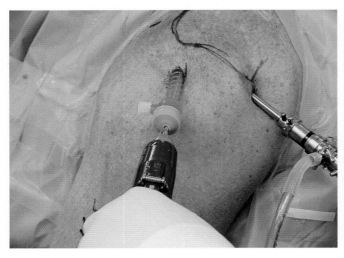

FIGURE 12–22. Bursectomy.

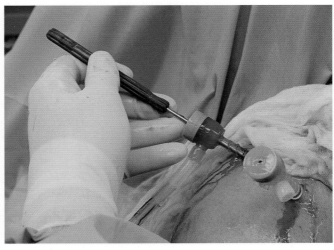

FIGURE 12–25. Introduce measuring probe.

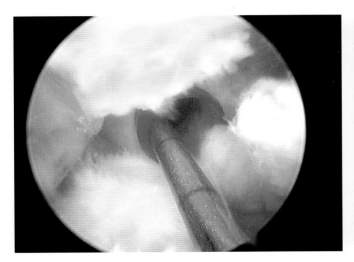

FIGURE 12–26. Measure rotator cuff tear.

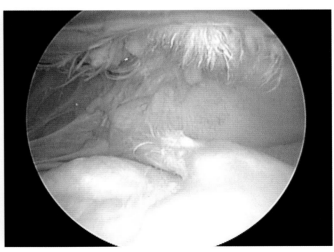

FIGURE 12–28. Transverse tear.

tears, the size and tear geometry are easily appreciated. The tear size is measured by comparing it with the known diameter of the lateral cannula or measuring it with an arthroscopic probe. The length of the tear from anterior to posterior and the amount of medial retraction are noted (Figs. 12–25 and 12–26).

Straight medial retraction and retraction in an elliptical shape are the most common findings. As tear size increases, the surgeon's ability to appreciate tear geometry becomes more difficult. In a right shoulder, reverse-L tears with a longitudinal component along the rotator interval will allow the tear to rotate posteriorly. L-shape tears have a longitudinal limb posteriorly, often at the junction of the

supraspinatus and infraspinatus, in addition to the lateral detachment at the greater tuberosity.

 — **Reverse-L Rotator Cuff Tear**

Longitudinal tears may occur in the area of the rotator interval and occasionally within the substance of the supraspinatus (Figs. 12–27 to 12–34). Only when tear geometry is appreciated can the surgeon perform an effective repair. I use a tissue grasper to pull on the tear edge, in an attempt to determine the repair site location. Varying

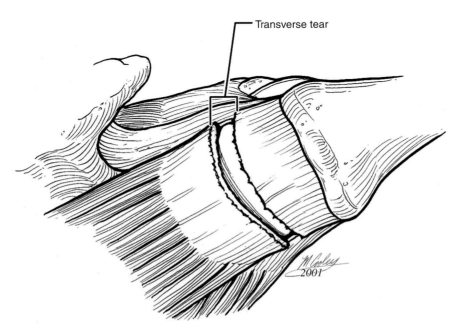

Transverse tear

FIGURE 12–27. Transverse tear.

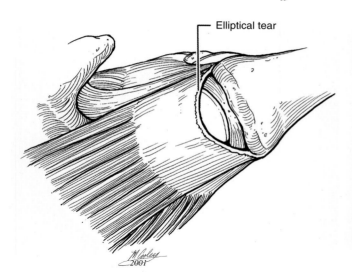

FIGURE 12–29. Elliptical tear.

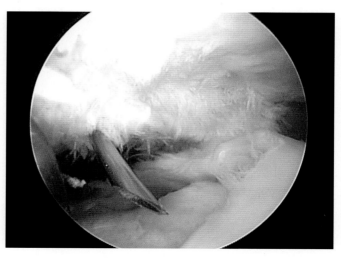

FIGURE 12–30. Elliptical tear.

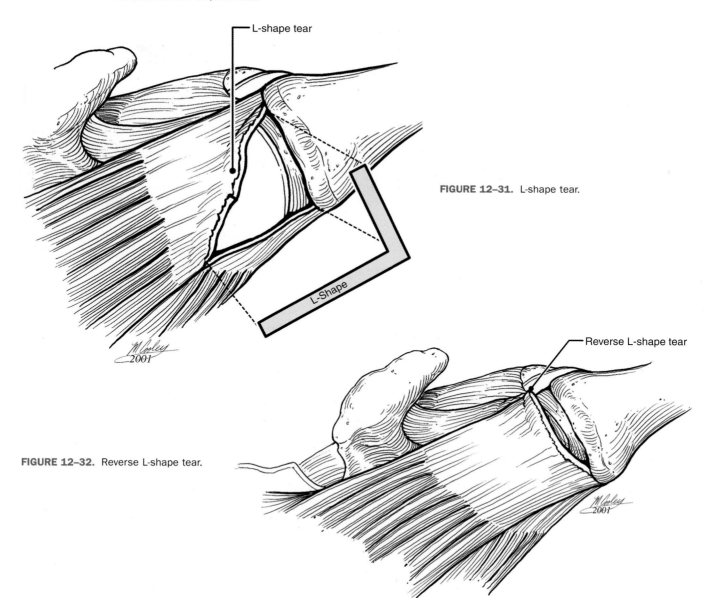

FIGURE 12–31. L-shape tear.

FIGURE 12–32. Reverse L-shape tear.

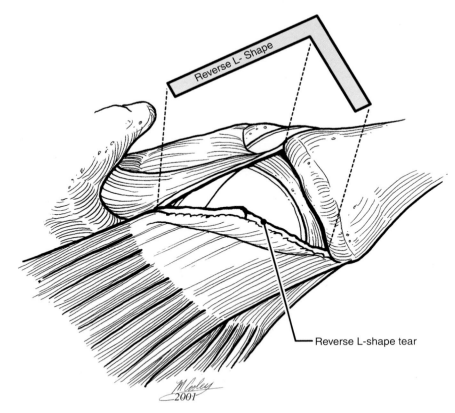

FIGURE 12–33. Reverse L-shape tear.

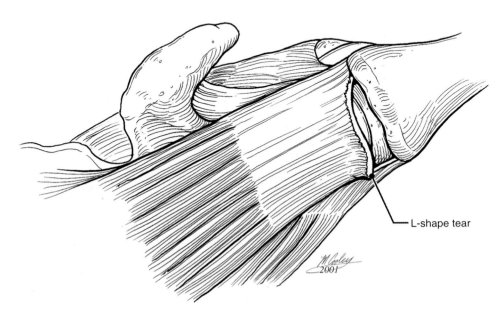

FIGURE 12–34. L-shape tear.

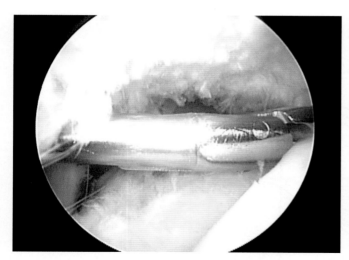

FIGURE 12–35. Grasper through lateral cannula to test tendon mobility.

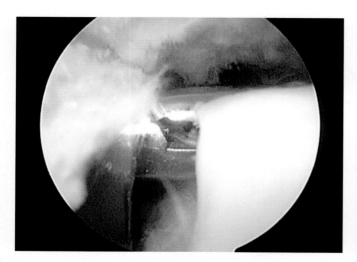

FIGURE 12–36. Grasper through lateral cannula to test tendon mobility.

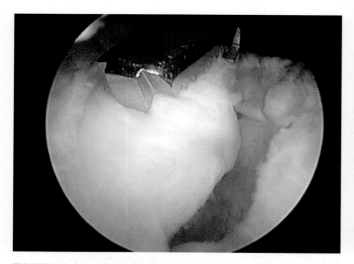

FIGURE 12–37. Grasper through anterior cannula to test tendon mobility.

both the direction of pull and the arm positions of elevation, abduction, and rotation are often required. Typically, the patient's arm is positioned in 20 degrees of elevation, 15 degrees of abduction, and 10 degrees of internal rotation (Figs. 12–35 to 12–42).

The arm is maintained in this position with the McConnell arm holder. Only when I determine that the tear is reparable do I begin the subacromial decompression. I prefer to maintain the static stabilizing effect of the coracoacromial arch (acromion and coracoacromial ligament) if the tear is not reparable or not likely to be durable, to protect against anterior superior subluxation or escape of the humeral head. With larger or retracted tears, I have found it helpful to move the arthroscope to the lateral portal to gain additional perspective.

Coracoacromial Ligament

If a full-thickness rotator cuff tear is reparable and the result of chronic impingement, I divide the coracoacromial ligament at its lateral insertion point on the acromion. I prefer to use the electrocautery device because of the inconvenient location of blood vessels in this area. Once the lateral margin of the ligament has been released, a power shaver resects the ligament to the medial acromial border (Fig. 12–43).

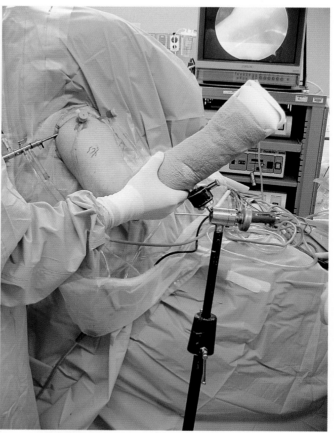

FIGURE 12–38. Maneuver arm until tear reduced and directly under lateral cannula.

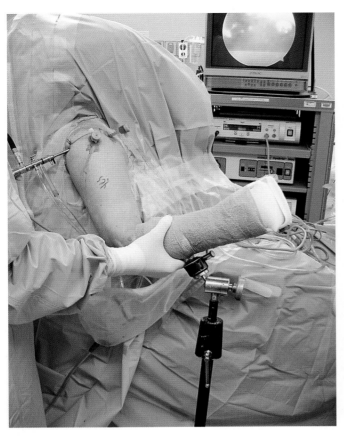

FIGURE 12–39. Maneuver arm until tear reduced and directly under lateral cannula.

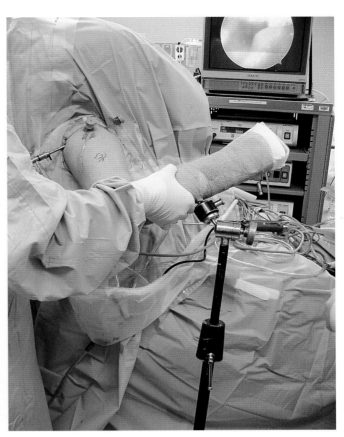

FIGURE 12–40. Maneuver arm until tear reduced and directly under lateral cannula.

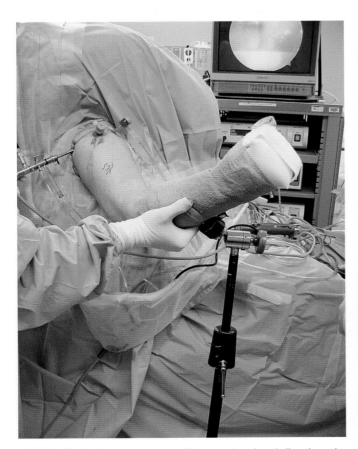

FIGURE 12–41. Maneuver arm until tear reduced and directly under lateral cannula.

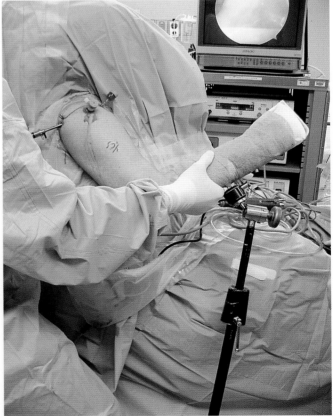

FIGURE 12–42. Maneuver arm until tear reduced and directly under lateral cannula.

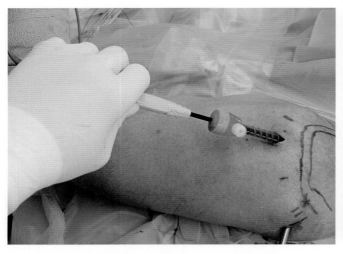

FIGURE 12–43. Identify anterolateral acromion.

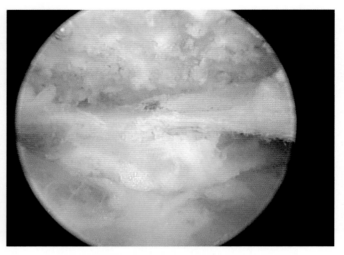

FIGURE 12–45. Completed acromioplasty.

Acromioplasty

The goal of the acromioplasty is to increase the size of the subacromial space. A type 2 or 3 acromion is converted to a flat, type 1 acromion. Unless the bone is extremely thick, there is no need to perform an acromioplasty of a type 1 acromion. I do not try to alter the medial lateral or anterior posterior dimensions of the acromion. If the acromion has a lateral slope as identified on MRI or plain radiographs, the inferior aspect of the lateral acromion is further thinned. I start the acromioplasty laterally and resect bone until the inferior portion of the medial acromion is removed and the soft tissue of the acromioclavicular joint is visible (Figs. 12–44 and 12–45).

Acromioclavicular Joint

After the medial acromion has been removed and the acromioplasty has been completed, the acromioclavicular

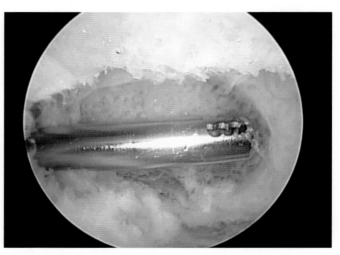

FIGURE 12–46. Completed acromioclavicular joint resection.

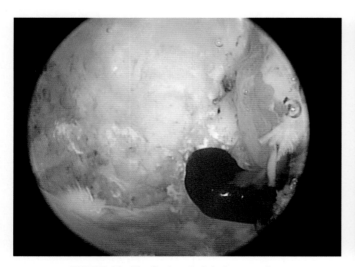

FIGURE 12–44. Cautery to inferior acromion.

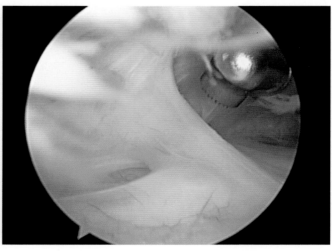

FIGURE 12–47. Subacromial adhesion.

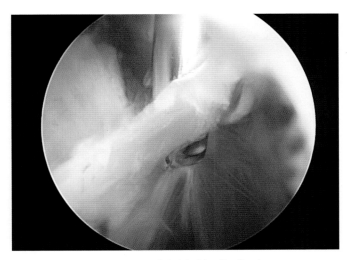

FIGURE 12–48. Subdeltoid-cuff adhesion.

joint comes into view. If preoperative imaging has detected inferior osteophytes, I coplane the joint by removing the inferior third of the distal clavicle with a power bur. Only if the patient has symptoms consistent with acromioclavicular joint arthritis on preoperative history and examination do I then perform an acromioclavicular joint resection (Fig. 12–46).

Cuff Mobilization

Adhesions may form within the subacromial space between the rotator cuff and the acromion or the rotator cuff and the deltoid, and they interfere with tendon mobilization. Adhesions to the coracoid or coracohumeral ligament contracture may restrict rotator cuff tendon excursion and may thereby falsely give the impression of irreparability (Figs. 12–47 and 12–48).

Posterior adhesions usually are not dense, and I can often release them by inserting a metal trocar and cannula through the lateral portal, by placing it superior to the anterior tear edge and sweeping posteriorly directly beneath the acromion.

Occasionally, electrocautery is used to divide adhesions if they are particularly thick. I have found it unwise to attempt to remove dense adhesions with a power shaver because bleeding will often result, and it is difficult to control because of the medial location of the bleeding vessels. Anterior adhesions to the coracoid are usually very thick and require release with electrocautery. This is particularly true in the area of the coracohumeral ligament (Fig. 12–49).

Repair Site Preparation

The next step is preparation of the bone surface at the repair site. A 4-mm round bur is used to prepare a cancellous bed for the tendon. The surgeon removes 1 to 2 mm

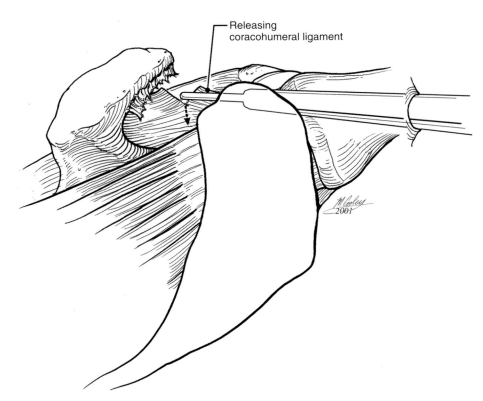

FIGURE 12–49. Coracohumeral ligament release.

Releasing coracohumeral ligament

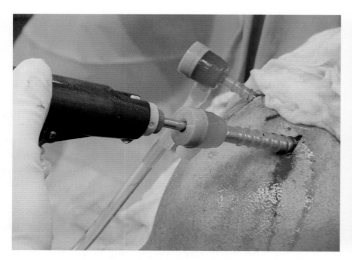

FIGURE 12–50. Prepare repair site.

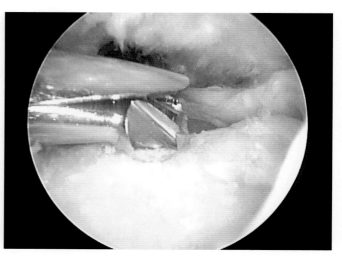

FIGURE 12–52. Bone abrasion.

of cortical bone until the cancellous bone is visible (Figs. 12–50 to 12–52).

I do not place the tendon in a trough. I consider this portion of the procedure a decortication and remove only 1 to 2 mm of bone. The site of bone preparation is based on tendon mobility. If an anatomic repair is possible, the bone is prepared from the articular margin of the humeral head to the greater tuberosity. The tendon tear length determines the length of the bone preparation site in its anterior to posterior dimension. The width is the distance from the articular cartilage of the humeral head to the medial margin of the greater tuberosity, a width of 1 to 2 cm. If anatomic repair is not possible without excessive tendon tension, I move the repair site. I prefer to repair the tendon up to 10 mm medially without tension rather than anatomically under excessive tension.

Anchor Selection

Anchor Design

The ideal suture anchor should have the following characteristics:

1. It should allow firm fixation in the greater tuberosity.

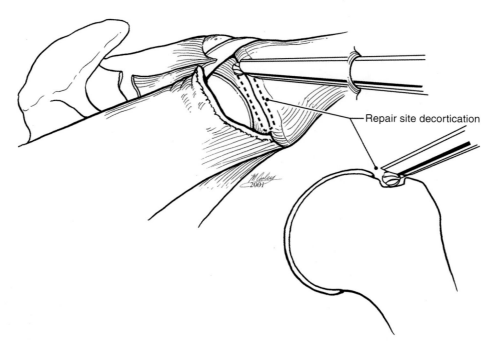

Repair site decortication

FIGURE 12–51. Width and depth of repair site.

2. The surgeon should be able to select which suture type is loaded on the anchor.
3. The anchor should be inserted manually without the need for predrilling or power instruments.
4. The suture should slide through the anchor.
5. The anchor should be removable from the bone in case of suboptimal placement or suture breakage.
6. The anchor must be attached securely to the inserting device so that it does not become dislodged during placement within the tight confines of the subacromial space.
7. The anchor must be able to penetrate the bone at an acute angle.
8. It should be biodegradable without any adverse effects.

No currently available suture anchor meets all these criteria. Each available anchor offers relative advantages and disadvantages when compared with the others, and the surgeon should select the anchor based on personal preference.

Currently, I use 5-mm anchors (Smith & Nephew Endoscopy, Andover, MA) for rotator cuff repair. These anchors have excellent pullout strength. The handle design and shaft length of the inserter are appropriate. The anchors are attached to the inserter shaft sufficiently so that they do not dislodge as the surgeon manipulates the anchors within the subacromial space. The anchors have a trocar tip so that predrilling is not necessary. I do not like to predrill during

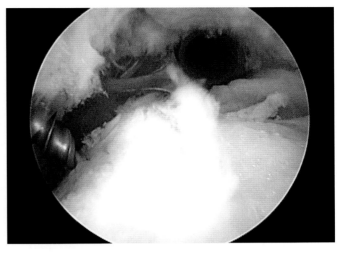

FIGURE 12–54. Anchor inserted perpendicular to greater tuberosity.

rotator cuff repair because the area lateral to the tuberosity is covered with soft tissue, and this makes it difficult to find the screw hole.

I also like an anchor I can insert with one hand because I prefer to hold the arthroscope simultaneously with the other hand. With tap-in anchors, it is necessary for the assistant to hold the arthroscope while the surgeon positions the anchor with one hand and uses the mallet with the other. The Smith & Nephew anchor has two preloaded No. 2 braided, nonabsorbable sutures. One suture is green and the other is white. This helps me to select the appropriate suture during the rotator cuff repair. The anchor eyelet is large enough to allow the sutures to slide freely during knot tying (Figs. 12–53 to 12–56).

Anchor Material

Anchors are available that are composed of four different materials: metal, nonabsorbable plastic, bioabsorbable plas-

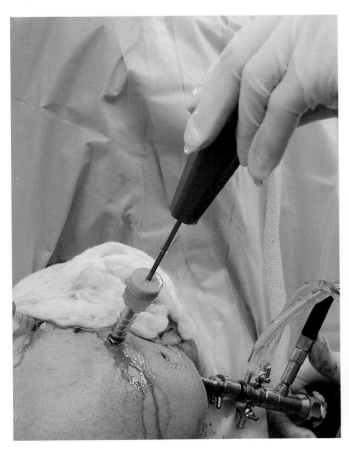

FIGURE 12–53. Insert anchor with fingertip pressure.

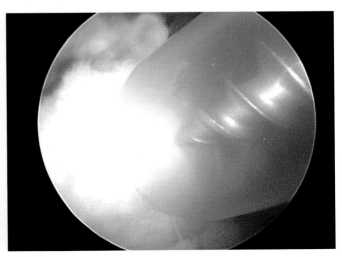

FIGURE 12–55. Slide cannula to greater tuberosity if soft tissue interfering.

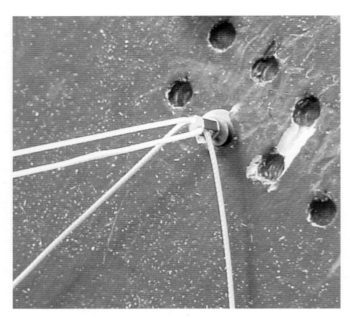

FIGURE 12–56. Order of sutures in anchor.

tic, and allograft bone. Currently, I prefer metal anchors because they offer secure fixation and lower cost. I also prefer that they are radiopaque. This feature allows me to visualize situations of anchor pullout or migration on a plain radiograph. The disadvantage of metal anchors is that they compromise postoperative MRI imaging even when specialized digital subtraction techniques are used.

I am not comfortable with the tissue reactions observed with currently available bioabsorbable anchors but remain confident that research in materials will alleviate this problem. I have had difficulty inserting plastic nonabsorbable anchors because of anchor deformation unless the anchor is inserted optimally. I have no experience with allograft bone anchors, although these anchors offer the advantage of bone graft to the proximal humerus.

Suture Selection

Because the management and identification of sutures within the subacromial space can be difficult, it is advantageous to use different colored sutures. The anchor is preloaded with one white and one green suture. This method allows the surgeon to identify more easily which suture corresponds to each suture anchor. I prefer braided, nonabsorbable No. 2 suture.

Anchor Placement

The number of anchors depends on the length and geometry of the rotator cuff tear. For all but the smallest tears, I place two anchors. I place the anchors lateral to the greater tuberosity for the following reasons:

1. The anchor is placed in bone with an intact cortical surface as compared with the prepared cancellous bed of the repair site.

2. Bone density is greater in this distal location than in the more proximal bone.
3. The angle of anchor insertion between the anchor and the bone is minimized, thus allowing straight-in anchor insertion.
4. The anchor can be inserted through the cannula without the need for percutaneous insertion.
5. Lateral anchor position places the vector of tendon pull approximately 90 degrees to the longitudinal axis of the anchor and thus minimizes anchor pullout.
6. The tendon can be repaired anatomically. If the anchors are positioned medially on the tuberosity, the ultimate tendon healing site also is moved medially.

The Smith & Nephew anchor inserter has two marks near the anchor end. The circumferential, transverse mark indicates the appropriate depth of insertion. I insert the anchor until this line is beneath the bone cortex.

The longitudinal lines on the inserter shaft indicate anchor eyelet orientation. The eyelet opening lies in the plane perpendicular to the plane that incorporates the two longitudinal lines. Understanding eyelet orientation is critical so that the sutures slide freely during knot tying. Theoretically, the eyelet should be parallel to the tendon edge, because this would allow the sutures to slide most easily. The problem the surgeon faces during the surgical procedure is that selecting the appropriate suture limb is both technically challenging and complicated by the anchor eyelet's subcortical location and by obscuring bursa. If the surgeon selects the suture limb nearest the tendon edge for passage through the tendon, the suture slides freely while tying; however, if the opposite limb is selected, the suture strands will cross after passage through the tendon and will encounter resistance to sliding. To eliminate this problem, I orient the eyelet perpendicular to the tendon edge. With the eyelet in this position, it does not matter which suture limb I select for passage, and the eyelet is large enough so that either suture limb will slide freely (Figs. 12–57 to 12–63).

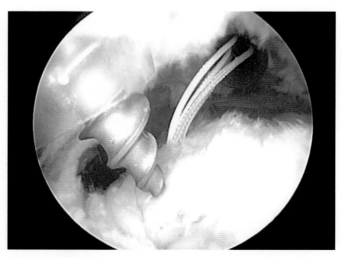

FIGURE 12–57. Anchor trocar tip penetrates bone without predrilling.

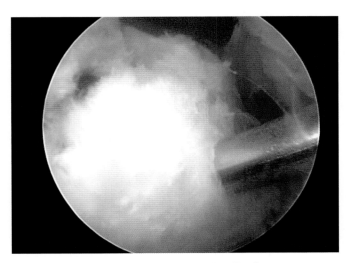

FIGURE 12–58. Insert anchor distally.

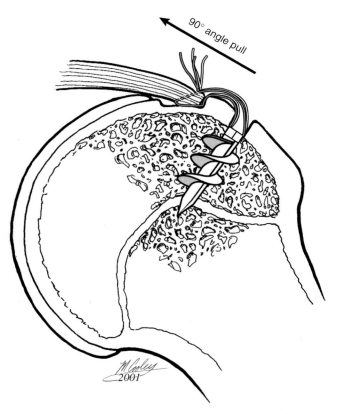

FIGURE 12–59. Right angle between tendon and anchor.

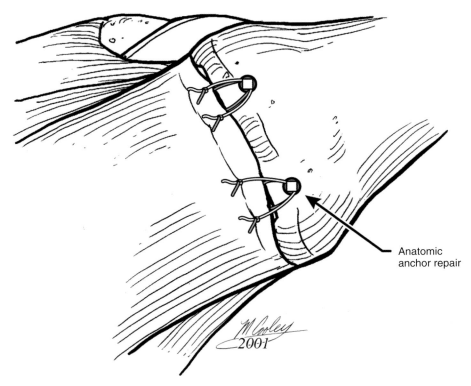

Anatomic anchor repair

FIGURE 12–60. Anatomic repair.

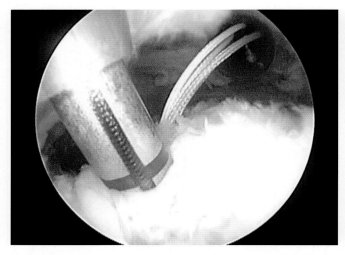

FIGURE 12–61. Horizontal mark indicates depth. Longitudinal mark indicates eyelet orientation.

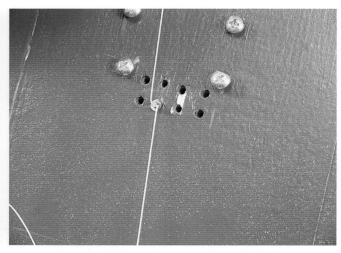

FIGURE 12–62. Either suture limb will slide freely.

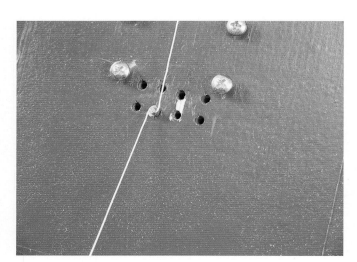

FIGURE 12–63. Either suture limb will slide freely.

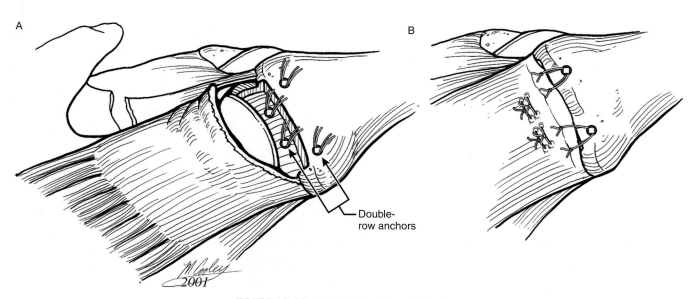

Double-row anchors

FIGURE 12–64. *A* and *B*, Double-row technique.

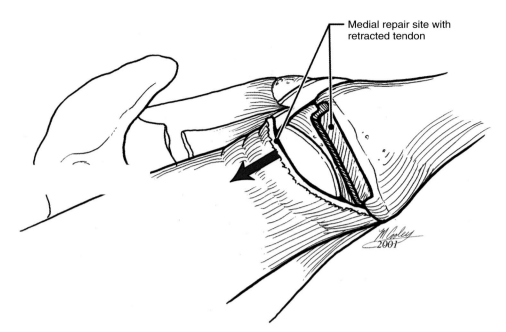

Medial repair site with
retracted tendon

FIGURE 12–65. Medial repair.

Alternative Technique 1

Some surgeons prefer to insert all anchors in the bed of the sulcus to repair the tendon more directly to the repair site. Others prefer a *double-row technique* with anchors inserted laterally to repair the tendon anatomically and an additional row of anchors medially for tendon-bone approximation. Theoretically, this technique should increase the tendon-bone contact area; however, investigators have not been able to demonstrate this in a laboratory setting (Fig. 12–64).

I repair the rotator cuff tear with the patient's arm in relative adduction. If the tendon cannot advance to its anatomic insertion point with the arm in adduction, I repair the tendon medially. I believe that function is not compromised by up to 10 mm of medialization. I do not believe that you can repair the tendon in abduction, brace it postoperatively, gradually lower the arm, and have the repair "stretch" (Figs. 12–65 and 12–66).

I place the most anterior anchor first and then proceed posteriorly with additional anchors as needed. I position the anchor trocar tip against the humeral cortex approxi-

FIGURE 12–66. Medial repair.

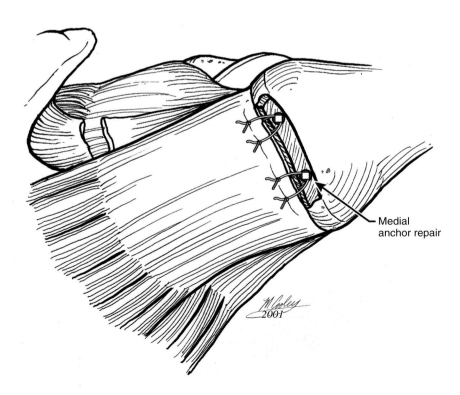

Medial
anchor repair

mately 5 mm distal to the greater tuberosity. I apply slight pressure until the trocar tip punctures the cortex. I then rotate the handle and let the anchor threads advance the anchor without pushing inward. I do not apply pressure to the anchor handle because the osteoporotic bone in some patients will allow the anchor to plunge into the humerus. After I insert each anchor, I pull on the suture strands to test anchor fixation. Ideally, one should be able to translate the humeral head (and patient) laterally when pulling on the sutures. This step assures me that the anchors are well inserted.

After the anchors are inserted, I pass the anchor sutures through the tendon. Passing the sutures independently of the anchor insertion allows me to determine the precise location of suture penetration through the tendon more easily.

Alternative Technique 2

Another technique is to insert an anchor, pass the sutures, and tie the knots before proceeding to the next anchor. If the surgeon is comfortable with this technique, it may produce good results. I find this approach difficult for two reasons. First, in large tears, it is often difficult to judge which suture goes where, and errors in anatomic repair are more likely. Second, in smaller tears, if the knots are tied and a portion of the tendon is repaired, it is possible to disrupt the repair when the suture-passing instruments are used for the remainder of the repair (Fig. 12–67).

After I insert each anchor, Dr. Hammerman inserts a crochet hook through the anterior cannula, pulls the four suture strands out the cannula, and clamps them with a hemostat so that each group of sutures is kept together. We find it helpful to use a differently sized hemostat for each group of four sutures to designate from which anchor they originate.

Suture Placement

Once suture anchor placement has been completed, the braided sutures are passed through the torn tendon. The soft tissue grasper is passed through the lateral cannula. Then the precise location for the tendon repair and the location and spacing of each suture are estimated. I space the sutures evenly from the anterior and posterior margins of the tear and place them approximately 5 to 8 mm proximal to the tendon edge. I insert the anchors from anterior to posterior and then pass the sutures through the tendon from anterior to posterior.

Suture Passing

The Caspari suture punch does not accept braided suture. I currently employ a 2-0 nylon suture, looped in half, as a suture relay. I prefer this over a wire shuttle because of its decreased cost and ready availability. The two free ends are passed into the suture punch, and the loop end exits from the handle.

I insert the Caspari punch through the lateral cannula and grasp the tendon at the point that I believe should be translated to the anterior anchor. I close the Caspari punch's jaws *slightly* but do not puncture the tendon, so that the instrument functions as a tissue grasper. I then pull the tendon toward the anterior anchor and determine whether this is indeed an anatomic repair. Often, it is apparent that some change in humeral position is necessary. Once I have assured myself that I have identified the appropriate site for the first suture, I then close the punch's jaws until I can see the needle tip of the suture passer exit from the tendon. The tendon is grasped and punctured, and the two paired suture ends advanced into the subacromial space. This seemingly simple step actually can prove quite difficult because of the tendon's thickness and the bursa

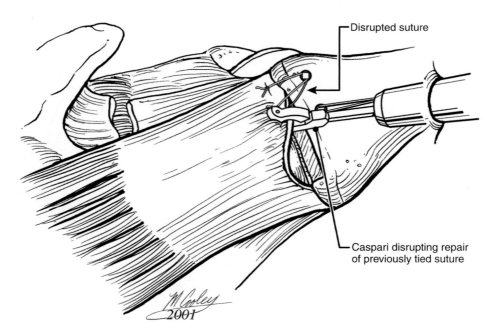

FIGURE 12–67. Caspari suture punch may disrupt previously tied sutures.

overlying the tendon surface. The needle on the Caspari punch is 4 mm, and if the tendon thickness is greater than 5 to 6 mm, it is hard to pass the needle tip completely through the tendon. My own solution to this problem was to ask Linvatec (Largo, FL) to modify the needle tip and to increase its length to 6 from 4 mm. This small modification has helped me greatly and is now available to any surgeon. Another technique I use is to twist the Caspari punch while I pull on the tendon so that I force the needle through the tendon. If I can see a thin layer of bursa or tendon covering the needle tip but I cannot advance the nylon sutures, Dr. Hammerman will insert a crochet hook through the anterior cannula, sweep away the bursa, and provide counterpressure. This technique allows the needle tip to penetrate the tendon fully.

The crochet hook is used to retrieve the free ends of the nylon suture out the anterior cannula, and a hemostat is applied to the suture ends. The hemostat prevents the nylon sutures from being pulled inadvertently through the anterior cannula as the Caspari punch is withdrawn laterally. The suture punch is then removed through the lateral cannula, and the loop is left protruding out the lateral cannula.

The hemostat on the anterior anchor sutures is removed. The crochet hook then is used to retrieve one of the anterior suture anchor strands and to bring it out the lateral cannula. To find the appropriate anchor, advance and rotate the arthroscope so that it points toward the anchor. Insert the crochet hook through the lateral cannula and identify the anterior anchor. Hook a limb of the green suture first and gently pull on it. If you have the correct suture, it will slide freely because the hemostat has been removed. If there is resistance, either you have selected the wrong suture (from a more posterior anchor) or it is entangled in the other sutures. Have your assistant tug on the correct suture exiting the anterior cannula to ensure that you have made the right choice. Another technique at this point in the operation is to have your assistant place the correct suture in the knot pusher and pass it down the anterior cannula into the subacromial space until you can visualize it.

To ensure that the nylon loop and the braided suture have not become entangled, suture retrieval forceps are passed through the lateral cannula into the subacromial space, and both strands of nylon suture are enclosed within the suture retrieval forceps' jaws. The braided suture should remain external to the forceps. The suture retrieval forceps' jaws are kept closed around the two nylon suture strands, and the retrieval forceps are removed from the cannula. This is a critical step and should be repeated for each suture.

The free end of the braided suture is placed within the loop of the 2-0 nylon external to the lateral cannula. Traction is placed on the two ends of the nylon suture anteriorly, and the braided suture is pulled from the lateral cannula, into the subacromial space, through the tendon, and out the anterior cannula. At this point, a simple suture has been placed through the anterior rotator cuff. Repeat these steps as necessary for the remaining anterior suture anchor strand and additional, more posterior, suture anchor strands. Some surgeons may find it helpful to apply a hemostat to each pair of suture strands immediately after passage through the tendon. This makes it impossible inadvertently

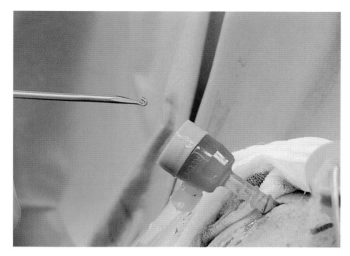

FIGURE 12–68. Retrieve anchor sutures out anterior cannula.

to pull the suture out from the tendon or from the anchor, and I believe is a critical point in suture management for the inexperienced surgeon (Figs. 12–68 to 12–93).

Text continued on page 224

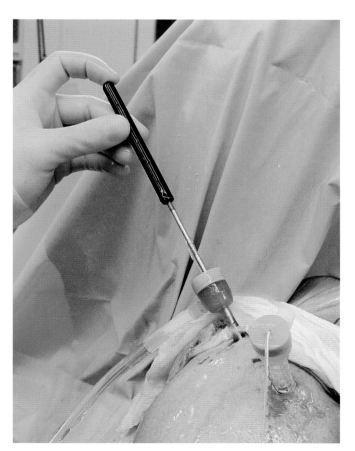

FIGURE 12–69. Retrieve anchor sutures out anterior cannula.

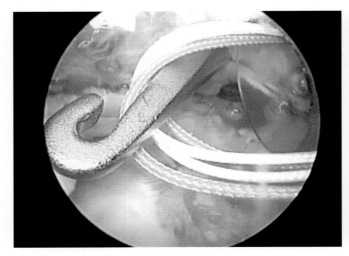

FIGURE 12–70. Retrieve anchor sutures out anterior cannula.

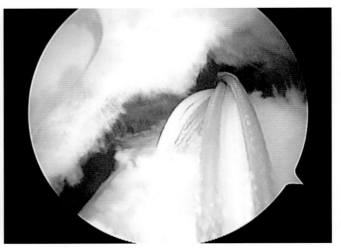

FIGURE 12–71. Retrieve anchor sutures out anterior cannula.

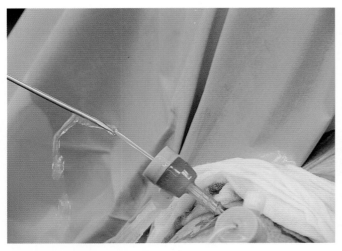

FIGURE 12–72. Retrieve anchor sutures out anterior cannula.

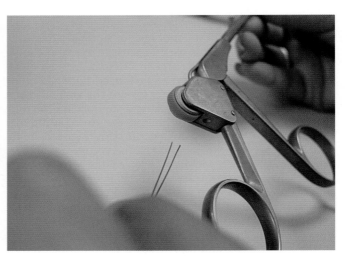

FIGURE 12–73. Load 2-0 nylon into Caspari suture punch.

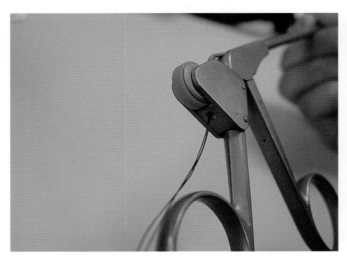

FIGURE 12–74. Load 2-0 nylon into Caspari suture punch.

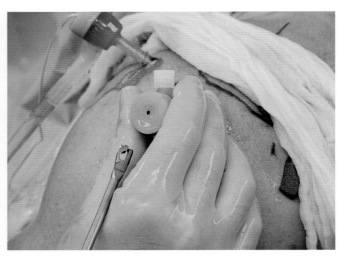

FIGURE 12–75. Insert Caspari suture punch through lateral cannula.

2

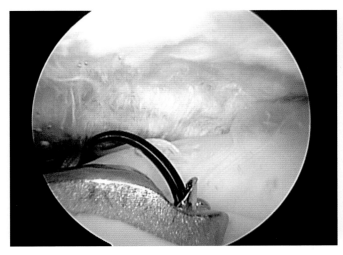

FIGURE 12–76. Puncture tendon.

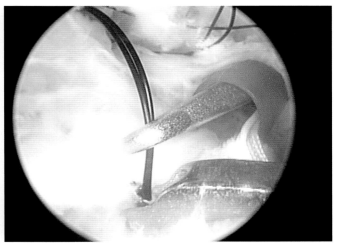

FIGURE 12–77. Retrieve two free ends of nylon out anterior cannula.

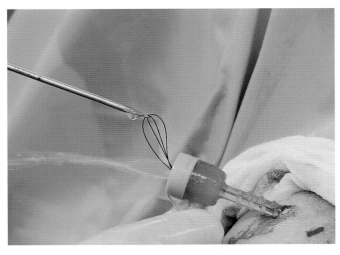

FIGURE 12–78. Retrieve two free ends of nylon out anterior cannula.

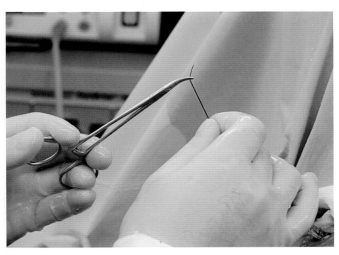

FIGURE 12–79. Apply hemostat.

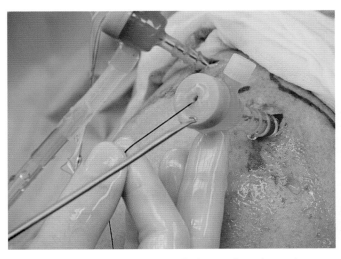

FIGURE 12–80. Looped end of nylon out lateral cannula.

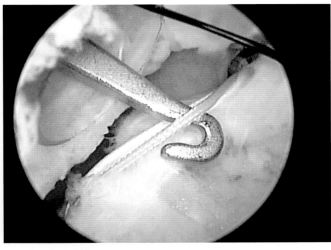

FIGURE 12–81. Retrieve one limb of anchor suture from anterior cannula.

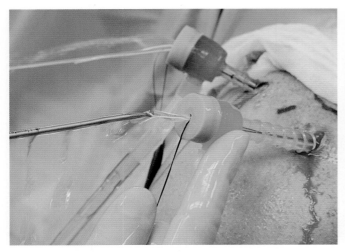

FIGURE 12–82. Withdraw suture out lateral cannula.

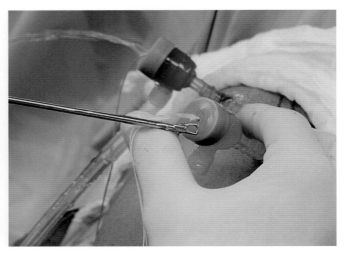

FIGURE 12–83. Use looped grasper to check for suture tangles.

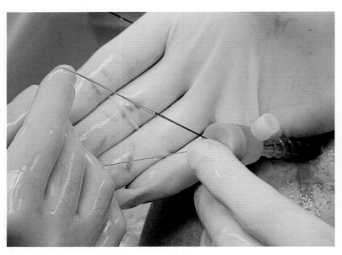

FIGURE 12–84. Insert 7.5 cm of anchor suture through nylon loop.

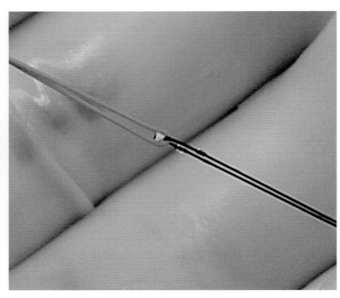

FIGURE 12–85. Close-up view.

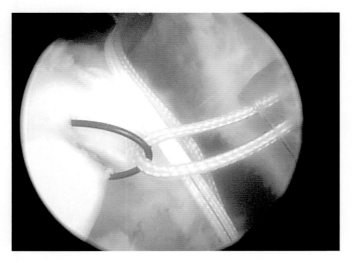

FIGURE 12–86. Pull on nylon sutures exiting anterior cannula and pull suture down lateral cannula in subacromial space.

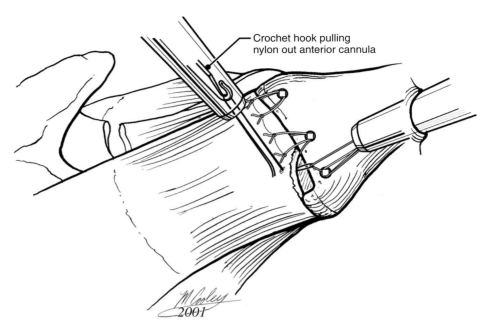

Crochet hook pulling
nylon out anterior cannula

FIGURE 12–87. Pull on nylon sutures exiting anterior cannula and pull suture down lateral cannula in subacromial space.

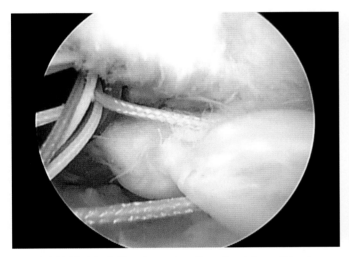

FIGURE 12–88. Pull anchor suture through rotator cuff tendon.

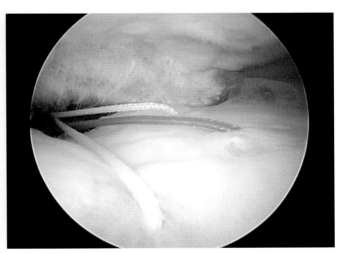

FIGURE 12–89. Remove slack in anchor sutures.

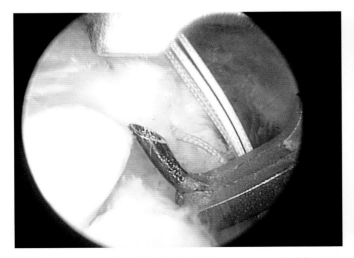

FIGURE 12–90. Alternative technique when space is tight.

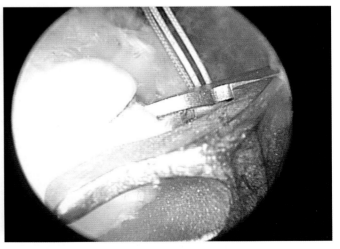

FIGURE 12–91. Rotate Caspari suture punch 90 degrees.

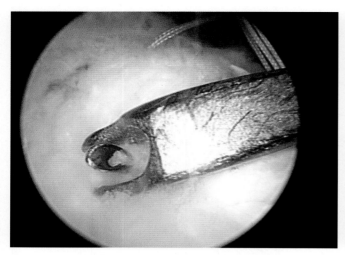

FIGURE 12–92. Slide under tendon.

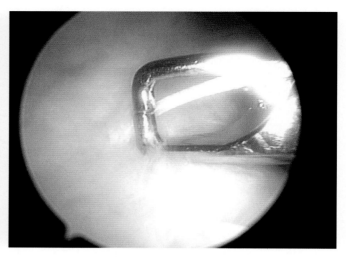

FIGURE 12–95. Check for tangles.

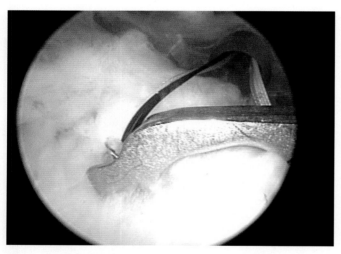

FIGURE 12–93. Advance nylon suture.

Knot Tying

Knot tying generally begins posteriorly and proceeds anteriorly, although the surgeon may modify this as determined by tear geometry. With a crochet hook, each pair of posterior anchor sutures is transferred from the anterior cannula to the lateral cannula and is tied individually. The anterior sutures are retrieved from the anterior cannula and brought out the lateral cannula, and these sutures tied in similar fashion. I have tried various suture techniques (mattress, modified Mason-Allen) but find them cumbersome and time consuming. Mattress sutures double the number of passes through the tendon and, because of their medial location on the tendon, cause the tendon edge to flip upward. I prefer to use simple (rather than mattress) sutures to repair all sizes of rotator cuff tears and have not experienced problems with suture pullout. Simple sutures pass over the tendon edge and hold it firmly against the bone (Figs. 12–94 to 12–100).

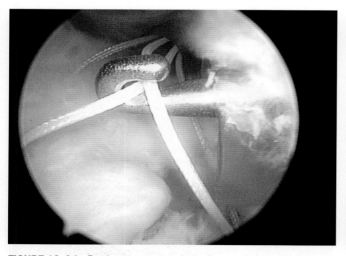

FIGURE 12–94. Retrieve two suture limbs from anterior cannula to lateral cannula.

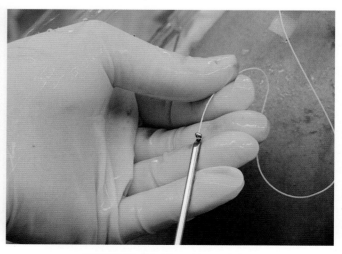

FIGURE 12–96. Thread knot pusher.

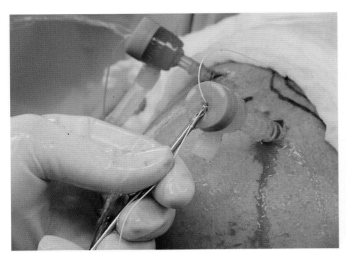

FIGURE 12–97. Advance knot pusher down lateral cannula.

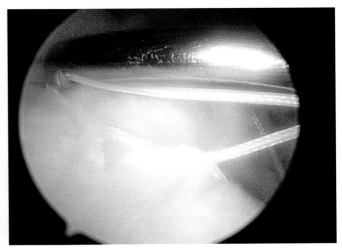

FIGURE 12–99. Second overhand throw.

— **Knot Tying**

— **Suture Technique Variations**

Horizontal Cleavage Tears

If the distal edge of the articular-sided layer is even with the distal edge of the more superficial bursal-sided layer, I repair the two layers together anatomically and incorporate both in the repair. First place a suture through the deeper layer using the Caspari suture punch and the technique previously described. Apply a hemostat to the corresponding limb of suture that was *not* passed through the deep layer. Repeat the process to pass the nylon shuttle suture through the superficial layer. Using the crochet hook, iden-tify the suture limb that was passed through the deep tendon layer and move it back to the lateral cannula. Pull this suture limb through the superficial tendon layer with the nylon shuttle suture, to complete passage through both layers. Remove the hemostat from the other limb of the suture and reapply it to both limbs.

If the deep layer is retracted medially (as is often the case) and will not advance laterally, I then repair it *in situ* with a mattress suture. Because the Caspari punch will not allow you to reach far enough medially to the superficial layer, I use the Cuff-Stitch to insert this suture.

After the repair is completed, I remove the patient's arm from the arm holder and move it through a range of motion. This allows me to document repair security and to examine the amount of clearance between the rotator cuff and the acromion.

Each incision is closed with a single subcutaneous, in-verted 3-0 absorbable monofilament suture and Steri-Strips. An absorbent sterile dressing is placed over the shoulder.

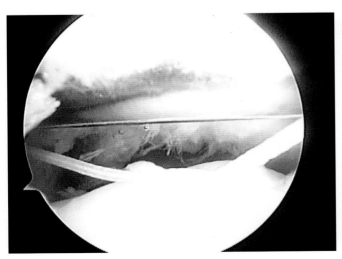

FIGURE 12–98. Overhand throw.

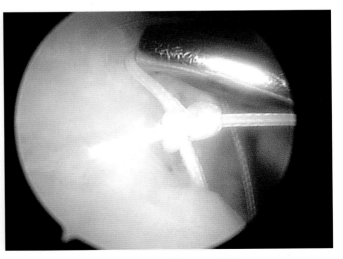

FIGURE 12–100. Slip second throw.

Postoperative Treatment

The postoperative management is identical to that of an open repair. I remove the dressing the morning after the operation and allow the patient to shower without any protection for the surgical wounds. The patient is placed in a sling, except for those periods when the continuous passive motion machine moves the arm in elevation and then into external rotation (Figs. 12–101 to 12–103).

The safe limits of movement are determined at the time of the surgical procedure and are documented. I have the patient use the continuous passive motion chair for 2 weeks. I evaluate the patient in the clinic after 2 weeks and obtain an anterior posterior radiograph to evaluate anchor position. I discontinue the continuous passive motion chair and have a physical therapist instruct the patient in passive range-of-motion exercises for elevation and external rotation with a dowel or pulley. The patient continues to wear the sling and is cautioned to avoid active range of motion with the operated shoulder. I next see the patient at 6 weeks after the operation. Passive range of motion continues, but active elevation and external rotation are allowed. Strengthening is instituted after 3 months, and the rehabilitation continues for 12 months.

Results

Because complete arthroscopic rotator cuff repair is a relatively recent procedure, there is little published literature to guide the surgeon. Our experience is that the results are equal to those of open repairs or mini-open repairs. I found that the average postoperative University of California at Los Angeles (UCLA) score was 31 out of 35, and 84% of patients were rated as good to excellent. Moreover, the UCLA, American Shoulder and Elbow Surgeons, and Constant rating systems all demonstrated an improvement in shoulder function (Tables 12–1 to 12–5). When the results were analyzed in terms of patient self-reporting, we found improvement in all the parameters of the 36-item Short Form Questionnaire (SF-36).

Effect of Associated Glenohumeral Lesions on Repair Strategies

In an early report on arthroscopic rotator cuff repair, we analyzed those patients with glenohumeral lesions (major labral tears, Bankart and SLAP lesions, and osteoarthrosis) as a subgroup. Mean preoperative UCLA scores were 23.7 for the normal group and 10.9 for the group with a major glenohumeral lesion. Postoperative UCLA scores were 31.2

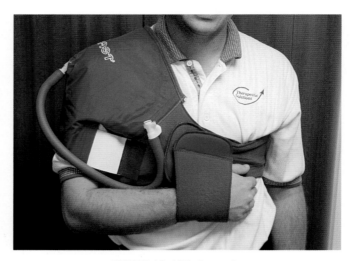

FIGURE 12–102. Ice pack.

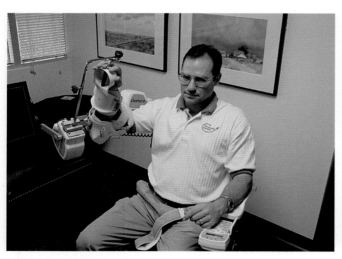

FIGURE 12–101. Continuous passive motion chair.

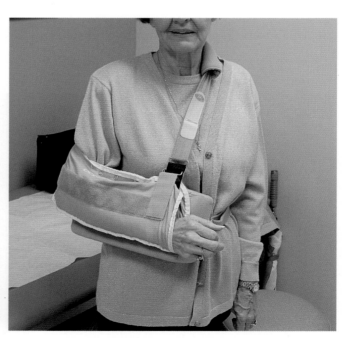

FIGURE 12–103. Shoulder immobilizer.

TABLE 12–1. RESULTS OF ARTHROSCOPIC REPAIR

System	Preoperative		Postoperative	
UCLA total	12.4	+/–4.2	31.1*	+/–3.2
Pain	2.4	+/–1.7	8.6*	+/–3.2
Function	3.7	+/–2.2	8.9*	+/–1.2
Flexion	3.6	+/–2.2	4.9*	+/–0.3
Strength	2.3	+/–1.0	4.1*	+/–0.9
Satisfaction	0.4	+/–0.5	4.6*	+/–0.9
ASES total	30.7	+/–15.7	87.6*	+/–12.8
Pain	7.7	+/–1.7	1.4*	+/–1.6
Function	11.4	+/–5.7	26.8*	+/–8.0
Constant (absolute)	41.7	+/–12.8	83.6*	+/–9.0
Constant (age-adjusted)	43.3	+/–11.6	84.0*	+/–7.5
Pain	3.58	+/–2.62	12.91*	+/–2.34
Function	3.37	+/–1.94	18.78*	+/–1.53
Elevation	7.62	+/–2.45	9.78*	+/–0.63
Abduction	6.15	+/–2.62	9.56*	+/–1.13
External rotation	6.82	+/–2.16	9.53*	+/–1.18
Internal rotation	6.66	+/–2.12	9.08*	+/–1.18
Strength	7.51	+/–4.69	14.00*	+/–5.41

*P = .0001
ASES, American Shoulder and Elbow Surgeons; UCLA, University of California at Los Angeles.

TABLE 12–2. AMERICAN SHOULDER AND ELBOW SURGEONS ACTIVITIES OF DAILY LIVING*

Activity	Preoperative		Postoperative	
Put on coat	1.55	+/–0.76	2.93	+/–0.30
Sleep	0.96	+/–0.95	2.62	+/–0.70
Reach up back	1.01	+/–0.76	2.70	+/–0.46
Toilet	2.39	+/–0.84	2.97	+/–0.16
Comb hair	1.59	+/–0.96	2.89	+/–0.36
Reach high shelf	0.96	+/–0.95	2.67	+/–0.58
Lift 10 pounds above shoulder	0.53	+/–0.78	2.22	+/–0.99
Throw overhead	0.55	+/–1.05	2.81	+/–0.99
Work	1.33	+/–1.05	2.81	+/–0.99
Sports	0.52	+/–0.82	2.67	+/–0.73

*All significant (P = .0001); Wilcoxon signed rank test used for difference between preoperative and postoperative scores.

TABLE 12–3. RESULTS OF ARTHROSCOPIC REPAIR ON RANGE OF MOTION*

Passive Range of Motion	Preoperative		Postoperative	
Elevation	135	+/–22	149	+/–4
External rotation	66	+/–12	78	+/–10
Internal rotation	L1	+/–4 levels	T9	+/–3 levels

*Differences significant (P = .001); Wilcoxon signed rank test used to test for significance.

TABLE 12–4. RESULTS OF ARTHROSCOPIC REPAIR*

Criterion	Preoperative		Postoperative	
Physical function	57.2	+/–25.7	76.6	+/–27.1
Role, physical	24.6	+/–37.4	75.7	+/–40.4
Bodily pain	27.2	+/–19.7	68.2	+/–24.1
General health	70.8	+/–28.7	72.4	+/–21.8
Vitality	50.6	+/–24.2	62.8	+/–18.4
Social functioning	57.5	+/–31.2	84.0	+/–25.5
Role, emotional	62.1	+/–43.8	82.4	+/–334.3
Mental health	70.3	+/–22.2	78.2	+/–19.3
Physical component summary	34.1	+/–9.1	46.6	+/–10.8
Mental component summary	48.7	+/–13.1	52.6	+/–9.4

*Differences in preoperative and postoperative SF-36 Health Survey Scores significant at $P = .0015$ for all scores except general health and mental component summary.

for the normal group and 29.9 for the group with a major glenohumeral lesion, differences that are not statistically significant. The comparison indicates that identification and treatment of intra-articular lesions resulted in outcomes similar to those in patients without intra-articular lesions.

Complications

The most common complications of arthroscopic rotator cuff repair are stiffness and recurrent tear or disruption of the repair. The treatment of these two complications is no different from when they occur after open rotator cuff repair. If stiffness persists 6 months after operation, I perform an arthroscopic contracture release as described in Chapter 6. If the patient has persistent pain and weakness, I obtain an MRI scan with gadolinium. Unfortunately, this often results in a false-positive study because of artifact from the prior operation. Nonetheless, persistent pain and weakness 6 months postoperatively are relative indications for revision operation. If a tear is identified at reoperation, it is repaired again. Occasionally, adhesions in the sub-acromial space produce a tethering effect and are responsible for the pain. The adhesions are usually easily removed. Most patients elect to have a second operation, but some, who are improved but have moderate pain and good function, accept their condition and decline further surgical treatment.

Anchor Retrieval

Occasionally, the surgeon will need to remove an anchor after it is inserted. Either the anchor is malpositioned or the surgeon has pulled the suture out of the anchor or had the suture break during knot tying. One option is to insert another anchor and ignore the empty anchor. If the surgeon wishes to remove the anchor, there are several techniques. If the sutures are still in the anchor, use the wire loop to replace the sutures in the inserter. Advance the inserter gently into the screw hole until it engages the anchor. Keep traction on the sutures so that the inserter maintains contact with the anchor and unscrew it.

If there are no sutures in the anchor, the situation is more difficult. If the bone quality is poor, there will be no resistance as you insert the inserter and try to engage the

TABLE 12–5. RESULTS OF ARTHROSCOPIC REPAIR

Criterion	Preop UCLA	Postop UCLA	Preop Strength	Postop Strength	Length	Width	Size	Age
Preoperative UCLA	1.00	0.081	0.417	0.067	0.067	–0.049	0.015	–0.157
Postoperative UCLA	0.081	1.00	0.309	0.515	–0.161	–0.092	–0.122	–0.04
Preoperative strength	0.417	0.309	1.00	0.456	–0.244	–0.131	–0.199	–0.448
Postoperative strength	0.067	0.515	0.457	1.00	–0.407	–0.310	–0.373	–0.368
Tendon tear								
Length	0.067	–0.161	–0.244	–0.407	1.00	0.676	0.906	0.336
Width	–0.049	–0.092	–0.133	–0.310	0.676	1.00	0.912	0.292
Size	0.015	–0.123	–0.199	–0.373	0.906	0.912	1.00	0.346
Age	–0.157	–0.043	–0.449	–0.368	0.336	0.292	0.346	1.00

UCLA, University of California at Los Angeles.

anchor. In this situation, I prefer to leave the anchor in position and simply insert another anchor. If the bone quality is good, you can place the inserter in the bone hole until it engages the anchor. Unscrew it until it is halfway out of the hole but the threads still engage the bone and the anchor is not loose. I then insert the loop grabber through the anterior portal and encircle the anchor around the thread. I use the inserter to unscrew the anchor completely out of the bone while the assistant holds onto the anchor by its threads. I then remove the inserter, and the assistant rotates the anchor so it is parallel to the lateral cannula. I insert a toothed grasper through the lateral cannula and grasp the anchor by the eyelet. The assistant loosens his or her grasp on the loop grabber, and I remove the anchor through the lateral cannula. Occasionally, the anchor will dislodge from the grasper as it is pulled through the rubber dam of the lateral cannula. This may result in a loose anchor that floats in the subacromial space. I generally avoid this complication by removing the lateral cannula with the anchor and grasper inside.

Discussion

Arthroscopic rotator cuff repair is currently performed in a limited number of centers around the world. The surgeons who have taken the repair from theory to practice are all expert arthroscopic technicians with a thorough understanding of rotator cuff repair fundamentals. Whether arthroscopic cuff repair has good long-term results comparable to open procedures remains to be seen, and I await the publication of studies with sufficient patient numbers and long-term follow-up. A separate issue is whether this technique has wide applicability among surgeons of varying arthroscopic skills. Each individual surgeon must consider the relative benefits of the arthroscopic repair and must decide whether the difficulty of this procedure, when compared with open technique, makes it worthwhile.

For the orthopedic surgeon considering the transition from open to arthroscopic technique, caution is appropriate. The orthopedic surgeon not only must master each of the individual elements described earlier but must also perform them in a precise and timely fashion. The surgeon must have a reasonable volume of patients with rotator cuff tears and must be proficient at arthroscopic subacromial decompression. Experience is required to recognize the patterns of tendon tear shapes as viewed through the arthroscope. Tendon mobilization of retracted tears can be difficult. Suture anchors must be placed accurately so that the repaired tendon rests in the desired location. The orthopedist must manage multiple strands of suture material within the tight confines of the subacromial space and must tie secure knots with the use of arthroscopic tools.

Bibliography

Blevins FT, Warren RF, Cavo C, et al: Arthroscopic assisted rotator cuff repair: Results using a mini-open deltoid splitting approach. Arthroscopy 12:50–59, 1996.
Burkhart SS: A stepwise approach to arthroscopic rotator cuff repair based on biomechanical principles. Arthroscopy 16:82–90, 2000.
Gartsman GM: Arthroscopic management of rotator cuff disease. J Am Acad Orthop Surg 6:259–288, 1998.
Gartsman GM: Arthroscopic assessment of rotator cuff tear reparability. Arthroscopy 12:546–549, 1996.
Gartsman GM, Brinker MR, Khan M, Karahan M: Early effectiveness of arthroscopic repair for patients with full-thickness tears of the rotator cuff. J Bone Joint Surg Am 80:33–40, 1998.
Gartsman GM, Brinker MR, Khan M, Karahan M: Self-assessment of general health status in patients with five common shoulder conditions. J Shoulder Elbow Surg 7:228–237, 1998.
Gartsman GM, Khan M, Hammerman SM: Arthroscopic repair of full-thickness rotator cuff tears. J Bone Joint Surg Am 80:832–840, 1998.
Gartsman GM, Taverna E: The incidence of glenohumeral joint abnormalities associated with full-thickness, reparable rotator cuff tears. Arthroscopy 13:450–455, 1997.
Gleyze P, Thomazeau H, Flurin PH, et al: [Arthroscopic rotator cuff repair: A multicentric retrospective study of 87 cases with anatomical assessment]. Rev Chir Orthop Reparatrice Appar Mot 86:566–574, 2000.
Grana WA, Teague B, King M, Reeves RB: An analysis of rotator cuff repair. Am J Sports Med 22:585–588, 1994.
Paulos LE, Kody MH: Arthroscopically enhanced "miniapproach" to rotator cuff repair. Am J Sports Med 22:19–25, 1994.
Snyder SJ: Technique of arthroscopic rotator cuff repair using implantable 4-mm Revo suture anchors, suture shuttle relays, and no. 2 nonabsorbable mattress sutures. Orthop Clin North Am 28:267–275, 1997.
Tauro JC: Arthroscopic rotator cuff repair: Analysis of technique and results at 2- and 3-year follow-up. Arthroscopy 14:45–51, 1998.
Zvijac JE, Levy HJ, Lemak LJ: Arthroscopic subacromial decompression in the treatment of full thickness rotator cuff tears: A 3- to 6-year follow-up. Arthroscopy 10:518–523, 1994.

13

Massive Rotator Cuff Tears

I define a massive rotator cuff tear as one involving at least two rotator cuff tendons and measuring 5 cm in length from anterior to posterior. It is difficult for surgeons to determine whether a massive, retracted rotator cuff tear is reparable. This is as true for arthroscopic technique as it is for conventional open technique. If the tendon is mobile and can be advanced to its anatomic location, or if it can be medialized within 10 mm of its anatomic location without shoulder abduction, the tear is reparable.

However, if on initial inspection, the tendon does not meet these criteria, it is not necessarily irreparable. Subacromial, subdeltoid, and intra-articular adhesions may limit cuff excursion. With arthroscopic technique, the surgeon can release these adhesions and can determine definitively whether the tear is reparable.

A question I am frequently asked is how I can repair massive tears arthroscopically. The answer, like the technique, is both simple and complex. The simple part is my attitude. I understand that massive tears will take more débridement and soft tissue releases before I can determine reparability and will require multiple movements of the arthroscope to different cannulas to help me understand the tear geometry, and suture management will prove challenging. I understand that I must move slowly, to minimize the possibility of technical error that will prolong an already complicated operation. I understand this will prove challenging because my desire is to move faster and to shorten a long operation. I also have to accept the reality that I will make technical errors during the operation and that I should be patient, correct the problem, and move on. The complex part is actually doing all this.

If you are now at the stage when you are about to undertake the repair of a massive rotator cuff repair, you already have the necessary technical skill, but I think it is helpful to spend some time detailing the challenges that lie ahead. You may find it helpful to review drill 3 outlined in Chapter 1.

Large or massive retracted rotator cuff tears differ from smaller tears in the following six aspects:

1. Quantity of sutures and anchors
2. Tear geometry
3. Variability of repair sequence
4. Suture management
5. Tendon-to-tendon repair
6. Muscle quality

The first and most straightforward aspect is quantity. Larger tears require more anchors, more sutures, and more time to complete.

Tear geometry is difficult to identify. Larger tears often assume distorted shapes because the tendons have detached, are rotated, and rest far from their insertion site. It is often difficult to understand how points on the retracted tendon attach to corresponding points on the humeral head. Identifying this relationship is understanding the geometry of the tear and thus the geometry of the repair (Fig. 13–1).

This is difficult enough when then tendon is mobile, but it becomes increasingly complex when the tear is retracted and fixed. It is only with thorough soft tissue releases that the surgeon can maneuver the tendon and can determine the precise repair site.

Third, the surgeon must often alter the normal repair technique of placing anchors from anterior to posterior and knot tying from posterior to anterior. The repair may require tying from anterior to posterior, or the repair may dictate that the surgeon repair the most anterior and posterior margins first and repair the central portion last.

Fourth, suture management is increasingly complex. As

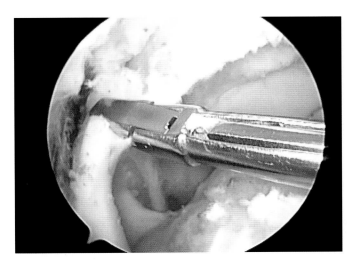

FIGURE 13–1. Massive rotator cuff repair.

patients) satisfactory results, satisfactory pain relief in 92% (56/61 patients), and mean gains in forward elevation of 76 degrees and external rotation of 30 degrees. Burkhart reported similar results with arthroscopic treatment of massive tears. Burkhart has also contributed greatly to our understanding of the biomechanics of massive rotator cuff tears and their repair. I find the concept of margin convergence particularly useful. The first principle of margin convergence is that the partial repair of a massive tear can reduce the patient's pain and can improve function. Complete, anatomic repair, although desirable, may not be possible in patients with massive rotator cuff tears, but with partial repair, a good outcome can be achieved. The second principle is that if the surgeon can establish anterior and posterior stability to the shoulder, good function is possible even if the supraspinatus is not reparable. Anterior stability may be achieved through a subscapularis repair, and posterior stability can be accomplished through an infraspinatus repair.

the numbers of anchors and sutures increase, the surgeon's difficulty seems to increase geometrically, and strict adherence to two principles is vital. Keep the working cannula free of sutures, and transfer suture strands so they do not cross the area of tendon repair.

Fifth, it is often necessary to combine longitudinal tendon-to-tendon repair with transverse tendon-to-bone repair. This may require that the surgeon select different suturing techniques, sutures, instruments, viewing portals, and knot-tying methods (Fig. 13–2).

Sixth, massive rotator cuff tears are diseases of tendon and muscle. These larger tendon tears are usually more chronic and are accompanied by significant muscle atrophy. The surgeon must be aware that heroic efforts to repair tendons will not produce a successful result if the corresponding muscles are not functional.

Literature Review

Bigliani and his coauthors reported on the open repair of massive rotator cuff tears. They reported 85% (52/61

Operative technique

 — **Large Rotator Cuff Tear**

Visualization

I inspect the glenohumeral joint and obtain full passive range of motion through gentle manipulation or contracture release (Fig. 13–3). I remove the arthroscope and redirect it into the subacromial space. I introduce the trocar and cannula through the subcutaneous tissue until I can palpate the posterior acromion. I then advance the cannula and trocar along the inferior acromion surface, not only to enter the subacromial space superior to any rotator cuff tendon adherent to the acromion but also to create the maximum distance between the arthroscope lens and the rotator cuff

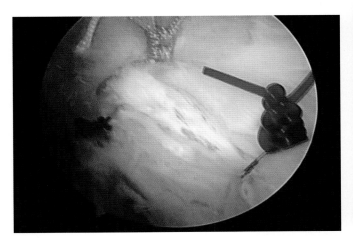

FIGURE 13–2. Tendon-to-tendon repair.

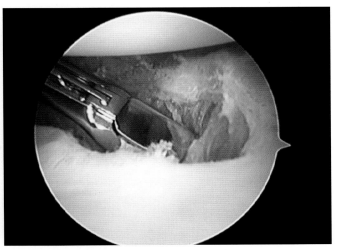

FIGURE 13–3. Contracture release.

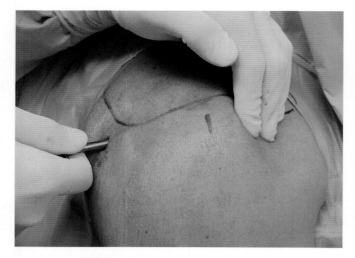

FIGURE 13–4. Palpate inferior acromion.

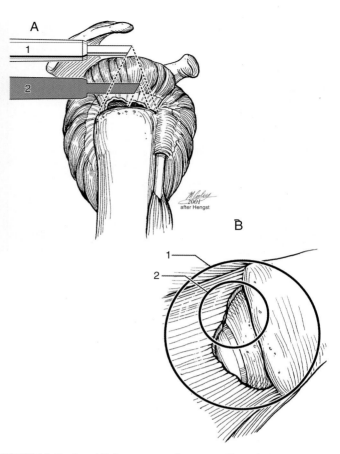

FIGURE 13–6. *A* and *B,* Appearance of rotator cuff repair changes with perspective.

tear (Figs. 13–4 to 13–6). I establish a lateral portal and use a motorized shaver to remove any bursal tissue that impedes a clear view of the tendon tear. Surprisingly, the subacromial space is often clearly visualized in massive full- thickness tears. The thick subacromial bursitis that characterizes stage 2 impingement usually is absent. When bursa is present, it is usually located posteriorly, and I remove it by inserting the arthroscope posteriorly and the soft tissue shaver laterally. I continue removing bursa until I can see the rotator cuff tear clearly. If I cannot obtain a clear view of the tendon, I move the arthroscope to the lateral portal and insert the shaver posteriorly (Fig. 13–7). At this point, I have the option of continuing the repair with the arthroscope laterally or moving it to its normal, posterior position.

Tear Classification

My preference is to work with the arthroscope in the posterior portal. I rotate the arthroscope so that it is pointed directly down at the rotator cuff tear (Figs. 13–8 and 13–9).

With small to medium tears, the size and tear geometry are appreciated easily, but such is not often the case with massive tears. I believe there are 13 factors that distinguish arthroscopic treatment of massive rotator cuff tears from smaller lesions, as follows:

1. Tear size
2. Muscle contraction
3. Muscle quality
4. Tendon retraction
5. Tendon substance loss

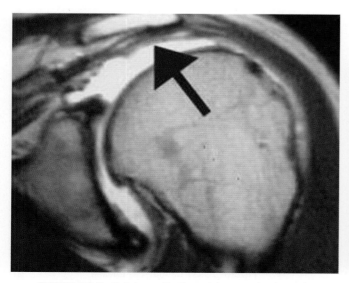

FIGURE 13–5. Rotator cuff adherent to acromion (*arrow*).

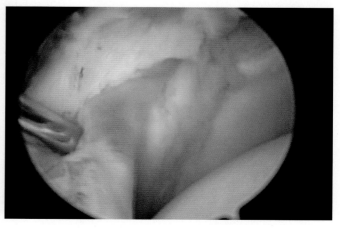

FIGURE 13–7. Thickened posterior bursa.

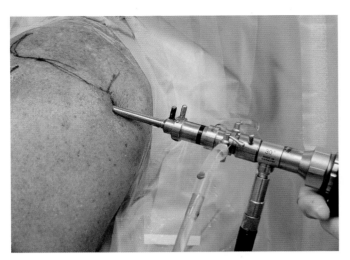

FIGURE 13–8. Arthroscope directed upward at acromion.

6. Tendon quality
7. Tendon rotation
8. Subdeltoid and subacromial adhesions
9. Coracohumeral ligament contracture
10. Capsular contracture
11. Greater tuberosity prominence
12. Superior humeral head migration
13. Repair without acromioplasty

Rotator cuff repair reduces fundamentally to a problem of what goes where. The size and retraction of massive tears often make implementing these repair steps difficult. Even when the surgeon understands the tear geometry, mobilizing the tendon is difficult. Because most of these lesions are chronic, muscle contracture limits the excursion of the tendon edge even when the surgeon has performed appropriate releases. Even if an anatomic repair is possible, the chronic nature of the lesion affects the muscle quality so that it does not function naturally. There is also the issue of tendon substance loss. Frequently, the surgeon identifies the musculotendinous junction and finds that there is very little tendon remaining for repair. The advanced age of

these patients and the longstanding duration of the lesion also adversely affect tendon quality and diminish repair security. With smaller tears, the tendon retracts medially. With larger tears, the tendon not only retracts medially but also rotates posteriorly or anteriorly and further complicates the repair.

Adhesions between the rotator cuff and the deltoid or the acromion limit mobilization. Contracture of the coracohumeral ligament and the glenohumeral joint capsule can also be significant. The greater tuberosity can enlarge and can encroach on the subacromial space, and these changes make the surgeon's choice of repair site difficult. Superior migration of the humeral head, seen in some patients with massive rotator cuff tears, diminishes the size of the subacromial space and complicates the task of maneuvering instruments during the repair.

Because of some or all of the factors cited earlier, I am not convinced that even with an anatomic repair, the rotator cuff will function normally and will centralize the humeral head into the glenoid during arm elevation. I consider these patients to have an anatomically intact but functional insufficient rotator cuff. If the passive superior restraints of the coracoacromial arch are removed with acromioplasty and coracoacromial ligament resection, the humeral head will escape the confines of the coracoacromial arch and will subluxate anteriorly, medially, and superiorly. Elevation will be limited and painful. Subacromial decompression with a nonfunctional rotator cuff repair (or an irreparable tear) transforms the patient from someone who has pain during elevation to someone with pain and no ability to elevate. For these reasons, during repair of a massive rotator cuff tear, I do not perform an acromioplasty or coracoacromial ligament resection. This further limits the maneuverability of instruments in the subacromial space.

I measure with a marked probe the length of the tear from anterior to posterior and the amount of medial retraction. Straight medial retraction and retraction in an elliptical shape are the most common findings (Figs. 13–10 and 13–11). As tear size increases, the surgeon's ability to appreciate tear geometry becomes more difficult. The following descriptions apply to a right shoulder and are reversed for a left shoulder. L-shape tears have a longitudinal limb posteriorly, often at the junction of the supraspinatus and infraspinatus, in addition to the lateral detachment at the greater

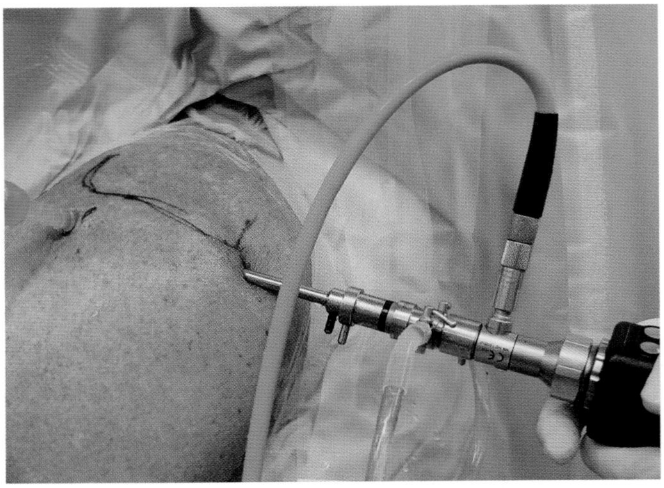

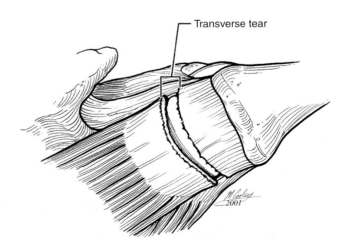

FIGURE 13–9. Arthroscope directed downward at rotator cuff tear.

Transverse tear

FIGURE 13–10. Transverse tear.

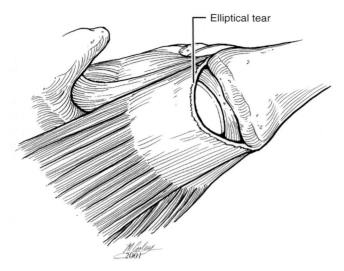

FIGURE 13–11. Elliptical tear.

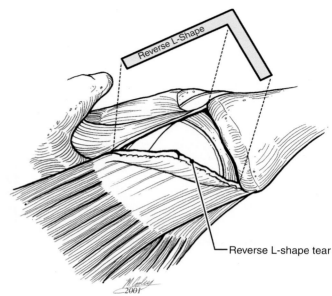

FIGURE 13–14. Reverse L-shape tear.

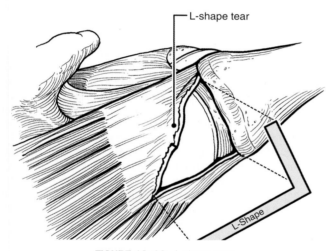

FIGURE 13–12. L-shape tear.

tuberosity. Reverse L-tears with a longitudinal component along the rotator interval will allow the tear to rotate posteriorly. Longitudinal tears may be present in the area of the rotator interval and occasionally within the substance of the supraspinatus (Figs. 13–12 to 13–15). V-shape tears have the longitudinal component in addition to a lateral detachment.

When the surgeon identifies a massive tear that will not reduce with straight lateral traction, I have found that grasping the posterior portion of the tendon and pulling anterolaterally can best accomplish tear reduction (Figs. 13–16 and 13–17).

This usually is more effective than pulling the anterior limb posteriorly or doing soft tissue releases. I use a grasper and pull on the tear edge, in an attempt to determine its anatomic location while varying elevation and rotation until a best fit is obtained. Only when tear geometry is appreciated can an effective repair be done. The McConnell arm holder then is secured to maintain the patient's arm position (Figs. 13–18 and 13–19).

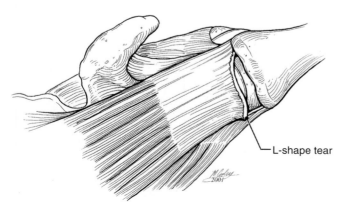

FIGURE 13–13. L-shape tear.

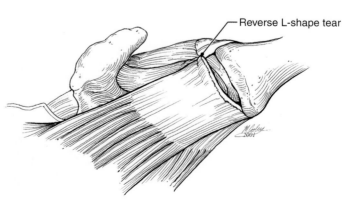

FIGURE 13–15. Reverse L-shape tear.

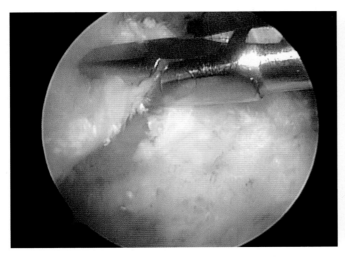

FIGURE 13–16. Grasping retracted tendon edge.

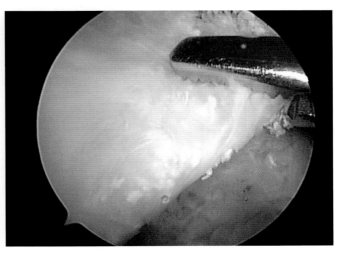

FIGURE 13–17. Advancing tendon edge.

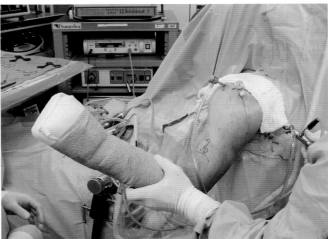

FIGURE 13–19. External rotation.

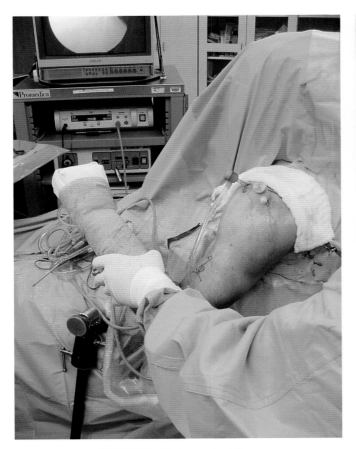

FIGURE 13–18. Internal rotation.

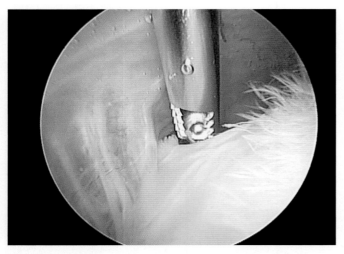

FIGURE 13–20. Adhesions, rotator cuff and deltoid fascia.

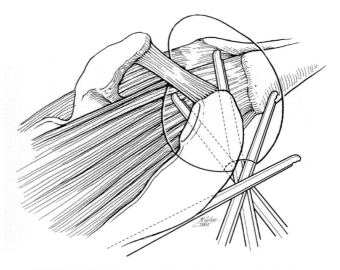

FIGURE 13–22. Sweep and disrupt subacromial adhesions.

Cuff Mobilization

Adhesions may have formed within the subacromial space between the rotator cuff and acromion or the rotator cuff and deltoid. They interfere with tendon mobilization and must be released to enable mobilization. I usually release anterior and lateral adhesions with a motorized shaver. Occasionally, electrocautery is used to divide adhesions if they are particularly thick (Figs. 13–20 and 13–21).

Posterior adhesions usually are not dense and often can be released by inserting a metal trocar and cannula through the lateral portal, by placing it superior to the anterior tear edge and sweeping posteriorly directly beneath the arthroscope (Fig. 13–22). It is unwise to remove these adhesions with a power shaver in that bleeding often will result that is difficult to control because of the posterior medial location of the bleeding vessels. Therefore, I release any remaining adhesions in this area with electrocautery.

Adhesions to the coracoid or coracohumeral ligament contracture may falsely give the impression of irreparability. Adhesions to the coracoid usually are thick and require resection with the electrocautery. This is particularly true in the area of the coracohumeral ligament. The coracohumeral ligament is not visualized clearly and is appreciated best by applying lateral traction to the tendon edge and observing a ridge of tissue that prevents mobilization. I grasp the tendon edge with a soft tissue grasper inserted through the lateral portal, insert the electrocautery device (or scissors) through the anterior portal, and divide the ligament (Figs. 13–23 and 13–24).

Coracohumeral ligament contracture is often accompanied by a contracture of the rotator interval. I palpate or visualize the superior border of the subscapularis and use scissors to divide the interval from the lateral tendon border to the coracoid (Figs. 13–25 to 13–27).

Occasionally, division of the intra-articular joint capsule is helpful. I release the capsule adjacent to the glenoid, begin-

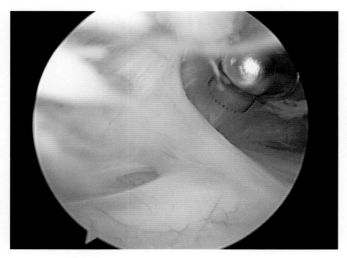

FIGURE 13–21. Adhesions, rotator cuff and acromion.

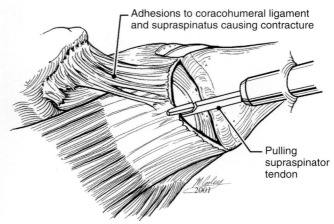

Adhesions to coracohumeral ligament and supraspinatus causing contracture

Pulling supraspinator tendon

FIGURE 13–23. Coracoacromial ligament contracture limits rotator cuff mobility.

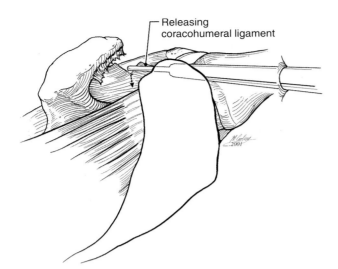

FIGURE 13–24. Coracohumeral ligament release.

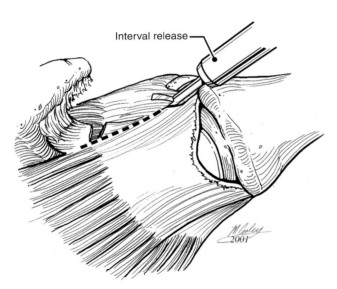

FIGURE 13–25. Interval release.

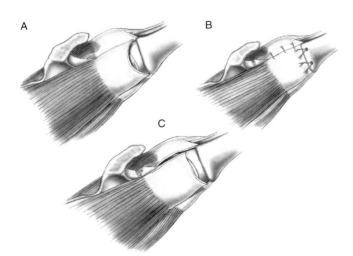

FIGURE 13–26. Interval slide.

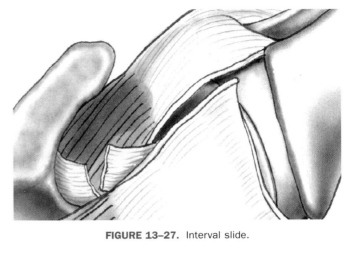

FIGURE 13–27. Interval slide.

ning posterior to the biceps-labrum attachment (Figs. 13–28 and 13–29). This maneuver increases tendon excursion slightly. I prefer to use arthroscopic scissors. The suprascapular nerve is located approximately 1 cm medial to the glenoid, and the surgeon must be careful during medial dissection not to injure this vital structure. This area is well visualized and is accessible with the arthroscope in the subacromial space in patients with massive tears. This is not the case with the inferior capsule and, to a lesser extent, the anterior capsule.

Subacromial and subdeltoid adhesions limit the tendon's ability to advance to the humeral head, but inferior capsular contracture can limit the ability of the humeral head to meet the tendon. These capsular contractures prevent the necessary humeral head movement required for tendon-bone apposition. Usually, I identify and correct the inferior contracture during the glenohumeral joint portion of the operation. I release inferior capsular contracture as necessary, as described in Chapter 6. If I cannot adequately release the anterior contracture with the arthroscope in the subacromial space, I remove the arthroscope and redirect it

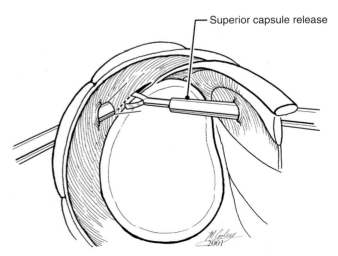

FIGURE 13–28. Superior capsule release.

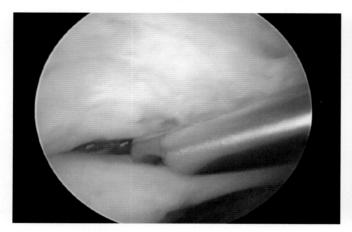

FIGURE 13–29. Superior capsule release.

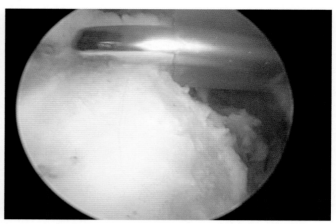

FIGURE 13–31. Greater tuberosity recession.

into the glenohumeral joint, release the anterior contracture, and then reposition the arthroscope in the subacromial space.

The greater tuberosity is often abnormal in patients with chronic, massive rotator cuff tears. The abnormalities include the presence of osteophytes and reactive enlargement of the greater tuberosity. These changes compromise the space available for instruments during the surgical repair and impinge against the acromion during arm elevation postoperatively. Because I do not perform acromioplasty in this setting, I recess the greater tuberosity. I insert the bur through the lateral cannula and remove the abnormal bony overgrowth from the greater tuberosity until I obtain adequate clearance between the proximal humerus and the acromion (Figs. 13–30 and 13–31).

Tendon reparability is based not only on tendon mobility but also on the quality of the tissue and its ability to hold sutures and thus be used in the repair. I gain a sense of tendon quality while I grasp and manipulate the tendon to determine repair geometry. This can affect the decision on how lateral or anatomic a repair is possible.

If anatomic repair is not possible without excessive ten-

don tension, the tendon is repaired medially, and the bone decortication site is adjusted accordingly. How medially can the tendon edge be repaired? You can repair the tendon as much as 10 mm medial to its anatomic insertion without a significant loss of overhead elevation.

Medial repairs require that the surgeon change the method of anchor insertion. An anatomic repair is best obtained with lateral anchor placement, but this is not possible for a medial repair. I identify the proper site and insertion angle with a spinal needle inserted percutaneously. The skin entry usually is immediately lateral to the acromion. I make a stab wound and insert the anchors percutaneously (Figs. 13–32 to 13–35).

If I cannot repair the tendon without further medialization, I repair the anterior and posterior margins anatomically and do not repair the central portion of the tear. A tendon repaired under appropriate tension in this manner is superior to an "anatomic, watertight" repair that is under excessive tension (Fig. 13–36).

I do not repair the tear with the patient's arm abducted because when the arm is brought back to the patient's side, the repair is under excessive tension and will fail.

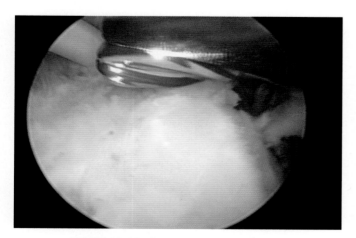

FIGURE 13–30. Prominent greater tuberosity.

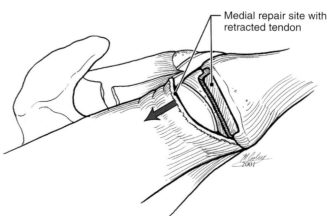

Medial repair site with retracted tendon

FIGURE 13–32. Medial bone preparation.

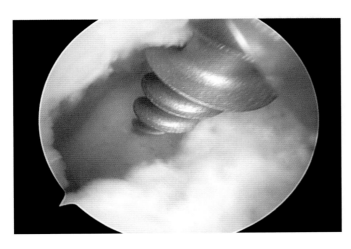

FIGURE 13–33. Percutaneous anchor insertion.

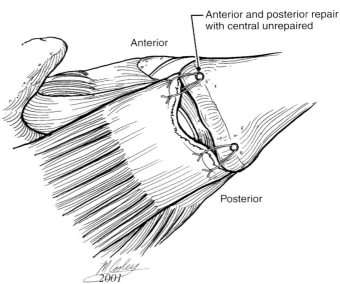

FIGURE 13–36. Anterior and posterior margin repair.

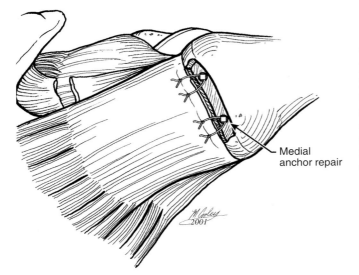

FIGURE 13–34. Medial repair.

Repair Sequence

It is often necessary to vary the repair sequence when one is faced with a large or massive rotator cuff tear. Because the tear is so large, it is possible to place anchors, insert sutures, and tie them before proceeding to the next anchor. For example, it may be helpful to place the most anterior anchor and two sutures first. Tie them and then place the most posterior anchor and sutures, and tie these. This approach converts the massive tear into a normal sized transverse tear (Fig. 13–37).

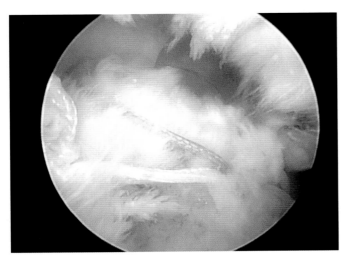

FIGURE 13–35. Medial repair.

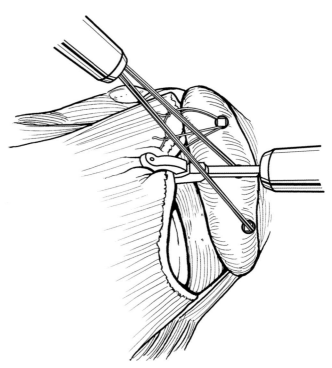

FIGURE 13–37. Anterior portion of tear repaired first.

Suture Management

There is a reason that the description that follows may appear complex to the reader. It *is* complex. It is possible, however. Write down every step of the procedure, and rehearse these steps with a practice board and the drills outlined in Chapter 1. Watch the videos that deal with larger rotator cuff repairs.

When three to four anchors are needed for the repair, it is helpful to alter the usual technique of suture management. Six to eight sutures within the subacromial space are difficult to manage. After I insert the anterior anchor, I withdraw the sutures through the anterior cannula as usual. I insert the next anchor posteriorly and withdraw these sutures out the anterior cannula. I internally rotate the arm and place the third anchor. At this point, if the sutures are pulled through the anterior cannula, there will be six sutures through this cannula, and six sutures are difficult to manage. Additionally, if the posterior sutures are through the anterior cannula, passing the anterior sutures through the tendon is difficult because the posterior sutures cross the tendon edge and may block access to the cuff tear. One option is to insert and then tie the anterior sutures before placing additional sutures or anchors. Often, however, the tendon tear is not quite large enough, and if the anterior sutures are tied, it is difficult to place more sutures without manipulating the tendon and possibly disrupting the repair. I modify the technique as follows: I insert the anterior anchor and withdraw the four suture strands out the anterior cannula. I insert the next anchor more posteriorly. I make a percutaneous stab wound anterolaterally, reach into the subacromial space with the loop grabber, and withdraw the four suture strands from the second anchor. I insert the most posterior anchor, make a percutaneous stab wound posterolaterally, and pull the posterior anchor sutures through this incision. The subacromial space is now relatively clear of sutures, and tendon repair can proceed naturally without having sutures cross the tendon edge (Figs. 13–38 to 13–49).

The next step is to pass the sutures through the tendon. I insert the Caspari suture punch through the lateral portal, grasp the most anterior portion of the cuff that corresponds to the anterior anchor, and pass the nylon through the rotator cuff tendon. I retrieve the two free ends of the nylon suture out the anterior cannula. I then insert the crochet hook through the lateral cannula, grasp the anterior anchor suture limb, and pull it out laterally. I insert the suture limb through the loop of nylon passing suture and, with traction on the two free ends that are external to the anterior cannula, pull them into the subacromial space, through the rotator cuff tendon, and out the anterior cannula. I repeat this with the second anterior suture. I then insert the crochet hook through the lateral cannula, pull one limb of the middle anchor sutures from the anterolateral stab wound, and insert this suture limb through the tendon as described earlier. You may withdraw this either out the anterior cannula or through the anterolateral stab wound. Repeat for the second suture of the middle anchor.

In order to place the posterior anchor sutures, I place the loop nylon suture through the most posterior portion of the rotator cuff tendon with the Caspari suture punch and withdraw the two free ends of the nylon suture out the

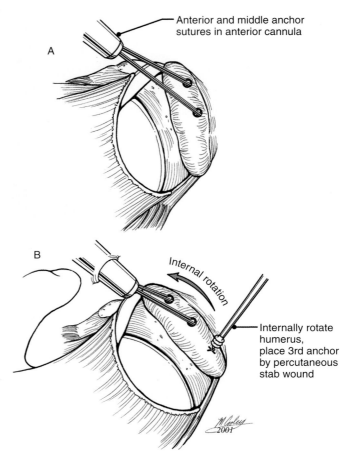

FIGURE 13–38. *A* and *B*, Internally rotate shoulder to place posterior anchors.

anterior cannula. I then insert the crochet hook through the lateral cannula and grasp one of the posterior anchor suture strands that are exiting the posterolateral stab wound. I place this through the loop end and pass it through the ten-

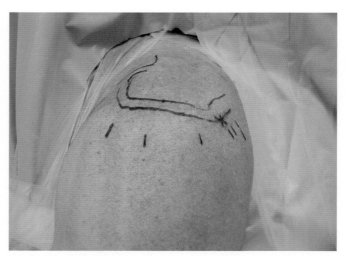

FIGURE 13–39. Lateral portal sites.

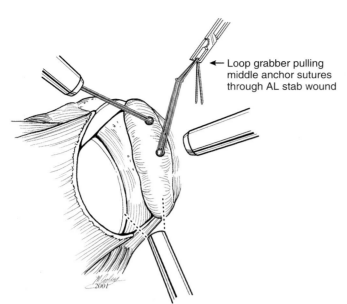

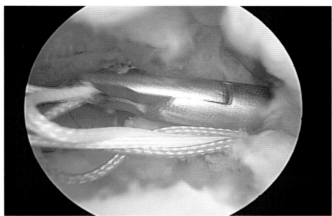

FIGURE 13–40. Withdraw middle anchor sutures out anterolateral stab wound.

Loop grabber pulling middle anchor sutures through AL stab wound

FIGURE 13–41. Sutures withdrawn out anterolateral stab wound.

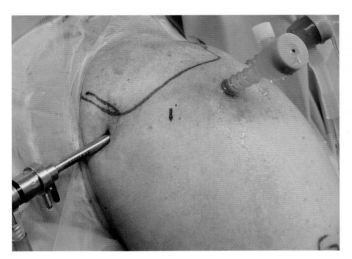

FIGURE 13–42. Posterolateral stab wound.

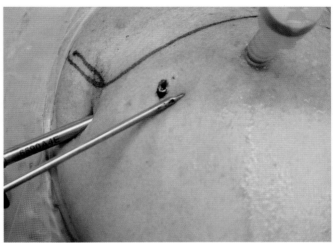

FIGURE 13–43. Small loop grasper.

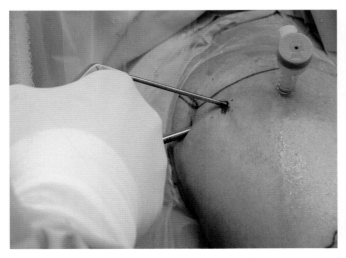

FIGURE 13–44. Insert grasper through posterolateral stab wound.

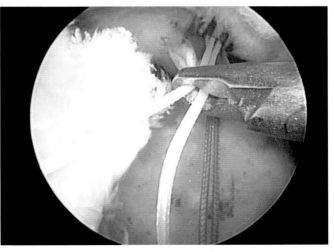

FIGURE 13–45. Grasp white sutures.

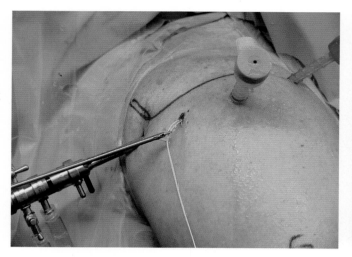

FIGURE 13–46. Withdraw sutures out stab wound.

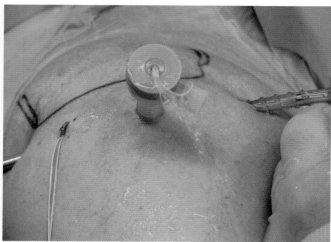

FIGURE 13–48. Withdraw sutures out stab wound.

don and out the anterior cannula. I then reach through the posterolateral stab wound and retrieve that strand of anchor suture and take it back out the posterolateral stab wound. If I leave it in the anterior cannula, it will cross that area of the rotator cuff where I want to place my next suture. I then use the Caspari suture punch to place the nylon suture for the second posterior anchor suture. I place the suture and pass the anchor suture as described earlier and bring it out the anterior cannula.

I am now ready to tie the sutures. I usually begin posteriorly and insert a crochet hook through the lateral cannula and retrieve the two suture limbs from the posterior anchor that exit the posterolateral stab wound. These are the suture limbs located in the most posterior portion of the torn tendon. I tie this set first because it is usually under the least amount of tension. I then retrieve the second set of posterior anchor sutures from the anterior cannula, and I tie and cut these. The rotator cuff repair is now smaller, and there are fewer sutures to manage. I tie the remaining sutures.

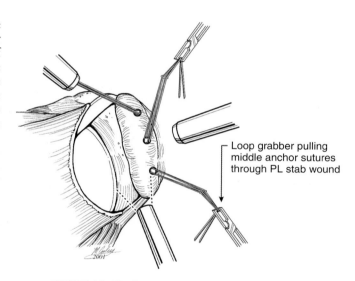

Loop grabber pulling middle anchor sutures through PL stab wound

FIGURE 13–49. Repair area free of crossing sutures.

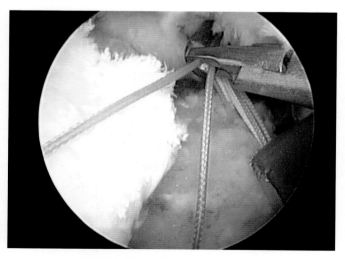

FIGURE 13–47. Grasp green sutures.

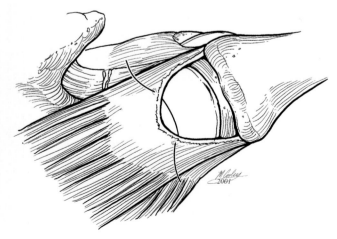

FIGURE 13–50. Margin convergence.

Margin Convergence

 — Massive Rotator Cuff Tear: Margin Convergence

 — Anterior Posterior Longitudinal Tears

 — Tendon-to-Tendon Longitudinal Repair

 — Suture Technique Variations

Margin convergence involves a tendon-to-tendon repair, beginning medially at the tear apex. I move the arthroscope to the lateral portal to gain a better understanding of tear geometry and establish anterior and posterior portals. I begin medially and place a suture approximately 5 mm lateral to the tear apex, tie the suture, and observe the change in tear size. I continue placing sutures from medial to lateral until I cannot further approximate the tear. At this point, if the lateral tendon margin is lateral to the articular cartilage, tendon-to-bone repair with suture anchors is appropriate (Figs. 13–50 to 13–55).

Certain modifications in repair technique are required. It is easier to repair the tendon by inserting the suturing instrument posteriorly, withdrawing the suture posteriorly, and then tying from either the posterior or anterior portal, depending on surgeon preference. I use the Smith & Nephew crescent Cuff-Stitch (Smith & Nephew Endoscopy, Andover, MA) or the Linvatec Spectrum (Largo, FL) crescent suture passer to place either a braided suture or a monofilament suture. Place the instrument through the posterior portal, and pierce the posterior limb of the rotator cuff. At this point, there are two options:

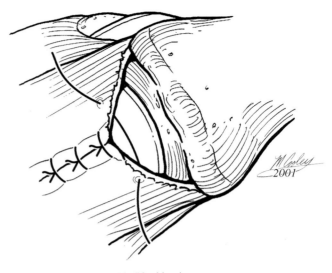

FIGURE 13–52. Margin convergence.

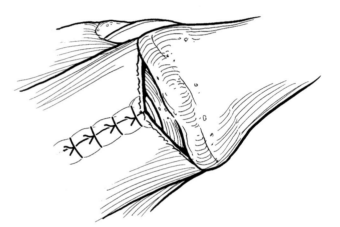

FIGURE 13–53. Margin convergence.

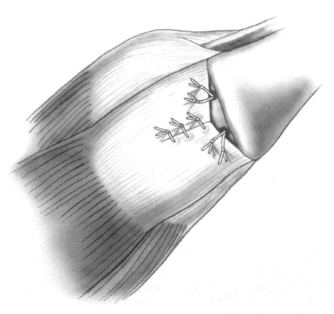

FIGURE 13–54. Margin convergence, medial anchor repair.

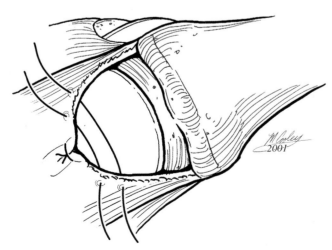

FIGURE 13–51. Margin convergence.

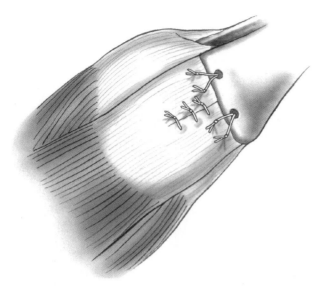

FIGURE 13–55. Margin convergence, anatomic repair.

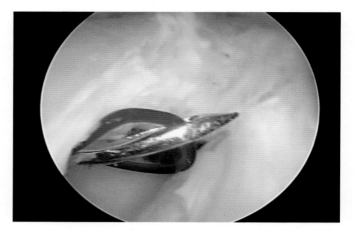

FIGURE 13–57. Cuff-Stitch.

1. Insert an instrument such as the Arthropierce (Smith & Nephew) through the anterior cannula and pierce the anterior limb of the rotator cuff. Grasp the suture, withdraw the instrument back through the anterior cannula, and pull the suture through the anterior tendon (Figs. 13–56 to 13–58).

2. Use a Spectrum crescent suture passer. Place this instrument through the anterior cannula, and pierce the anterior tendon limb. Feed the posterior suture into the end of the anterior suture passer. Use the wheel to pull the suture through the anterior instrument. Withdraw both the instrument and the suture through the anterior cannula.

I use a crochet hook to pull both suture limbs out the posterior cannula, and I tie the knot.

Subscapularis Tears

Subscapularis tears are often identified in patients with massive supraspinatus and infraspinatus tears. The sub-

scapularis tears may be partial-thickness or full-thickness tears. The full-thickness lesions are usually confined to the superior portion of the subscapularis and are easily repaired with standard arthroscopic rotator cuff repair technique. More substantial lesions require that I move the arthroscope to the lateral portal and introduce instruments through the anterior and posterior portals. However, the repair techniques are similar to those I discuss in the treatment of full-thickness supraspinatus tears.

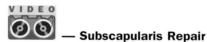 **— Subscapularis Repair**

Postoperative Management

The perioperative management of these patients is similar to that of patients who undergo a routine rotator cuff repair. I use continuous passive motion for 2 weeks and then start supine dowel exercises in elevation and external rotation for the next 4 weeks. The patients protect the arm in a sling

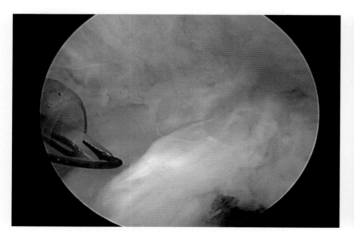

FIGURE 13–56. Cuff-Stitch.

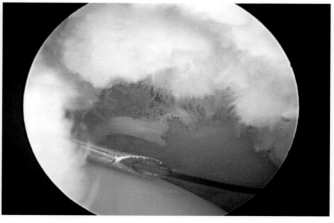

FIGURE 13–58. Spectrum suture passer.

for the first 6 weeks. I allow active range of motion for the next 6 weeks.

My normal practice is to have a physical therapist instruct the patient in appropriate exercises, but in those with massive rotator cuff tears and a complex repair, I prefer to educate the patients myself. The rehabilitation is so individualized and variable because of the repair quality that I believe the surgeon is in the best position to monitor the patient's progress. I use the term *three-phase active elevation program* to describe this part of the rehabilitation. Dr. Charles Rockwood, who I believe learned this approach from an even higher authority, instructed me in these exercises.

The program consists of three stages: (1) passive elevation and then actively holding the arm overhead, (2) passive elevation and then actively lowering the arm, and (3) active elevation. Patients must satisfactorily complete each stage before advancing to the next. This gentle and graduated program provides enough stress to strengthen the rotator cuff tendons and muscles but does so in a safe and controlled manner. The easiest activity is holding the arm directly overhead after raising it passively. The next easiest movement is actively lowering the arm because gravity is helping the movement. The most difficult action is to raise the arm against gravity. I have patients use their unaffected arm to raise the operated shoulder to maximal elevation passively. Patients then remove their affected hand from the affected wrist but keep the hand ready to catch the operated arm in case the muscles fatigue and the arm drops. Patients actively maintain their shoulder in maximum elevation starting with 5 seconds and progressing at their own pace until they can hold the elevated position for 30 seconds. I ask them to do these exercises in front of a clock that has a second hand so that they can monitor the time precisely. Once they can hold the position for 30 seconds, they increase the number of repetitions until they can do 10 repetitions 3 times daily. When this is accomplished, they move to stage 2.

In stage 2, the patients passively elevate their shoulder, hold it for 10 seconds, and then actively lower it in a slow, controlled fashion. Again, the contralateral hand is placed 4 inches below the forearm of the operated shoulder, so that if the arm falls because of muscle fatigue, it can be protected. When patients can do 10 repetitions of this exercise, they move to stage 3.

In stage 3, patients actively elevate the operated shoulder. With slight pressure from the nonoperated hand, they begin active assisted elevation. They gradually decrease the pressure from the contralateral hand until they can actively elevate the operated arm in a slow, controlled fashion. Throughout this process, I stress to the patient that recovery takes months rather than weeks, and gradual progress is the goal. Once patients can actively elevate the arm (or 3 months after operation), they return to the office for strengthening exercises using rubber tubing (Figs. 13–59 to 13–62).

Three months after the surgical procedure, I start the patients with rubber tubing strengthening exercises for the scapular rotators, deltoid, and internal rotators. Because of the large tear and muscle atrophy, I do not start external rotation or elevation strengthening until 5 to 6 months after operation. If pain relief, function, and range of motion are

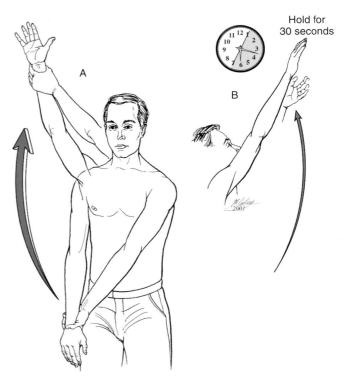

FIGURE 13–59. *A* and *B,* Passive elevation. Maintain actively.

satisfactory, then I never introduce resisted elevation or external rotation strengthening exercises.

Rotator cuff surgery in patients with massive tears is complex and technically demanding. Patient satisfaction is high, however, because pain relief is excellent and function is satisfactory.

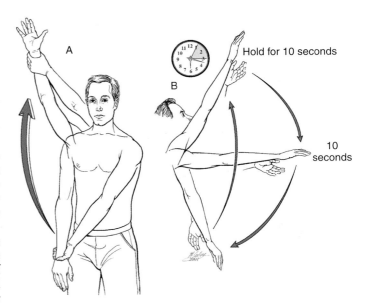

FIGURE 13–60. *A* and *B,* Passive elevation. Lower actively.

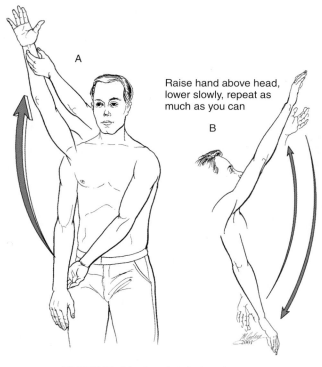

Raise hand above head, lower slowly, repeat as much as you can

FIGURE 13–61. *A* and *B,* Active elevation.

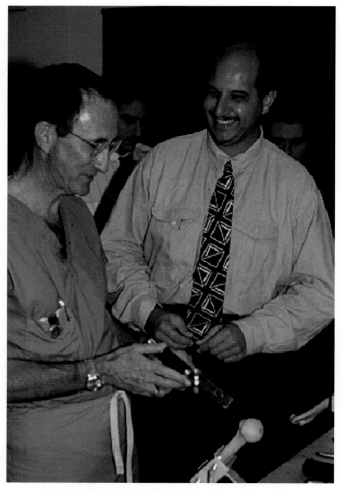

FIGURE 13–62. Charles Rockwood and author.

Bibliography

Burkhart SS: Partial repair of massive rotator cuff tears: The evolution of a concept. Orthop Clin North Am 28:125–132, 1997.

Burkhart SS, Athanasiou KA, Wirth MA: Margin convergence: A method of reducing strain in massive rotator cuff tears. Arthroscopy 12:335–338, 1996.

Burkhart SS, Danaceau SM, Pearce CE, Jr: Arthroscopic rotator cuff repair: Analysis of results by tear size and by repair technique-margin convergence versus direct tendon-to-bone repair. Arthroscopy 17:905–912, 2001.

Cordasco FA, Bigliani LU: The rotator cuff: Large and massive tears. Technique of open repair. Orthop Clin North Am 28:179–193, 1997.

DiGiovanni J, Marra G, Park JY, Bigliani LU: Hemiarthroplasty for gleno-humeral arthritis with massive rotator cuff tears. Orthop Clin North Am 29:477–489, 1998.

Gartsman GM, Khan M, Hammerman SM: Arthroscopic repair of full-thickness tears of the rotator cuff. J Bone Joint Surg Am 80:832–840, 1998.

14

Irreparable Rotator Cuff Tears

The greatest difficulty with arthroscopic treatment of an irreparable cuff tear is the possibility of misdiagnosis. Often, a massive cuff tear is retracted and appears irreparable, but after soft tissue release, the defect is reparable. I overcame this difficulty through careful study. I practiced estimating arthroscopically both the size and reparability of tears and then opening the shoulder for comparison until I became comfortable making accurate decisions arthroscopically.

If the lesion is truly irreparable, then arthroscopic treatment allows thorough débridement while retaining all the advantages of arthroscopic surgery. These advantages include glenohumeral joint inspection and correction of intra-articular abnormalities, preservation of the deltoid insertion, and complete inspection and manipulation of the rotator cuff without the need for acromioplasty (Fig. 14–1).

Literature Review

When a massive, irreparable defect in the rotator cuff tendons is identified at operation, the surgeon must decide among various treatment options. Local tissue transfer from the remaining intact rotator cuff, using the upper portion of the subscapularis or incorporating the intra-articular portion of the biceps tendon, supraspinatus advancement, deltoid muscle flap, synthetic materials, and tendon allograft have been proposed. A latissimus dorsi transfer was described by Gerber and others, but questions remain about the morbidity caused by this procedure as well as about the dynamic function of the graft.

One of the most widely used options for an open procedure, described by both Rockwood and me, includes débriding edges of the necrotic tendon, thoroughly decompressing the subacromial space by performing an anterior and inferior acromioplasty, resecting the coracoacromial ligament, and removing the subacromial bursa. The deltoid is meticulously repaired. Postoperatively, the patient is started on an immediate rehabilitation program. Using this technique, we obtained good results, with patients gaining pain relief and marked improvement in function.

Since these reports appeared, Flatow and Nirschl have taught us to avoid acromioplasty in these patients. Preserving the coracoacromial arch helps to keep the humeral head centered in the glenohumeral joint and prevents the disastrous complication of anterior superior humeral head subluxation.

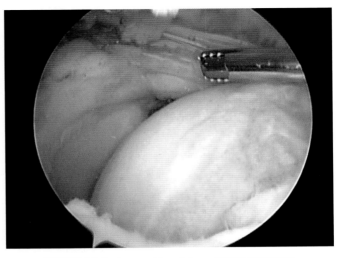

FIGURE 14–1. Irreparable rotator cuff tear treatment.

Less has been written about the arthroscopic treatment of patients with irreparable tears. Ellman and I both achieved good pain relief with arthroscopic treatment in a limited number of patients, with reasonable pain relief documented in most patients at up to 5-year follow-up. We emphasized thorough débridement and synovectomy accompanied by removal of any downward-protruding acromial or acromioclavicular joint spurs as necessary. Burkhart reported that 25 patients with massive irreparable tears had 88% good or excellent results after arthroscopic treatment; those results have not deteriorated with the passage of time.

Diagnosis

Physical examination usually demonstrates normal or near-normal passive range of motion, but sometimes there are limits because of capsular contractures. Active range of motion is decreased. Supraspinatus and infraspinatus atrophy may be observed. Manual muscle testing demonstrates grade 3 or less strength with external rotation and elevation. Carefully examine the patient's subscapularis function using either the belly press test or the lift-off test with the patient's arm internally rotated to the back.

Plain radiographs may show the humeral head centered in the glenoid, but superior migration may be present. Magnetic resonance imaging (MRI), which some surgeons do not use routinely in older patients, is often of great value in this clinical setting. The amount of tendon retraction is more clearly defined than on arthrography, and, perhaps more important, the degree of atrophy and fatty degeneration or substitution in the rotator cuff muscles can be appreciated (Fig. 14–2).

If a patient has grade 3 rotator cuff strength or less and the MRI study demonstrates humeral head superior migration and retraction of the tendon to the glenoid rim with severe muscular atrophy, the cuff defect is almost certainly irreparable.

Subscapularis status requires close attention. Patients

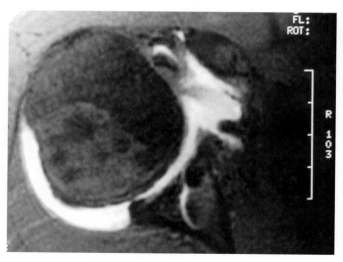

FIGURE 14–3. Subscapularis tear.

with an irreparable, retracted subscapularis tear can be treated with arthroscopic débridement. However, Burkhart showed us that patients with a repairable subscapularis tear benefit from subscapularis repair even in the presence of superior humeral head migration (Fig. 14–3).

Nonoperative Treatment

Nonoperative treatment consists of activity modification, nonsteroidal anti-inflammatory medications, cortisone injections, and a physical therapy program designed to maintain or improve shoulder range of motion and to strengthen the deltoid, scapular rotators, biceps, and intact rotator cuff muscles. I continue nonoperative treatment for at least 6 months, because a surprising number of patients will have reduced pain as the inflammation decreases, and they regain adequate function with muscle-strengthening exercises. Stretching can often improve capsular contracture and can further diminish pain.

Indications

Indications for the operation include pain interfering with work and activities of daily living and/or night pain unresponsive to the conservative care program discussed earlier. Patients should have a well-preserved glenohumeral joint space on plain radiographs and should have relatively pain-free passive external rotation with the arm at the side.

Contraindications

Because the goal of this procedure is pain relief, patients who require strength for overhead work usually will not be satisfied with débridement. In my practice, this is an unusual situation because most of my patients with this condition are older and less active. Patients with painful passive external and internal rotation and advanced gleno-

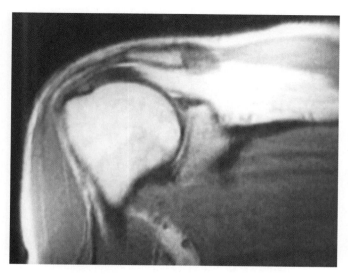

FIGURE 14–2. Fatty infiltration, supraspinatus.

humeral joint arthritis are not candidates for arthroscopic débridement. I prefer to treat these patients, or those with true rotator cuff arthropathy, with arthroplasty.

Operative technique

 VIDEO — Irreparable Rotator Cuff Tear

Examine the shoulder for range of motion and compare it with the contralateral shoulder. Perform a gentle manipulation to correct losses of motion in abduction, elevation, and external and internal rotation.

Glenohumeral joint

A standard posterior portal is used to enter the glenohumeral joint, and an inspection is performed. Because there is no infraspinatus tendon, the joint is entered easily. Patients with irreparable rotator cuff tears are often older, and multiple glenohumeral abnormalities are identified. I ignore areas of minor labral fraying or cartilage thinning on the glenoid or humeral head because I do not believe they are responsible for the patient's pain.

If I find labral flap tears that can cause mechanical abnormalities, a glenoid surface abnormality such as a step-off, or capsular contracture, I create an anterior portal with a spinal needle. I try to place the anterior portal as laterally as possible. If the anterior portal is placed normally (more medially and inferiorly) so that it enters the glenohumeral joint adjacent to the superior border of the subscapularis tendon, it will not be useful for the subacromial portion of this procedure, and you will have to create an additional portal.

Débride labral flap tears with a motorized shaver. Correct areas of contracture as describe in Chapter 6 (Fig. 14–4). I then remove all instruments and cannulas from the glenohumeral joint.

Subacromial Space

It may appear that this technique of cannula removal and reinsertion is unnecessary because with the irreparable tear, the surgeon can view both the glenohumeral joint and the subacromial space. I have found a subtle, but critical difference in the angle of the arthroscope between the two views. When I enter the glenohumeral joint, the arthroscope is angled slightly inferiorly. This allows a better view of the structures within the glenohumeral joint. If you want to view the subacromial space and direct the arthroscope superiorly, the arthroscope is too close to the humeral head, and its angle of approach tends to distort the view.

I use the same posterior skin incision to enter the subacromial space; however, after the trocar passes through the skin and subcutaneous tissue but before it enters the deltoid muscle, I translate the cannula and trocar superiorly until the trocar tip touches the posterior acromion. I then direct the cannula and trocar until they are parallel to the acromion. I advance the cannula and trocar and palpate the acromion's inferior surface. Then I slide along the inferior surface until the trocar tip is 2 cm posterior to the anterior edge of the acromion. This technique has three beneficial effects: (1) the trocar tip can be used to dissect any rotator cuff tendon that is adherent to the acromion; (2) the cannula will be positioned parallel to the inferior surface of the acromion and not directed superiorly; (3) the arthroscope will be positioned at the maximum distance from the humeral head, and this improves my perspective of the size and shape of the rotator cuff lesion. I remove the trocar, insert the arthroscope, and establish a lateral, working portal. I perform a bursectomy to view the rotator cuff defect clearly, and then I insert a cannula for outflow through the anterior portal (Figs. 14–5 and 14–6). I insert a grasper through the lateral portal and pull on the tendon edges to determine their quality and mobility (Figs. 14–7 and 14–8).

I usually move the arthroscope to the lateral portal and obtain a different view of the rotator cuff tear. Some surgeons prefer to view laterally and instrument from posteri-

FIGURE 14–4. Anterior inferior capsular release.

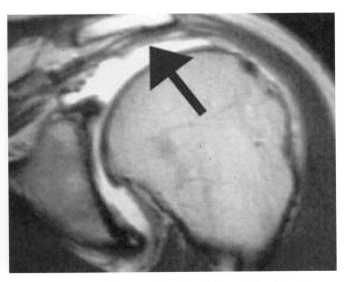

FIGURE 14–5. Rotator cuff adherent to acromion (*arrow*).

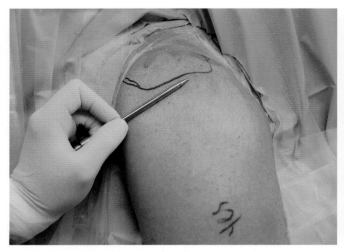

FIGURE 14–6. Cannula parallel to acromion.

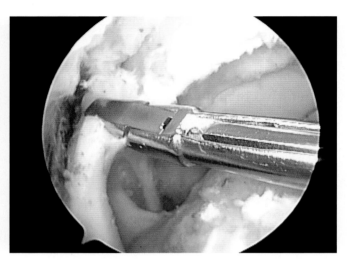

FIGURE 14–9. Lateral view.

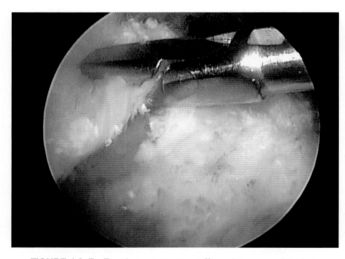

FIGURE 14–7. Traction on rotator cuff tendon, posterior view.

orly, whereas others prefer to leave the arthroscope in the posterior portal and insert the instruments laterally. I use whichever portal gives me the best view of the subacromial space (Fig. 14–9).

If the tear is massive and MRI or physical examination does not demonstrate significant atrophy, perform soft tissue releases and consider repair (Figs. 14–10 to 14–15). In these patients, the posterior bursa can be quite hypertrophic and may appear to be the posterior tendon. I palpate and débride with a shaver to separate the bursa from the tendon (Fig. 14–16). I carefully examine the subscapularis. Débridement of irreparable supraspinatus tears combined with an arthroscopic subscapularis repair will often lead to surprisingly good shoulder function. I discuss the details of this procedure in Chapter 13. If the rotator cuff tendons are absent or excessive tension is necessary to affect a repair, I proceed to débridement.

I use the motorized shaver to remove rotator cuff remnants from the greater tuberosity. If the greater tuberosity is prominent, I smooth it with the bur. I inspect the anterior,

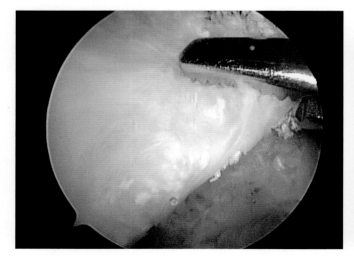

FIGURE 14–8. Traction on rotator cuff tendon, posterior view.

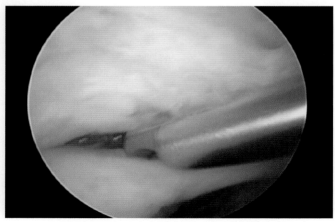

FIGURE 14–10. Superior capsule release.

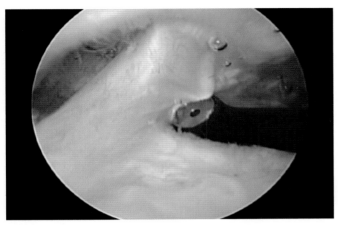

FIGURE 14–11. Medial adhesions, rotator cuff tendon.

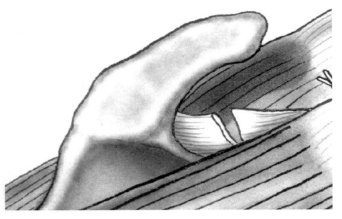

FIGURE 14–12. Coracohumeral ligament release.

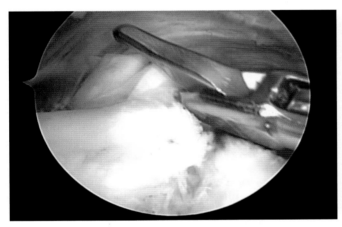

FIGURE 14–13. Coracohumeral ligament release.

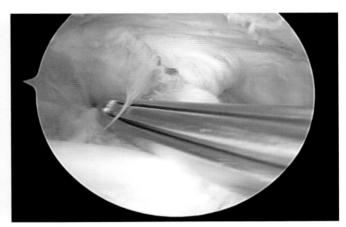

FIGURE 14–14. Coracohumeral ligament release.

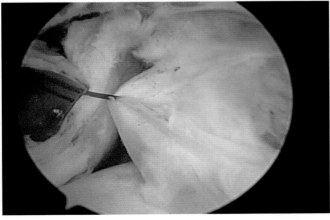

FIGURE 14–15. Excessive tension.

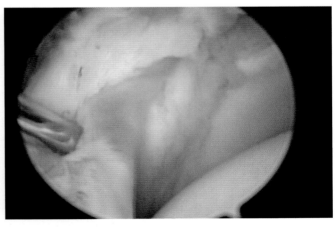

FIGURE 14–16. Thickened posterior bursa.

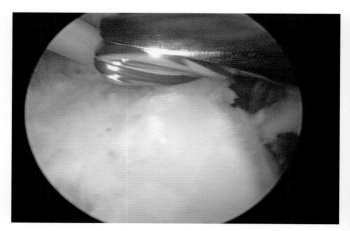

FIGURE 14–17. Tuberosityplasty.

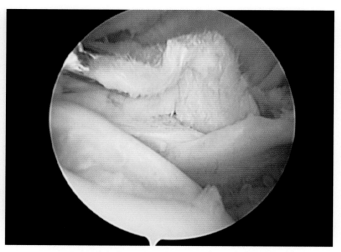

FIGURE 14–19. Medial dislocation, biceps.

lateral, and posterior gutters for adhesions that can restrict motion between the deltoid and the rotator cuff, and I remove them with arthroscopic scissors, an electrocautery device, or a power shaver (Figs. 14–17 and 14–18).

As Nirschl and Flatow reported, removal of the coracoacromial arch in patients without any functioning rotator cuff can result in the devastating complication of superomedial humeral head dislocation. The coracoacromial ligament is not resected, and I do not perform an acromioplasty.

An important source of pain in patients with irreparable rotator cuff tears can be the biceps tendon. I consider tenotomy if the biceps tendon quality is poor, it has a greater than 50% tear, or it is dislocated medially. Another relative indication for biceps tenotomy is a lack of tendon excursion. I grasp the tendon with a tendon grasper that I insert through the lateral cannula and try to translate it. Often, the tendon is adherent to bone or soft tissue distal to the bicipital groove and will not glide. My interpretation of this finding is that the biceps is already effectively tenodesed, and the intra-articular portion may be sacrificed without any apparent negative effects. I discuss the option of tenotomy with the patients preoperatively and caution them about

potential deformity. I have been pleased with the amount of pain relief tenotomy provides (Figs. 14–19 to 14–25).

Postoperative Treatment

I start patients on immediate passive range of motion with a continuous passive motion chair, dowel, or pulley. Active range of motion for routine activities of daily living can be started once the patient recovers from the interscalene block. I do not place the patient in a sling. Once passive range of motion has recovered, the patient may begin active assisted range-of-motion exercises. The active range of motion has three phases. First, I have the patient elevate the arm passively and try to maintain it in elevation actively. I advise the patient to keep the contralateral hand under the operated forearm. This provides some emotional support because most patients have not had their arm in this position for some time. Moreover, if they cannot control the operated shoulder, the contralateral hand is there to prevent the operated arm from falling to the side. Once they can

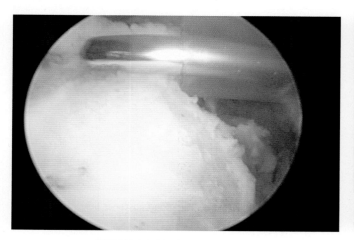

FIGURE 14–18. Tuberosityplasty.

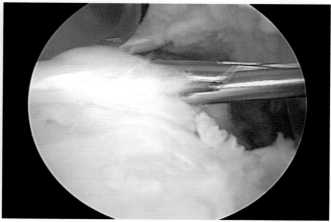

FIGURE 14–20. Test biceps excursion.

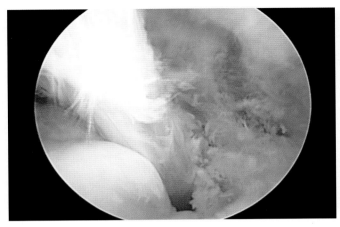

FIGURE 14–21. Test biceps excursion.

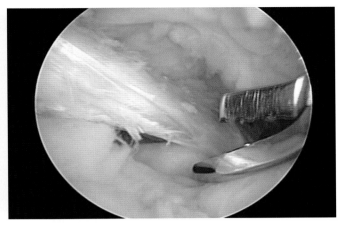

FIGURE 14–22. Distal biceps tendon release.

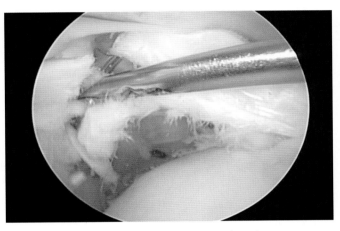

FIGURE 14–23. Proximal biceps tendon release.

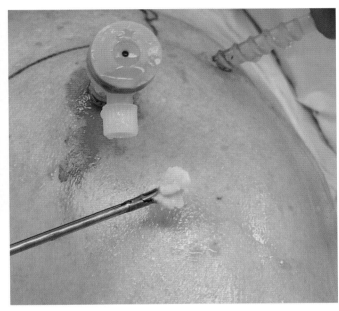

FIGURE 14–24. Biceps tendon removed.

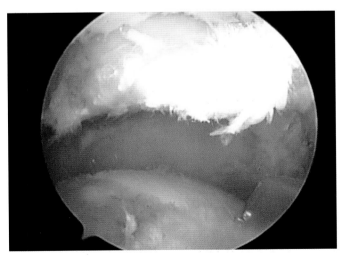

FIGURE 14–25. Biceps stump débrided.

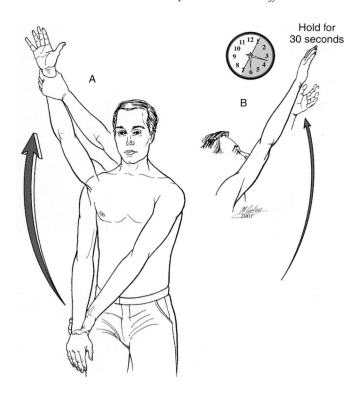

Hold for
30 seconds

FIGURE 14–27. *A* and *B*, Three-phase rehabilitation program.

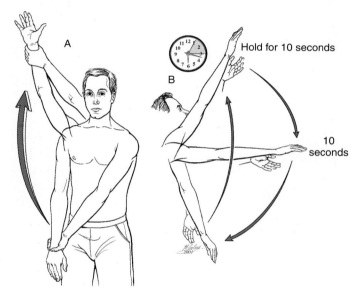

FIGURE 14–26. *A* and *B*, Three-phase rehabilitation program.

Hold for 10 seconds

10
seconds

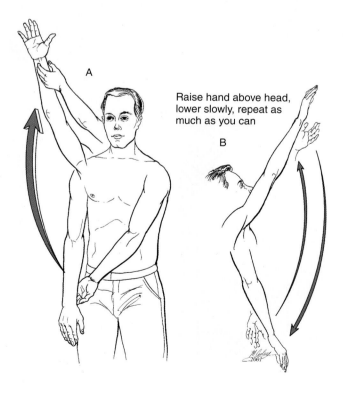

Raise hand above head,
lower slowly, repeat as
much as you can

FIGURE 14–28. *A* and *B*, Three-phase rehabilitation program.

hold this position comfortably for 30 seconds (I have patients perform the exercise in front of a clock with a second hand), I have them raise the arm passively, hold it there for 5 seconds, and then lower it slowly. Again, the contralateral hand is there for support as needed. Once they are comfortable with phase 2, they start active elevation. Patients begin by assisting the operated arm with fingertip pressure from the contralateral arm until they can achieve full elevation. I gradually have the patients decrease the use of the unoperated arm, until full, slow, controlled active elevation is possible (Figs. 14–26 to 14–28).

Once postoperative pain has diminished, patients begin a strengthening program and use light surgical tubing to strengthen the deltoid and the scapular rotators. I believe it is critical to provide encouragement to this group of patients and to educate them that it will take many months to achieve the goals of the operation.

Complications

The most devastating complication is superior medial humeral head instability with subluxation. I have avoided this problem by leaving the coracoacromial ligament intact and not performing an anterior acromionectomy or anterior inferior acromioplasty.

Bibliography

Budoff JE, Nirschl RP, Guidi EJ: Debridement of partial-thickness tears of the rotator cuff without acromioplasty. Long-term follow-up and review of the literature. J Bone Joint Surg Am 80(5):733–748, 1998.

Burkhart SS: Arthroscopic treatment of massive rotator cuff tears: Clinical results and biomechanical rationale. Clin Orthop 267:45–56, 1991.

Burkhart SS, Nottage WM, Ogilvie-Harris DJ, et al: Partial repair of irreparable rotator cuff tears. Arthroscopy 10:363–370, 1994.

Ellman H: Arthroscopic subacromial decompression: Analysis of one- to three-year results. Arthroscopy 3:173–181, 1987.

Flatow EL: Coracoacromial ligamant preservation in rotator cuff surgery. J Shoulder Elbow Surg 3:573, 1994.

Gartsman GM: Arthroscopic acromioplasty for lesions of the rotator cuff. J Bone Joint Surg Am 72:169–180, 1990.

Gartsman GM: Massive, irreparable tears of the rotator cuff: Results of operative debridement and subacromial decompression. J Bone Joint Surg Am 79:715–721, 1997.

Gartsman GM: Arthroscopic assessment of rotator cuff tear reparability. Arthroscopy 12:546–549, 1996.

Gerber C: Latissimus dorsi transfer for the treatment of irreparable tears of the rotator cuff. Clin Orthop 275:152–159, 1992.

15

Acromioclavicular Joint

A cromioclavicular joint pain is a common shoulder condition that may result from a specific injury, repetitive minor traumas, or over time. When the source of pain is articular incongruity, the lesion is amenable to arthroscopic treatment (Fig. 15–1).

This incongruity may be seen in post-traumatic arthritis, type 2 acromioclavicular dislocations with less than 25% subluxation, primary osteoarthritis, rheumatoid arthritis, septic arthritis, and osteolysis of the distal clavicle. In my experience, patients with type 3 to 6 acromioclavicular dislocations are not suitable candidates for arthroscopic surgery because their pain is the result of acromioclavicular joint instability. Currently, I treat these patients with open reconstruction of the coracoclavicular ligaments (Fig. 15–2).

Literature Review

My colleagues and I demonstrated that an adequate acromioclavicular resection can be performed arthroscopically in a laboratory setting and that satisfactory results are obtained in a clinical setting. Snyder and Flatow and colleagues also reported good results in 90% of patients. T. Neviaser (personal communication) demonstrated the efficacy of resecting only the medial acromion, without resecting the distal clavicle.

Diagnosis

Patients complain of pain in the area of the acromioclavicular joint during cross-body adduction (washing the opposite axilla or reaching for a seatbelt) or behind-the-back internal rotation (fastening a bra or pulling a belt through its loops). Weightlifters experience pain during a flat or incline bench press. Physical examination demonstrates normal active and passive range of motion, with the exception of limited adduction or internal rotation. There is pain on direct palpation of the anterior or superior aspects of the acromioclavicular joint. Selective injections are a useful adjunct and are described later.

Plain anterior posterior radiographs demonstrate joint space narrowing, joint incongruity, inferior osteophytes, or distal osteolysis. A 15-degree apical tilt view may show the acromioclavicular joint more clearly. Magnetic resonance imaging (MRI) studies demonstrate and MRI reports note changes that are interpreted as acromioclavicular arthritis, so the surgeon should be careful to interpret such studies in light of an appropriate patient history and physical examination (Fig. 15–3).

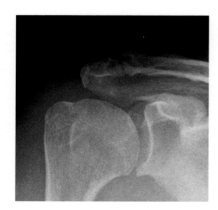

FIGURE 15–1. Acromioclavicular joint arthritis.

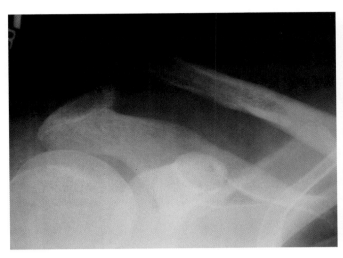

FIGURE 15–2. Type 5 acromioclavicular joint dislocation.

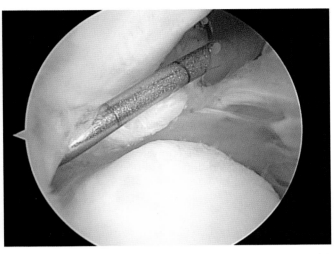

FIGURE 15–4. SLAP lesion.

Some patients with SLAP (superior labrum from anterior to posterior) lesions have a presentation similar to those with acromioclavicular arthritis. Patients localize their pain deep to the acromioclavicular joint and have pain with adduction and with behind-the-back internal rotation. Specific acromioclavicular tenderness to palpation is absent. Adduction is a movement similar to that performed during the O'Brien test and may misdirect the surgeon (Fig. 15–4).

Nonoperative Treatment

Nonoperative treatment is usually successful and consists of avoidance of painful positions and activities and the use of nonsteroidal anti-inflammatory medication. Because the pain from this condition is rarely disabling, I try to counsel patients to wait 6 to 12 months before they consider surgery.

Injection

Lesions of the acromioclavicular joint and subacromial space are difficult to differentiate because acromioclavicular arthritis can cause irritation of the underlying cuff, and the altered shoulder mechanics that accompany rotator cuff disease may aggravate an otherwise normal acromioclavicular joint. Acromioclavicular joint injection may have two benefits in that selective injection may be diagnostic in determining the primary source of pain, and it can also prove therapeutic if the cortisone diminishes the joint inflammation. I use a 25-gauge short-barrel needle because a longer needle can inadvertently penetrate the inferior acromioclavicular joint capsule and can enter the subacromial space. Palpate the sulcus between the distal clavicle and medial acromion. Because the acromioclavicular joint may slope or tilt in different directions, study the anterior posterior radiograph and try to orient yourself to the joint inclination. Clean the skin overlying the superior aspect of the joint with an antibacterial preparation. Advance the needle through the skin while you maintain gentle pressure on the plunger, and when the joint is entered, you can feel the change in resistance. I inject 1 to 2 mL of 2% plain lidocaine and 1 mL of methylprednisolone (Depo-Medrol).

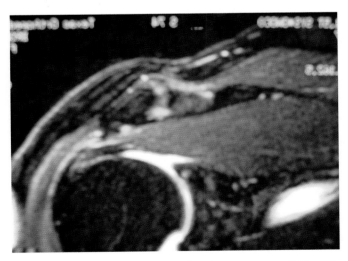

FIGURE 15–3. Magnetic resonance imaging scan, acromioclavicular joint arthritis.

Indications

The indication for surgical treatment is acromioclavicular joint arthritis that has been identified as the source of shoulder pain by patient history, physical examination, plain radiographs, and, when appropriate, MRI. Patients who have pain interfering with activities of daily living, work, or sports that has not responded to conservative care for a minimum of 6 months are good candidates for arthroscopic acromioclavicular joint resection.

Operative Technique

— Acromioclavicular Joint Resection

The two goals of arthroscopic acromioclavicular resection are to remove the abnormal distal portion of the clavicle and to create enough space between the medial acromion and distal clavicle so that physical contact is eliminated during shoulder motion. Traditionally, open resection involves removal of 1 to 1.5 cm of distal clavicle. Arthro-scopic acromioclavicular resection accomplishes this by removing 5 to 8 mm of distal clavicle and 5 mm of medial acromion (Fig. 15–5).

Patient setup and diagnostic glenohumeral arthroscopy are performed routinely. However, I move the posterior incision 2 to 3 mm laterally from its normal location. This allows me to have a better view of the distal clavicle when I enter the subacromial space. The instruments are removed, and attention is turned to the subacromial space.

The cannula and trocar are inserted through the posterior incision into the subacromial space. The arthroscope is inserted, and a subacromial inspection is performed. If the space is not seen clearly, a bursectomy is performed as

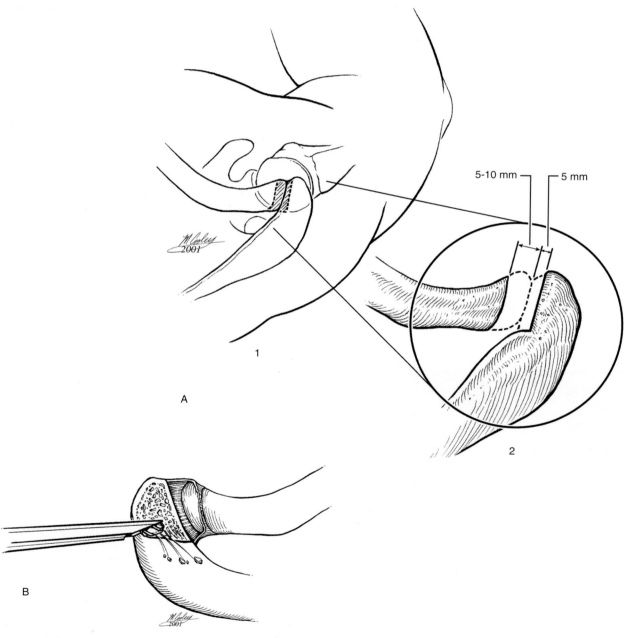

FIGURE 15–5. *A,* Area of desired bone removal. *B,* Acromioplasty. *(Figure continues on next page.)*

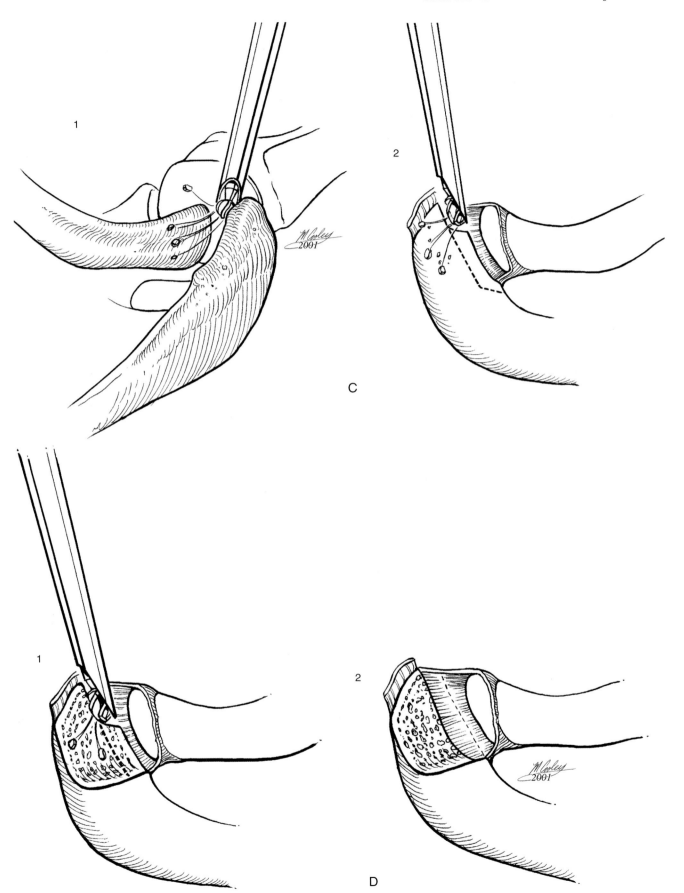

FIGURE 15–5 *Continued.* *C,* Resect anterior portion medial acromion. *D,* Complete medial acromion resection.
(Figure continues on next page.)

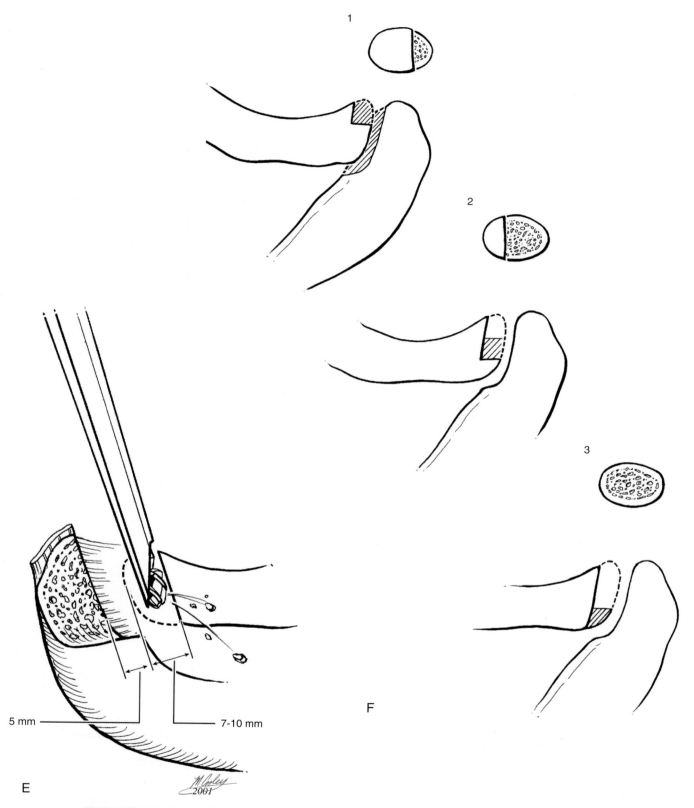

1

2

3

F

5 mm

7-10 mm

E

FIGURE 15–5 Continued. *E*, Resect distal clavicle. *F*, End-on view showing sequence of distal clavicle resection.

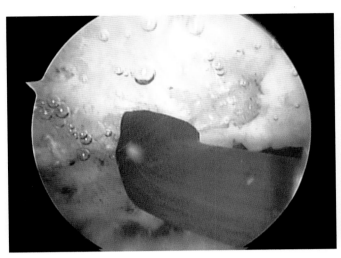

FIGURE 15–6. Cautery to expose bone surface and cauterize blood vessels.

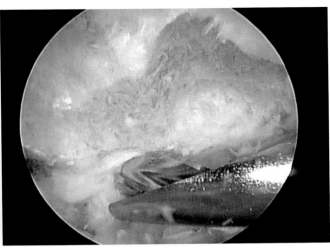

FIGURE 15–7. Resect medial acromion inferior aspect. Bur in lateral portal.

described in Chapter 10. If arthroscopic subacromial decompression is required, the procedure is performed as described in Chapter 10. I modify the arthroscopic subacromial decompression when I combine it with an acromioclavicular resection. I completely resect the medial acromial wall adjacent to the acromioclavicular joint from anterior to posterior.

If arthroscopic subacromial decompression is not necessary, I establish a lateral portal. I use a soft tissue resector to remove any bursa that obscures the view of the medial acromion and use electrocautery to coagulate the soft tissue and vessels on the acromion. The cutting or ablation setting on the electrocautery device can effectively expose acromion bone. I use a soft tissue resector until the medial acromial surface is free from soft tissue, and then I insert a power bur through the lateral portal and remove the medial acromion until soft tissue or distal clavicle is visible (Figs. 15–6 and 15–7).

If I have a good view of the distal clavicle with the arthroscope positioned in the posterior cannula, there is no need to change the location of the arthroscope. Usually, I can angle the cannula medially and rotate the arthroscope to obtain a good view. In most patients, I routinely move the arthroscope to the lateral portal (Figs. 15–8 and 15–9).

I then establish an anterior portal directly anterior to the acromioclavicular joint. The precise location is critical, and I use a spinal needle to localize the cannula site. The anterior portal should be located in the center of the acromioclavicular joint. If the location is too lateral, it is difficult to remove distal clavicle, and if it is too medial, it is difficult to remove medial acromion (Figs. 15–10 and 15–11).

I cauterize the soft tissue at the anterior, inferior, and posterior borders of the distal clavicle. This technique decreases the likelihood of bleeding during bone and soft tissue removal (Figs. 15–12 and 15–13).

At this point, I usually move the arthroscope to the lateral portal and the outflow cannula to the posterior portal. This position allows an end-on view of the distal clavicle.

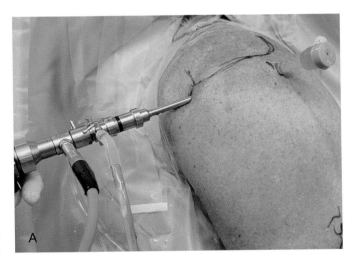

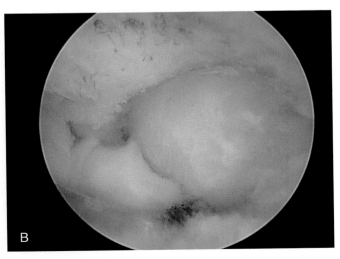

FIGURE 15–8. *A,* Arthroscope rotated medially. *B,* Distal clavicle viewed from posterior portal.

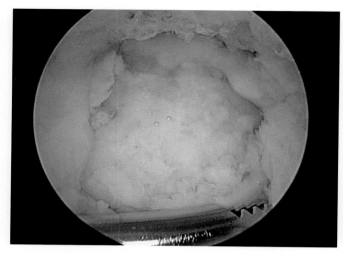

FIGURE 15–9. Distal clavicle viewed from lateral portal.

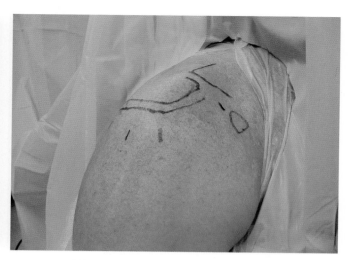

FIGURE 15–10. Location of anterior portal.

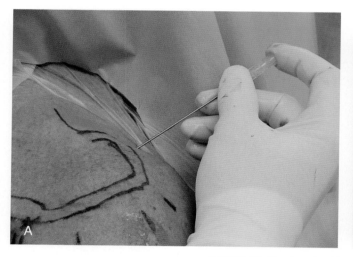

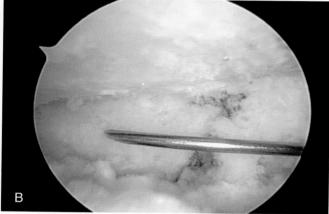

FIGURE 15–11. *A* and *B,* Needle localizing anterior portal.

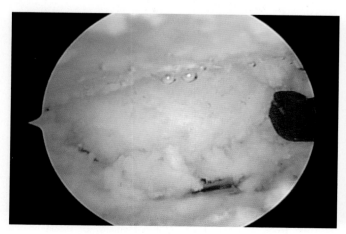

FIGURE 15–12. Cautery, anterior clavicle.

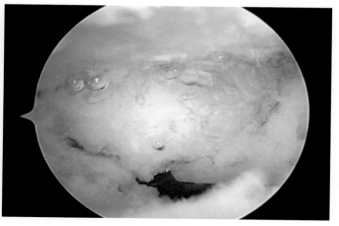

FIGURE 15–13. Cautery, inferior clavicle.

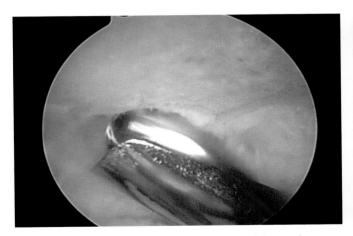

FIGURE 15–14. Resect superior portion medial acromion.

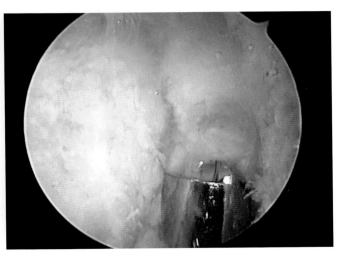

FIGURE 15–16. Resect superior portion medial acromion, arthroscope rotated superiorly.

I tilt the arthroscope superiorly and rotate the camera until I have the best view of the anterior portion of the medial acromion. I use the bur to remove the superior surface of the medial acromion from anterior to posterior (Figs. 15–14 to 15–17). I am careful not to violate the superior capsule of the acromioclavicular joint (Fig. 15–18). At this point, I have removed 4 to 5 mm of bone from the medial acromion (Fig. 15–19). I then withdraw the arthroscope and rotate it so that I am looking directly at the distal clavicle. I remove one bur width of distal clavicle from anterior to posterior and begin by removing bone from the anterior half of the distal clavicle. I remove bone equal to the depth of the acromionizer (5 mm) or the metal guard around the bur (7.2 mm). I move the bur posteriorly and remove the same amount of bone from the posterior half of the distal clavicle until the clavicle surface is flat (Figs. 15–20 and 15–21). I rotate and tilt the arthroscope until I can see the posterior border of the distal clavicle and the posteromedial acromion, I inspect the posterior aspect

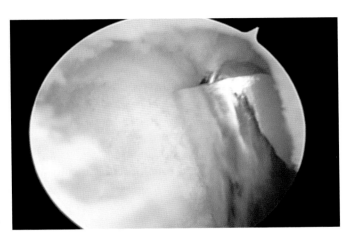

FIGURE 15–17. Resect superior portion medial acromion, arthroscope rotated superiorly.

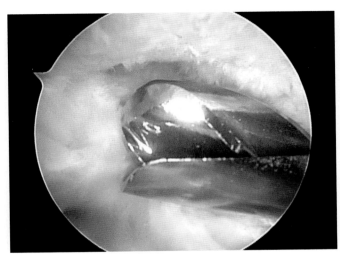

FIGURE 15–15. Resect superior portion medial acromion.

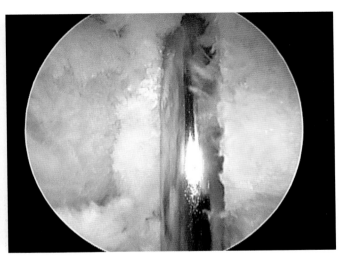

FIGURE 15–18. Superior capsule acromioclavicular joint.

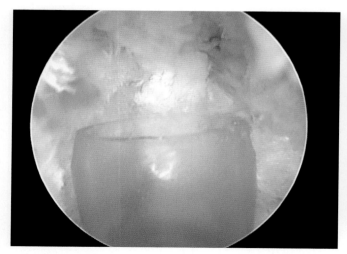

FIGURE 15–19. Remove 4 to 5 mm of bone from medial acromion.

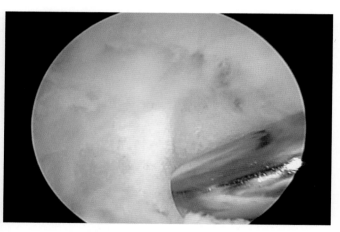

FIGURE 15–21. Anterior clavicle resection.

of the acromioclavicular joint, and I remove any remaining posteromedial acromion that may impinge during shoulder extension or abduction (Fig. 15–22). At this point, I have removed 10 to 15 mm of bone (5 mm medial acromion and 5 to 10 mm distal clavicle). I advance the cannula or shaver (an instrument with a known size) into the resected area to ensure that there is adequate space between the distal clavicle and the acromion (Figs. 15–23 to 15–25).

Cannula Position

Cannula position is critical. Small errors significantly prolong operative time and diminish the quality of the resection.

Posterior Portal

If the posterior portal is placed in the "soft-spot," it is too medial and inferior to allow a good view of the distal clavicle. My standard portal for an arthroscopic subacromial decompression is 1 cm inferior and 1 cm medial to the pos-

terolateral acromial margin. For an acromioclavicular joint resection, I move the posterior portal 2 to 3 mm more laterally. This position allows me to angle the arthroscope medially and to obtain a better view of the distal clavicle.

Lateral Portal

If the lateral portal is too far anterior, the anterior clavicle and acromion are not well visualized, and this can cause inadequate bone resection. If the lateral cannula is too far superior, the superior aspect of the distal clavicle and medial acromion cannot be seen.

Postoperative Management

An ice pack decreases swelling, inflammation, and pain postoperatively and is worn 1 hour, four times daily for the first 2 weeks. Active and passive range of motion is started on the first postoperative day. Strengthening is started when examination demonstrates pain-free manual muscle testing. Work and sports are allowed as tolerated by the patient.

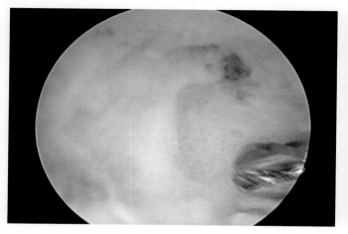

FIGURE 15–20. Anterior clavicle resection.

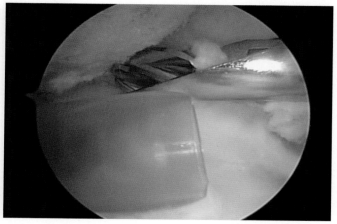

FIGURE 15–22. Evaluate posteromedial acromion for contact.

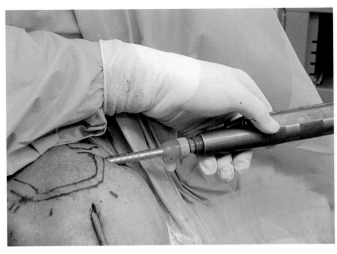

FIGURE 15–23. Outside view of bur in anterior cannula.

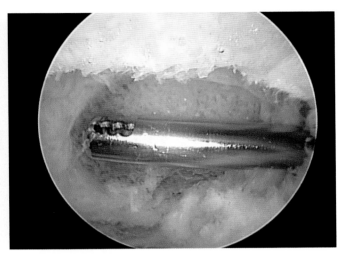

FIGURE 15–25. Check final acromioclavicular joint resection.

Maximum improvement occurs 6 to 12 months after operation.

Complications

Acromioclavicular instability is a concern after acromioclavicular resection. I limit distal clavicle resection to

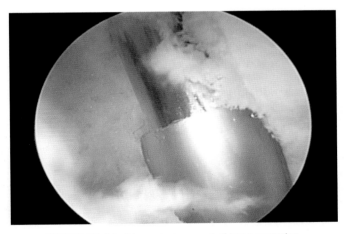

FIGURE 15–24. Measuring amount of bone resection.

10 mm to avoid violating the coracoclavicular ligaments. When I remove the superior distal clavicle osteophyte, I do not resect any superior acromioclavicular ligament.

Bibliography

Berg EE, Ciullo JV: The SLAP lesion: A cause of failure after distal clavicle resection. Arthroscopy 13:85–89, 1997.

Buford D Jr, Mologne T, McGrath S, et al: Midterm results of arthroscopic co-planing of the acromioclavicular joint. J Shoulder Elbow Surg 9:498–501, 2000.

Flatow EL, Duralde XA, Nicholson GP, et al: Arthroscopic resection of the distal clavicle with a superior approach. J Shoulder Elbow Surg 4:41–50, 1995.

Gartsman GM: Arthroscopic resection of the acromioclavicular joint. Am J Sports Med 21:71–77, 1993.

Gartsman GM: Extra-articular uses of the arthroscope—acromioclavicular arthroplasty. Clin Sports Med 12:111–121, 1993.

Gartsman GM, Combs AH, Davis PF, et al: Arthroscopic acromioclavicular joint resection: An anatomical study. Am J Sports Med 19:25, 1991.

Petchell JF, Sonnabend DH, Hughes JS: Distal clavicular excision: A detailed functional assessment. Aust NZ J Surg 65:262–266, 1995.

Snyder SJ: Shoulder Arthroscopy. New York, McGraw-Hill, 1994, pp 87–113.

Stein BE, Wiater JM, Pfaff HC, et al: Detection of acromioclavicular joint pathology in asymptomatic shoulders with magnetic resonance imaging. J Shoulder Elbow Surg 10:204–208, 2001.

16

Calcific Tendinitis

One of the most painful acute conditions affecting the shoulder is calcific tendinitis. Patients note the sudden, atraumatic onset of severe pain that is present at rest and increases with any shoulder movement. The pain is often severe enough to cause the patient to present at a local emergency room or the orthopedist's office. Patients often appear to be in distress and cradle the affected arm.

Diagnosis

The diagnosis of calcific tendinitis is radiographic. The plain radiograph shows single or multiple calcium deposits, usually located in the supraspinatus tendon. These deposits also can occur in the subscapularis tendon or, more rarely, in the infraspinatus or teres minor. The size, density, and location of the deposit must be evaluated closely to distinguish this condition from the calcific densities that occur incidentally in rotator cuff tendinitis. These findings are summarized in Table 16–1 and are shown in Figures 16–1 to 16–4.

The shoulder is often swollen, and the overlying skin is sensitive to touch. The slightest pressure applied over the supraspinatus insertion may elicit severe pain. Active and passive range of motion is painful and restricted. Another cause of acute shoulder pain is cervical radiculopathy, and the surgeon should carefully examine the patient for neck pain, radicular pain, and paresthesias. A review of the radiographs confirms the diagnosis. Because of persistent, severe pain, patients often present with a magnetic resonance imaging scan taken to evaluate the rotator cuff tendons (Fig. 16–5).

Literature Review

The etiology of acute calcific tendinitis is not precisely known, but Uhthoff and Loehr have made the best analysis of this condition. They consider calcific tendinitis a self-healing tendinopathy and believe there is a precalcifying

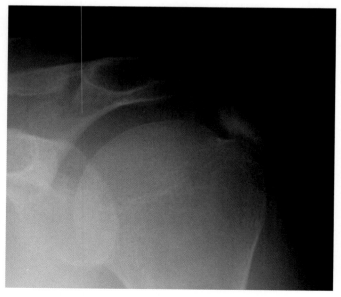

FIGURE 16–1. Calcific tendinitis, shoulder externally rotated.

TABLE 16–1. RADIOGRAPHIC FINDINGS		
Feature	Calcific Tendinitis	Rotator Cuff Tendinitis
Size	5–15 mm	< 5 mm
Location	10–15 mm medial to greater tuberosity	Adjacent to tuberosity
Density	Less opaque	Dense
Character	Soft	Hard

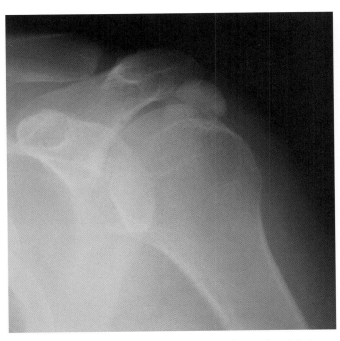

FIGURE 16–2. Calcific tendinitis, shoulder internally rotated.

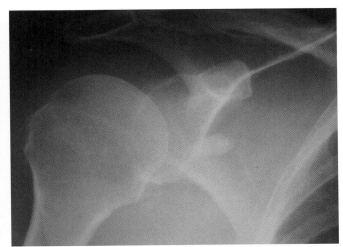

FIGURE 16–4. Calcific tendinitis in subscapularis, shoulder internally rotated.

phase during which a reduction in oxygen tension transforms a portion of the tendon into fibrocartilage. In this phase, the chondrocytes mediate the deposition of calcium. After the formative phase, the calcium may exist for an indefinite period and may not produce any symptoms. At some point, phagocytic cells accumulate around these calcium foci, and vascular proliferation occurs. The resorptive phase begins when these new vascular channels provide a pathway for resorption and restore normal perfusion and oxygen tension to the tissues. After the calcification is resorbed, the tendon is capable of normal function. The

acute pain experienced by the patient begins with the resorptive phase.

Ellman and I reported on a multicenter study of 131 patients treated with an arthroscopic technique. The average constant functional score was 69.4 out of a possible 75. There was no correlation with patient age, size of the calcification, or duration of symptoms. Acromioplasty was not shown to be of any benefit.

Nonoperative Treatment

I believe that patients presenting with an attack of acute calcific tendinitis are in the resorptive phase, and the condition is self-resolving. Therefore, my nonoperative care is supportive and consists of an explanation of the condition's natural history, narcotic analgesics, rest, and ice. The application of heat increases blood flow to an inflamed area and

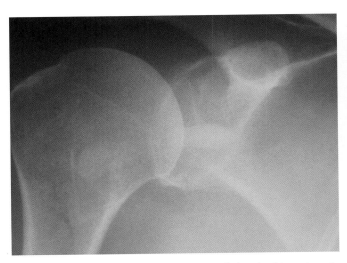

FIGURE 16–3. Calcific tendinitis in subscapularis, shoulder externally rotated.

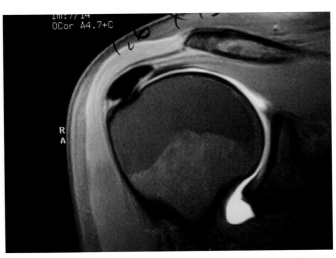

FIGURE 16–5. Calcific tendinitis, magnetic resonance imaging scan.

is contraindicated. Because I believe that nonsteroidal anti-inflammatory medication decreases the patient's ability to resorb the calcium, I do not prescribe these medications, nor do I inject cortisone into the subacromial space. Occasionally, I will inject a local anesthetic (bupivacaine 0.25%) into the subacromial space to provide temporary pain relief, but I do not make any attempt to needle the calcium deposit. Once the severe pain has subsided, I instruct the patients in gentle stretching exercises and allow them to resume activities as tolerated. If the calcific tendinitis attack is prolonged and muscular atrophy develops, then I have the patient begin a series of home exercises with surgical tubing to improve the strength of the shoulder girdle muscles.

Indications

I have not found it necessary to operate on a patient with a first-time, acute attack of calcific tendinitis because the nonoperative care program described earlier is successful. The indication for operation is a history of repeated episodes of acute calcific tendinitis. I do not require a set number of attacks before considering operation, but after the second episode I offer arthroscopic surgery as a treatment option to the patient. The patient's ability to tolerate episodes of severe pain varies greatly; some patients do not desire operation for a yearly attack, whereas others welcome the opportunity for surgical correction.

Operative Technique

VIDEO — Calcific Tendinitis

The location of the deposit is determined by review of radiographs taken with the patient's arm in different positions. On an anterior posterior radiograph, deposits in the supraspinatus tendon move medially when the arm is internally rotated. Lesions in the infraspinatus move laterally as the arm is moved into internal rotation. Also note how far medially the calcium is located from the greater tuberosity. Study the axillary radiograph to note the location of the calcific deposit.

Calcium excision usually produces a vigorous inflammatory response, and many patients experience an acute attack in the postoperative period. For this reason, unless there are medical contraindications such as diabetes or hypertension, I have the anesthesiologist administer 100 mg of methylprednisolone (Solu-Medrol) intravenously before the operation and place the patient on a methylprednisolone (Medrol) dose pack after surgery. Interscalene block anesthesia is extremely helpful in the treatment of these patients.

I establish routine anterior and posterior glenohumeral joint portals and perform a complete glenohumeral joint inspection. I try to inspect the rotator cuff for areas of erythema or increased vascularity because these areas correspond to the location of the calcium deposit. Most com-

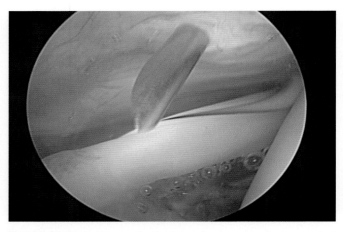

FIGURE 16–6. Erythema of articular surface, supraspinatus marked with spinal needle.

monly, these areas of erythema are located anteriorly in the rotator cuff, within the supraspinatus tendon.

While viewing from within the glenohumeral joint, I insert a needle percutaneously into the area of increased vascularity (Fig. 16–6). I thread an absorbable monofilament suture through the needle, gently remove the needle, and leave the suture in the glenohumeral joint. However, the articular surface of the rotator cuff often appears normal. If the rotator cuff and the remainder of the glenohumeral joint appear normal, I immediately proceed to the subacromial space.

I insert the arthroscope into the subacromial space through the posterior portal and establish a lateral subacromial portal. I insert the motorized shaver, identify the monofilament suture (if previously inserted), and perform a bursectomy so that I can see clearly within subacromial space. Calcium deposits may appear as whitish discolorations or as bulges in the tendon (Fig. 16–7). If the tendon appears normal and no deposit is seen, I insert a blunt trocar through the lateral cannula and palpate the tendon for areas of increased hardness. I am careful not to confuse

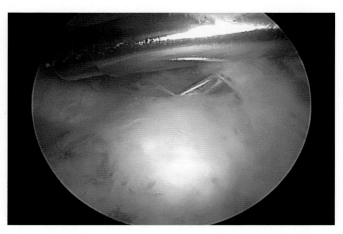

FIGURE 16–7. Calcium deposit viewed from subacromial space.

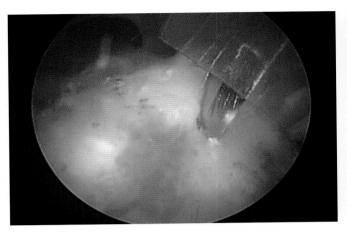

FIGURE 16–8. Knife to incise bursal covering of calcium.

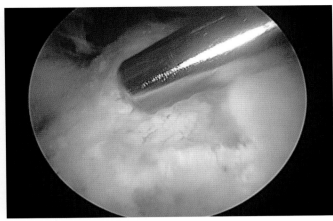

FIGURE 16–10. Shaver removing calcium.

the firm supraspinatus insertion into the greater tuberosity with a calcium deposit. If I cannot detect any calcium through inspection or palpation, I insert a spinal needle and puncture the tendon in multiple areas of the suspected lesion. If no abnormal areas are identified with this approach, I insert a spinal needle into the most likely area of the tendon and use intraoperative radiographs or fluoroscopy. Once the calcium deposit is identified with the foregoing techniques, I can begin the process of calcium removal.

I insert arthroscopic scissors or a knife through the lateral portal and incise the deposit (Figs. 16–8 and 16–9).

The deposit often resembles toothpaste or is granular. Pressure on the tendon expresses the calcium, and you visualize it filling the subacromial space. I increase the rate of pump flow (not the pump pressure) to maintain visualization. Commonly, a portion of the calcium remains adherent to the tendon fibers or interspersed within the tendon substance. I insert a motorized shaver and gently remove calcium while maintaining tendon integrity. The shaver tip can also be used as a probe to apply pressure to the calcium deposit (Fig. 16–10).

If the deposit is hard or bone-like, I use the shaver to remove as much calcium as possible without excising tendon fibers. I prefer to leave some calcium rather than sacrifice tendon integrity. Once the deposit is opened and most of the calcium has been removed, the resorption process is unimpeded. The postoperative radiograph almost always demonstrates a complete absence of calcium.

If a defect exists in the tendon after calcium removal, I do not repair the tendon (Fig. 16–11). The protected motion that is required after rotator cuff repair often results in profound shoulder stiffness. I have never had to repair a supraspinatus defect that became a full-thickness tear.

I do not perform an acromioplasty, because I believe the exposed bone surface increases the risk of postoperative stiffness. This approach is supported by Ellman's data.

Postoperative Treatment

I have patients start immediate passive range of motion in elevation and external rotation the afternoon of the surgical procedure. I find the continuous passive motion chair a most effective mechanism that patients appreciate. Patients are encouraged to use the shoulder actively and to perform

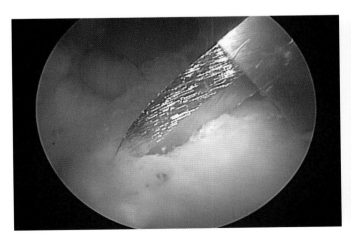

FIGURE 16–9. Knife to incise bursal covering of calcium.

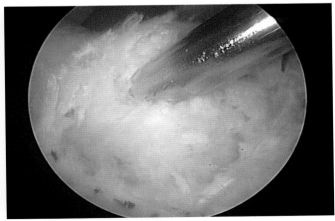

FIGURE 16–11. Rotator cuff defect after calcium removal.

routine activities of daily living within the limits of their discomfort. I do not allow patients to use a sling. I see patients in the office 2 weeks after operation and obtain a postoperative anterior posterior radiograph to observe the change in the calcium deposit.

I stop continuous passive motion and have the patients instructed in supine dowel passive range of motion in the same planes. Two months after the operation, patients return to the office, and if they have no pain with resisted muscle testing, I have them start a home strengthening program with rubber tubing.

Bibliography

Ark JW, Flock TJ, Flatow EL, Bigliani LU: Arthroscopic treatment of calcific tendinitis of the shoulder. Arthroscopy 8:183–188, 1992.

Ellman H, Gartsman GM: Arthroscopic Shoulder Surgery and Related Procedures. Philadelphia, Lea & Febiger, 1993, pp 219–231.

Jerosch J, Strauss JM, Schmiel S: Arthroscopic treatment of calcific tendinitis of the shoulder. J Shoulder Elbow Surg 7:30–37, 1998.

Uhthoff HK, Loehr JW: Calcific tendinopathy of the rotator cuff: Pathogenesis, diagnosis, and management. J Am Acad Orthop Surg 5:183–191, 1997.

Fractures

Arthroscopic techniques are rarely used in the treatment of shoulder fractures; however, in a few situations, I have found arthroscopy beneficial. Displaced greater tuberosity fractures and greater tuberosity nonunions can be treated arthroscopically. I have also identified significant partial-thickness rotator cuff tears in patients who have persistent pain after satisfactory bone union.

Literature Review

Acute greater tuberosity fractures occur both with and without glenohumeral dislocation. The association of a greater tuberosity fracture and an acute anterior inferior glenohumeral dislocation is well known. Operative treatment for displaced greater tuberosity fractures using an open surgical approach has been described. My colleagues and I have documented our experience with arthroscopic repair for acute greater tuberosity fractures associated with glenohumeral dislocation and greater tuberosity nonunion.

Diagnosis

The diagnosis of a greater tuberosity fracture is usually made on the basis of plain radiographs. Accurate anterior posterior and axillary films are mandatory. Computed tomographic scans may be helpful to determine precise fracture anatomy. The patient's history often indicates whether a glenohumeral dislocation occurred at the time of injury.

Nonoperative Treatment

Nonoperative treatment is the mainstay for nondisplaced greater tuberosity fractures and for almost all fractures with less than 5 mm of displacement. If pain or weakness persists longer than 3 months after injury, a magnetic resonance imaging scan may demonstrate an associated partial-thickness or full-thickness rotator cuff tear. Because greater tuberosity fractures usually heal quite readily, persistent pain may also signal a fracture nonunion. Tomograms or computed tomographic scans will demonstrate the nonunion.

Indications

Minimally displaced greater tuberosity fractures may be treated nonoperatively; however, more recent evidence suggests that even as little as 5 mm of superior displacement may produce shoulder dysfunction. Patients can usually tolerate greater degrees of posterior rotation than superior migration of the fractured tuberosity.

The two typical clinical situations described in the following sections represent examples of cases with indications for arthroscopic treatment.

Acute Fracture

A 46-year-old right-handed man was involved in a polo accident and sustained an anterior inferior glenohumeral dislocation along with a greater tuberosity fracture. The dislocation was reduced in the emergency room, but because of the displacement of the greater tuberosity fracture, the treating orthopedist referred the patient to our office. The patient's medical history revealed no prior significant shoulder problems. Physical examination was limited by pain from the shoulder injury but demonstrated normal neurovascular status. Plain radiographs demonstrated prereduction and postreduction views of the dislocation and displaced greater tuberosity fracture. Because the patient wished to pursue his avocation of competitive polo, we advised operative arthroscopic treatment.

Nonunion

A 63-year-old woman fell and sustained a minimally displaced greater tuberosity fracture. In spite of appropriate nonoperative treatment, her fracture progressed to nonunion. Physical examination demonstrated painful, limited active shoulder motion in elevation and abduction. Plain radiographs showed a nonunion. Based on the patient's clinical presentation, we advised operative arthroscopic treatment.

Contraindications

Insufficient bone stock, significant displacement, or tuberosity retraction may preclude the reduction and fixation of a greater tuberosity fracture using arthroscopic techniques.

Operative Technique

After the successful induction of general anesthesia with interscalene block supplementation, place the patient in the sitting position and prepare and drape the patient's arm. A standard entry into the glenohumeral joint is made. Inspect the joint for any associated injuries, and repair these as indicated. Remove the arthroscope, and insert it into the subacromial space. Identify the lateral portal site with a spinal needle, and insert a large, self-sealing cannula and trocar. Introduce an arthroscopic probe to identify the fracture site. Probe palpation can detect any movement in the greater tuberosity, because soft tissue covering the fracture site usually makes it impossible to view to the bone directly. If the fracture is acute, hemorrhage will also be visualized around the fracture area. Establish an anterior portal, and introduce a cannula. Use a curette or power shaver to remove the soft tissue covering the fracture site laterally, and lift up the fragment to expose the fracture bed. Lightly abrade the fracture (or nonunion) site with a power bur. Reduce the greater tuberosity using a trocar (placed through the anterior portal). Either through the lateral cannula or percutaneously, insert a Kirschner wire through the tuberosity fragment into the humeral head under arthroscopic guidance. I use a partially threaded, cannulated, 6.5-mm screw inserted over the guidewire to obtain firm, compressive fixation of the tuberosity. Reinsert the arthroscope into the glenohumeral joint, and verify that the screw has not penetrated the humeral articular surface and has no cartilage penetration. Check the reduction and screw placement with an intraoperative radiograph. Fluoroscopic imaging or intraoperative radiographs are suggested to ensure appropriate screw position (Figs. 17–1 to 17–5).

Postoperative Treatment

Postoperative treatment is similar to that for a full-thickness rotator cuff tear. Place the patient's arm in a sling for 6 weeks. Start passive range of motion in elevation and external rotation the afternoon after the surgical procedure and continue for 6 weeks. At the 2-week, 6-week, and 3-month visits, radiographs should be taken to verify healing and position of both the bone fragment and the screw. Active range of motion is started at week 6, and strengthening is initiated at 3 months. If the patient complains of pain in the

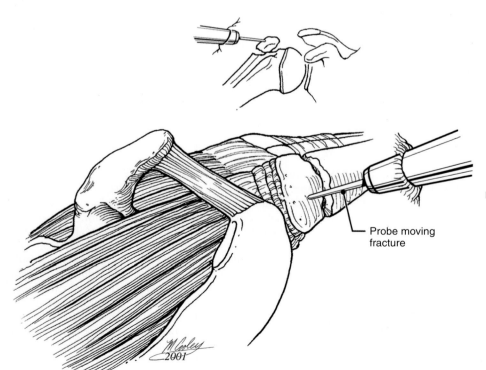

Probe moving
fracture

FIGURE 17–1. Identify fracture site.

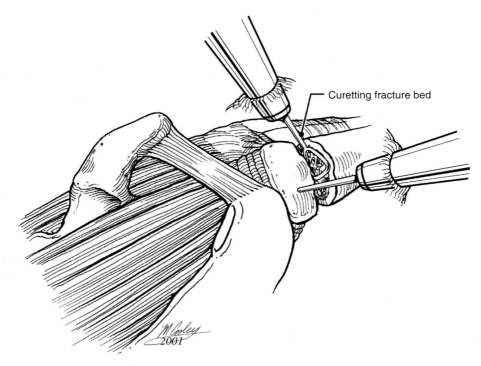

FIGURE 17–2. Curette fracture bed.

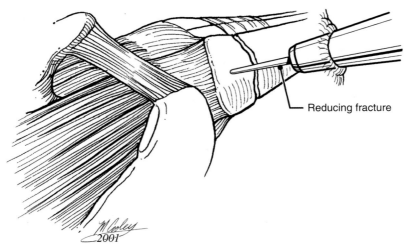

FIGURE 17–3. Reduce fracture with probe or Kirschner wire.

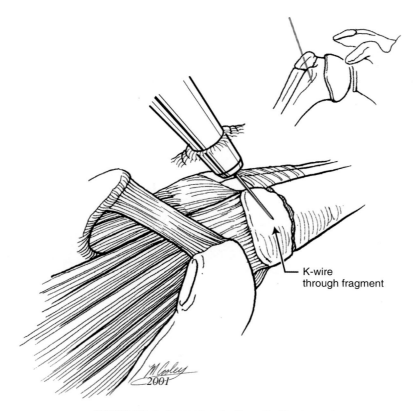

FIGURE 17–4. Temporary fixation with Kirschner wire.

K-wire
through fragment

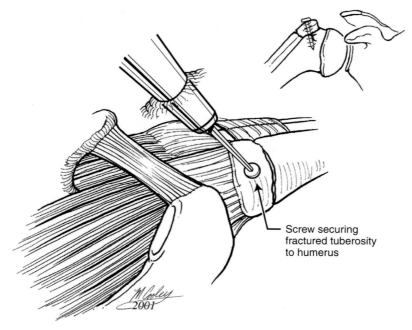

FIGURE 17–5. Permanent screw fixation.

Screw securing
fractured tuberosity
to humerus

area of the screw head, I remove the screw once fracture consolidation is demonstrated on radiographs.

Bibliography

Flatow EL, Cuomo F, Maday MG, et al: Open reduction and internal fixation of two-part displaced fractures of the greater tuberosity of the proximal part of the humerus. J Bone Joint Surg Am 73:1213–1218, 1991.

Gartsman GM, Taverna E: Arthroscopic treatment of rotator cuff tear and greater tuberosity fracture nonunion. Arthroscopy 12:242–244, 1996.

Gartsman GM, Taverna E, Hammerman SM: Arthroscopic repair of acute, traumatic glenohumeral dislocation and greater tuberosity fracture. Arthroscopy 15:648–650, 1999.

Kim SH, Ha KI: Arthroscopic treatment of symptomatic shoulders with minimally displaced greater tuberosity fracture. Arthroscopy 16:695–700, 2000.

McLaughlin HL: Dislocation of the shoulder with tuberosity fracture. Surg Clin North Am 43:1615–1620, 1963.

Index

Note: Page numbers followed by the letter f refer to figures; those followed by the letter t refer to tables.